HANDBOOK OF
PSYCHIATRIC CONSULTATION

HANDBOOK OF PSYCHIATRIC CONSULTATION

JOHN J. SCHWAB, M.D.

Professor of Psychiatry and Medicine
University of Florida College of Medicine
Gainesville, Florida

With a foreword by

HENRY W. BROSIN, M.D.
Professor and Chairman, Department of Psychiatry
Director, Western Psychiatric Institute and Clinic,
University of Pittsburg School of Medicine
President, American Psychiatric Association (1967–68)

APPLETON-CENTURY-CROFTS
Division of Meredith Corporation
NEW YORK

FOREWORD

This volume was written primarily for psychiatric residents who are furnishing consultation on other medical services and medical students working on those services. It should be useful to all physicians and our colleagues in the other health professions because of its wide theoretical scope and down-to-earth practical suggestions on the consultation process in many different clinical situations, including consultation to agencies.

The author is drawing upon a rich and varied clinical experience to furnish the reader with attitudes and policy positions as well as many hints and instructions for the guidance of the psychiatric consultant in specific situations. The text is often frankly didactic with explicit directions about the procedures which are recommended and those to be avoided. This approach will be welcome to students and residents who want detailed instructions during the early phases of their training. To supplement this aspect of the training, the author has also provided much explanatory material at several levels to provide integration of information over a wide spectrum of medical practice. This includes an historical review with a discussion of concepts of disease; full sections of the fundamentals of the consultation process and useful procedures, techniques and practices; a full section on diagnosis and management. There is also appendices outlining the differential diagnosis of acute psychiatric disorders; possible medical sources of emotional symptoms; psychiatric symptoms accompanying medical illness; and a brief section on the use of medications. In these ways, this volume becomes a true handbook as it is called in the title as well as a specialty text.

There are also sections on "The Surgical Consultation," The Pediatric Consultation" (by Paul Adams), and "The Community Consultation of the Psychiatrist" (by Rufus M. Vaughn) which will be most helpful to the student because they exhibit the extensive experience of the authors

v

in dealing with real problems in all their complexity. They portray many of the barriers and pitfalls which make the consultation process difficult, because it is, ultimately, an intimate relation between two people, even though all professional safeguards against a psychotherapeutic or other types of nonprofessional relationships are observed. The request for technical guidance and advice by one professional worker from another in a peer relation, and the ways it can be best nurtured are carefully described.

Teachers as well as students will welcome this "Handbook" because it will ease the task of introducing young physicians to many of the principles of dealing with patients and colleagues in complex settings. There are numerous references to other current authors whose writings are helpful in gaining better understanding of the many different facets of the consultation process. During these days of increasing publication of technical articles in all areas of professional work, all workers welcome abstracts, critical reviews, and well-written texts with selected bibliographies which can save many man-hours in the library.

Doctor Schwab has attempted a comprehensive task in trying to bring together so many different subjects related to the general theme of "the psychiatric consultation." Only experience through usage will demonstrate the major strengths and weaknesses. It seems probable that this "Handbook" should become popular for the purposes for which it is designed, not only because there is a great need in our rapidly changing society with its new patterns of medical care, but because the author has written clearly and frankly about many sensitive areas which are often not well defined.

The section entitled "A Teaching Program" will be of interest to all teachers who are developing new programs even though their schedules and curricula differ in various respects. Only by experimenting with different programs and adapting them to different local needs will we be able to furnish our colleagues with the uniform high level of patient care to which we aspire. Doctor Schwab furnishes us with an example from his school at the University of Florida which makes fruitful comparison and research possible.

HENRY W. BROSIN, M.D.
Pittsburgh, 1968

PREFACE

Since the first chapters of this volume were started two years ago, Psychiatric Consultation has come of age. The term "Psychiatric Consultation Work" is now used widely, and there is an increasing amount of writing on the subject. In recently reviewing the literature of consultation psychiatry and psychosomatic medicine, Lipowski notes that psychosomatic medicine is developing vigorously in two directions: toward laboratory based psychophysiological research and clinically based consultation-liaison services for hospitals and clinics. Mendel and Solomon recently edited a multi-authored volume, *The Psychiatric Consultation*, which emphasizes the need for liaison services, discusses the consultation process, and describes techniques for training psychiatric residents in this work.

I believe that this flurry of interest in psychiatric consultation work should not generate a subspecialty; the term is only descriptive of psychiatric activities with patients who complain of somatic distress or seek the help of physicians, surgeons, or general hospitals for treatment. Another aspect of consulting work involves the psychiatrist's service to others in the health and related professions, particularly community agencies. These various consulting activities should be complimentary. A psychiatric consultant is not a subspecialist; in fact, a major purpose in writing this book is to discuss some of the features of the consultation, so that all psychiatrists can glean from our experiences as they are increasingly called upon for these endeavors. Because most of the consultant's work will be with patients in medical settings, he will be better equipped for his job when he enlarges his knowledge of people and their distress by recalling his medical education and by seeing man in a social perspective. The consulting psychiatrist should be a specialist only in the sense that he is dedicated to comprehensive medicine, with a view of man as a creature of biology, a social being, and a part of his culture. To do this well, as Garner says, "The physician must search in the recesses of the spirit, as well as the fossae of the skull, for the meaning of symptoms and for the clues to the curative process."

I began this book with the thought of providing a manual for psychiatric residents on the Consultation-Liaison Service at the University of Florida College of Medicine. When I first organized this program in 1961, after leaving the practice of internal medicine and completing my training in psychiatry, I needed a textbook to support my teaching, but none was available. Our instruction relied too heavily on personal experience, intuition, and anecdote. Many writers had described with insight particular aspects of the psychiatric consultation, but I could not find a textbook which presented the theoretical basis and furnished practical guidance for students, residents, and psychiatrists engaged in this work. Moreover, available material supplied little substantive data answering the questions posed by the new resident as he anxiously began his duties as a consultant and specialist, unsheltered by the familiar inpatient or outpatient setting. Residents would ask, "What will I do if medical patients refuse to see me?" "What do I tell the consultee?" and, "How do I handle problems with diagnosis when a patient is both physically and emotionally ill?" Therefore, as part of our teaching program, we arranged for seminars in which the faculty and residents could share clinical experiences and discuss the problems in our work. We taped and summarized these seminars in order to document and organize our clinical knowledge about the consultation. In other conferences we compared our work with that described in the literature. This book developed from the core of our clinical experiences with patients in the consultation setting.

Since 1961 my colleagues and I have also worked on a series of systematized studies focused on consultation procedures and practices: How can patients needing referral be identified? How do the staff (physicians, nurses, students, and others) perceive, affect, and respond to their patients' emotional distress and the referral for psychiatric consultation? How do patients react to psychiatric consultants? How does referral affect patients' attitudes toward their physicians? And, are the current psychiatric concepts of anxiety and depression applicable to general medicine? This book is a synthesis of our clinical experiences, the research findings, and the literature in the field.

As this work progressed, we enlarged its scope so that it could be presented as a textbook rather than as a manual. It includes sections addressed to physicians in other specialties and deals with the relationships between psychiatry and the other health-related professions. The contents will be helpful to psychologists, nurses, social workers, and occupational and physical therapists.

Because it was designed to be used by students, certain parts are didactic. The section on techniques and practices outlines methods for routine as well as difficult care. The recommendations are offered to illustrate concrete steps which can be taken in given situations. Of course, neither dogma nor codified procedure supplant empathy and the desire to take on the care of these patients. For efficient learning one must draw on others' experiences, modifying and refining this knowledge by personal observation and reflection; then there is more time to develop that particular sensitivity which marks the good physician.

This volume may be used as a handbook, not necessarily to be read from cover to cover, but for reference and guidance as specific problems arise in consultation work. Most of the sections contain guidelines; there are outlines for differential diagnosis and medications; and, we have provided a complete index with cross-references. At critical points the reader is advised to consult specific references. We have also compiled a comprehensive bibliography.

The most pleasurable part in preparing a book is that of expressing one's acknowledgments to the many persons who have helped with it, though I realize that such expressions are seldom adequate.

When writing a book of this sort, one learns how little of his own thought is original. Time and again, in reviewing others' works and in searching the writings of the past, I learned that few if any ideas are really new; at best, they are shared. One can only hope to synthesize, embellish, add a note, and not detract.

I have had an unusual opportunity to draw from the work of others and to learn from their experiences. As an NIMH Career Teacher I visited over 30 Consultation-Liaison Programs in the United States and Canada in 1962–64. On those visits, more than 100 faculty members at the different universities and medical centers gave me their time, spoke freely of their experiences, shared their problems, and assisted my endeavors with advice and encouragement. Many of the ideas which I have expressed in this volume are the fruits of those visits. It is impossible to name every one with whom I consulted, but I would be remiss not to list Knight Aldrich, Klaus Berblinger, Henry Brosin, George Engel, Shervert Frazier, Thomas Hackett, W. E. Meyer, and Erich Wittkower.

This book is dedicated to my teachers, especially Doctors Peter F. Regan III, Robert L. Williams, and Paul L. Adams, and to my colleagues, students, and patients. Their stimulation was a necessary precondition. The greatest debt is to my assistants, Mrs. Linda Bialow and Mrs. Judith Brown, who not only toiled with me during the preparation of the manuscript, but provided critical advice, steadfast encouragement, and a dedication to the work which went beyond conventional working hours and wages. Mrs. Brown assisted with every phase and contributed so substantially to the chapters on Hospitalization and Depression that she will have to share the responsibility for them as a co-author. Others, particularly Miss Marilyn Sokolof, Mary Helen Giron, and Mrs. Nancy McGinnis assisted with the arduous editing, indexing, and typing. Mrs. Mary T. Ring searched the library indefatigably for needed references. Mrs. Felice Pralle and Mrs. Esther Hudson did most of the typing; they cheerfully accepted the seemingly endless job of typing revisions and correcting errors.

The Department of Psychiatry, headed by Doctor Robert L. Williams, was helpful; the members looked upon my labors sympathetically and hopefully. On many occasions they gave specific advice; on all occasions I felt that the spirit of our department was cooperative and supportive—conducive to the preparation of this book. Knowing of my involvement in the writing, they shared some of my teaching and clinical responsibilities and overlooked many of my shortcomings. My colleagues, Doctors Paul L. Adams and Rufus M. Vaugh, wrote special chapters which round out the volume and give it broader range. Two other colleagues, Doctors Roy S. Clemmons and Leon Marder assisted with specific chapters; their help is gratefully acknowledged. Many others helped and encouraged me. My wife reviewed and edited the manuscript scrupulously; her objectivity added clarity and logic; and her understanding during the two years of preparation has been invaluable. My daughter's lively presence, and witticisms, during these last two years when I often felt afflicted by overwork, helped me maintain some sense of humor.

I wish to thank Doctor William Steiger and the American Sociological Association for permission to reproduce an excerpt from his paper entitled, "Medical Science and Things" which was published in The Journal of Health and Human Behavior. Much of our research which has been cited throughout the book was supported in part by NIMH Grant No. MH 2152-02.

CONTENTS

HANDBOOK OF
PSYCHIATRIC CONSULTATION

SECTION ONE   The Background for Consultation Work

1   ORIGIN

For where there is love of man there is also love of the art of medicine.
Hippocrates: (Decorum VII, Precepts 11)

In recent years there has been a surge of interest in the psychiatric consultation. This developed in response to a problem: the lack of comprehensive patient care. The problem is not new; but, changing concepts of illness and sociocultural, historical, and scientific influences are increasing our awareness of the need for comprehensive medical care. A summary of these developments provides a background for understanding consultation work.

SOCIOCULTURAL INFLUENCES

The population explosion, urbanization, greater mobility, speed of communication, and the breakdown of extended family relationships are fundamental sociocultural factors contributing to the dire need for improved mental health resources. Also, public attitudes toward medicine have changed (see references listed under CHANGES IN ATTITUDES TOWARD PSYCHIATRY, p. 5). In the past, the physician could do little more than alleviate discomfort. Now patients also seek medical help for dilemmas which are sociologic in nature. These problems in living are given a medical slant, and the physician is expected to provide solutions.

Using the family as an example of these developments, Bittner (1967) specifies four features of modern life which lead to the demand for comprehensive medical care.

1. The modern family is radically reduced in size compared with the larger kinship systems of the American past. Increasing numbers of people are cut off fairly early in life from nurturing sources of guidance

1

and support. Newly married couples highly value their independence. Reliance on the extended family has diminished, and instead: "When a problem in living will have even the slightest health aspect associated with it, the physician will be chosen as the proper remedial agent."

2. The family emphasizes romantic love, rather than the more traditional social, economic, and religious bonds. This premium on feelings has medical implications: "Given the fact that feelings are closely tied to the perception of bodily states, it is a foregone conclusion that the physician will be called upon to advise, help, and counsel."

3. The breakdown of the family as a production unit leads to separation. The stresses of the husband's employment, removed from the home and often highly specialized, are almost incommunicable to his wife. The importance of the man's employment stands in contrast to the drudgery of housekeeping and contributes to emotional disturbances that are often somatized, causing occupational illness in one and the housewife syndrome in the other.

4. New parents are unprepared for child rearing. Older family members no longer live nearby and cannot serve as authorities. Today's young woman does not learn first-hand from her mother's experience. Thus, the pediatrician becomes the sole guide for child raising.

Bittner concludes this excellent essay: "As once we have searched the heavens for signs to tell us our fate, so we are now attuned to the quivers of our body."

On a larger scale, governmental influences cannot be underestimated. Governments now respond to expectations that they ensure general health and well-being in addition to economic stability. Preventive medicine is the goal; public health programs and even remedial medical facilities are demanded.

The Riot Commission Report, a landmark in recent history, describes our urgent social problems and testifies to their magnitude. In the Negro center-city ghettos, a vicious cycle operates: unemployment, poverty, family breakdown, deprivation, exploitation, and crime. We surmise that this is a breeding ground for mental illness, but we lack epidemiologic studies and evaluations of the influence of social forces on the development of mental illness. In the future, the psychiatrist will have to think in terms of social engineering and will have to serve as a consultant to groups who are grappling with such dilemmas.

HISTORICAL INFLUENCES

Our present emphasis on comprehensive medical care is a return to concepts once accepted as indisputable. The essential unity of mind and body, a fundamental tenet of Greco-Roman medicine, was artificially divided by Christian theology. As medicine progressed through the nineteenth century, psychiatrists became custodians of the mentally ill, separated from the currents of the emerging scientific medicine.

With the development of psychoanalysis at the end of the century, psychiatry underwent a profound change; interest in the new knowledge about psychodynamics, psychopathology, and psychotherapy supplanted the concern with descriptive psychiatry. However, these two major accomplishments, scientific medicine and psychoanalysis, contributed to the further isolation of psychiatry. A mechanistic concept of disease was the unfortunate concomitant of magnificent discoveries, and the view of the patient was fragmented. As a reaction to specialization, psychosomatic medicine developed.

Early psychosomatic medicine was based on the little-known works of Groddeck, Ferenczi, and Deutsch. Then, in 1939, the American Psychosomatic Society was founded. Its stated purpose was "to study in their interrelation, the psychological and physiological aspects of all normal and abnormal bodily functions" (*Psychosomatic Medicine*, 5 [No. 1]: 3–5, January, 1939). World War II provided a medical laboratory for this new approach. Psychiatrists were brought into close association with their medical colleagues in the war environment, and within five years psychosomatic concepts were popularized and accepted. Unfortunately, psychosomaticists fell prey to the very problems that afflicted the fields they rejected; they also specialized, appropriating a few diseases of unknown etiology, such as hypertension and peptic ulcer, as their special province.

There were no spectacular achievements in this field; disillusionment followed. However, it did become apparent that psychosomatic influences contributed skills and knowledge which benefit medical and surgical patients with emotional distress. Also, the increasing contacts between psychiatrists and other physicians continued to break down existing barriers. Psychiatry entered the general hospital. The medical practitioner's responsibility for his patients' psychiatric problems was emphasized by the pioneer work of Kubie (1948, 1950, 1964), Kaufman and Margolin (1948), Levine (1942, 1945), Bibring (1956), and others.

SCIENTIFIC INFLUENCES

The impact of continued technological advances cannot be totally assessed. But in general, technology is transforming our national character, while in particular, it is invading every aspect of day to day living. With the progressing scientific revolution, illness itself is changing. For example, while automation reduces many occupational hazards, it creates others, psychological as well as physiological.

In the medical world the changes are great. Physicians now have access to complex diagnostic equipment, which works with unparalleled precision, and to new therapeutic skills for organ transplantation and cardiopulmonary surgery. Psychiatrists are being called upon to screen patients prior to these procedures and to make life-death decisions, for example, in the selection of patients for chronic hemodialysis. Soon we will meet the "artificial man," who contains numerous organs once belonging to others and who is attached by various life lines to apparatuses which perform vital mechanical and metabolic functions. Abrams (1967, 1968) et al. are writing about adaptation to these procedures; vast areas for research on changes in body image and object relationships with machines lie ahead.

Computerized medicine is fact not science fiction (Rome et al., 1962). Already, multiphasic screening centers are processing thousands of patients, rapidly diagnosing their physical and chemical disabilities. Freed from many technical tasks, the physician is given the opportunity—and the responsibility—for comprehensive patient care. Psychiatrists are devising measures and techniques which can be introduced into the multiphasic screening so that patients needing psychiatric consultations can be readily identified. Because of these developments, the humanizing function of the consultation assumes even greater importance. As Brosin (1968) says: "The automated assembly lines are often effective and efficient, but lack that emotional communication input so necessary to sustain the doctor as an altruistic professional worker. The psychiatric consultation has the potential of giving him an overall view of the patient and his family in a psychological dynamic setting, and can also help revive his more humanistic impulses and resist the dehumanizing process."

Knowledge is accumulating so rapidly that specialization is a way of life. Specialists are required not only to keep the new machines operating, but also to comprehend the vast amounts of new data, amassed facts, and concepts. Improved communication brings the news of these advances to the public who clamor for tangible benefits.

IMPLICATIONS

Against this sociocultural, historical, and scientific background the character of medical practice is evolving. Specialization is an inevitable result; and consultations between specialists are necessary to pool knowledge and skills for total patient care. As Mendel and Solomon (1968) state in their preface to *The Psychiatric Consultation*, psychiatry is developing a "new concept of the role of its specialty." In the summary Solomon says:

"The increasing importance of psychiatry in many aspects of modern life has brought about the emergence of a new psychiatric discipline, consultation psychiatry."

REFERENCES

ABRAM, HARRY S. The psychiatrist, the treatment of chronic renal failure, and the prolongation of life. Amer. J. Psychiat., 124 (10): 1351, April, 1968.
——— The psychiatrist, the treatment of chronic renal failure, and the prolongation of life, II. Delivered at the 124th Annual Meeting of the American Psychiatric Association, May 15, 1968, Boston.
BIBRING, G. L. Psychiatry and medical practice in a general hospital. New Eng. J. Med., 254:366, 1956.
BITTNER, E. Social institutions and medical care. Psychosomatics, 8 (3): 126–129, May/June, 1967.
BROSIN, HENRY. Communication systems of the consultation process. In The Psychiatric Consultation. W. M. Mendel and P. Solomon, eds. New York, Grune and Stratton, 1968.
DEUTSCH, F. Psychoanalysis at the bedside. Int. J. Psychoanal., 5:394, 1924.
——— The choice of the organ in organ neurosis, (Read before the Amer. Psychiat. Assoc., Chicago, May 8, 1939), Int. J. Psychoanal., 20:3, 1939.
——— et al., eds. Training in Psychosomatic Medicine. New York, Hafner Publishing Co., Inc., 1964.
Editorial. Psychosom. Med., 5(1):3, 1939.
FERENCZI, S. Further Contributions to the Theory and Technique of Psychoanalysis, Selected Papers. New York, Basic Books, Inc., Publishers, 1952.
GRODDECK, G. Book of the It. New York, Vintage, 1965.
——— Psychische Bedingtheit und Psychoanalytische Behandlung Organischer Leiden. (Psychic conditioning and the psychoanalytic treatment of organic disorders.) Leipzig, Hirzel, 1917.
——— Psychical treatment of organic disease. Brit. J. Med. Psychol., 9:179, 1929.
KAUFMAN, M. R., and MARGOLIN, S. G. Theory and practice of psychosomatic medicine in a general hospital. Med. Clin. N. Amer., 32:611, 1948.
KUBIE, L. S. The future of preventive psychiatry. Ment. Hyg. News (NH Conn), 24:1, 1948.
——— Practical and Theoretical Aspects of Psychoanalysis. New York, International Universities Press, Inc., 1950. (A revision of Practical Aspects of Psychoanalysis.)
——— A school of psychological medicine within the framework of medical school and university. J. Med. Educ., 39:476, 1964.
LEVINE, M. A. Psychotherapy in Medical Practice. New York, The Macmillan Company, 1942.
MENDEL, W. M., and SOLOMON, P. The Psychiatric Consultation. New York, Grune and Stratton, 1968.
——— Psychosomatic medicine. J. Kentucky Med. Ass., 43:39, 1945.
ROME, H. P., et al. Symposium on automation technique in personality assessment. Mayo Clin. Proc., 37:61, 1962.

CHANGES IN ATTITUDES TOWARD PSYCHIATRY

ALTROCCHI, J., and EISDORFER, C. Changes in atttudes toward mental illness. Ment. Hyg., 45:563, 1961.

BACKNER, B., and KISSINGER, R. D. Hospitalized patients' attitudes toward mental health professionals and mental patients. J. Nerv. Ment. Dis., 136:72, 1963.

BRADY, J. P., REZNIKOFF, M., and ZELLER, W. W. The psychiatric attitudes battery: A procedure for assessing attitudes toward psychiatric treatment and hospitals. J. Clin. Psychol., 15:260, 1959.

———— ZELLER, W. W., and REZNIKOFF, M. Attitudinal factors influencing outcome of treatment of hospitalized psychiatric patients. J. Clin. Exp. Psychopath., 20:326, 1959.

BRODSKY, C. A social view of the psychiatric consultation. Psychosomatics, 8(2): 61–68, March/April, 1967.

GYNTHER, M. D., REZNIKOFF, M., and FISHMAN, M. Attitudes of psychiatric patients toward treatment, psychiatrists, and mental hospitals. J. Nerv. Ment. Dis., 136:68, 1963.

JONES, N., KAHN, M., and MacDONALD, J. Psychiatric patients' views of mental illness, hospitalization, and treatment, J. Nerv. Ment. Dis., 136:82, 1963.

KLOPFER, W., WYLIE, A., and HILLSON, J. Attitudes toward mental hospitals. J. Clin. Psychol., 12:361, 1956.

NUNNALLY, J. The communication of mental health information: A comparison of the opinions of experts and the public with mass media. Behav. Sci., 2:222, 1957.

———— KITTROSS, J. M. Public attitudes toward mental health professions. Amer. J. Psychol., 13:589, 1958.

REZNIKOFF, M., BRADY, J. P., ZELLER, W. W., and TOOMEY, L. C. Attitudinal change in hospitalized psychiatric patients. J. Clin. Psychopath., 21:309, 1960.

2   CONCEPTS OF ILLNESS

Disease is a biographical event
Meerloo (1964)

Historically there have been separate mechanistic, biologic, psychosomatic, and ecologic concepts of illness. A comprehensive approach to illness, grounded on the principles of ecology, is imperative for the consultant. The comprehensive-ecologic model, recognizing that ideas change, embraces various concepts of disease and unites them into a working system. Consequently, any single approach may be utilized with maximal effectiveness when appropriate, without dislocating others. It always insists on patient orientation rather than disease orientation. Alan Gregg (1956) stated: "Possibly the next major development in the interpretation of disease will stress the ecologic approach—that is the recognition of the intimate yet extensive interrelatedness of the organism and its environment."

THE MECHANISTIC CONCEPT

The mechanistic concept implies that the human being is a machine composed of mutually adjusted parts and systems; disease results when a part is injured or defective, when a system is faulty, or when an adjustment fails. Halliday (1948) says: "Illness corresponds to a breakdown in this machine." He emphasizes that mechanistic principles are useful primarily in therapeutics, and states: "Mechanistic etiology provides no direct guidelines about the measures that will keep people from becoming ill. It is not an etiology suitable for prevention." He believes that a logical extension of the mechanistic concept of illness would be the proliferation of medical specialties.

7

Mechanistic principles were overvalued in the past; recently they have been attacked because of their inherent limitations and consequent reductionism. Obviously, the mechanistic approach is opposed to the holistic. The law of parsimony was a logical corollary of the mechanistic concept. This law states that all of a patient's symptoms should be explained by as few diagnoses as possible, preferably a single diagnosis. It emphasized the organic-versus-functional dichotomy, and, at times, even led to an outright disregard of the patient's emotional distress. Further, the focus on single-factor etiology is scientifically invalid and at variance with clinical experience. Nevertheless, mechanistic concepts underlie many of the advances in modern medicine, notably the development of microbiology and skilled surgery.

THE BIOLOGIC CONCEPT

Biologic concepts are fundaments of medicine. They furnish more than a knowledge of processes, e.g., physiology; they generate principles of the etiology of disease and also provide a scientific perspective on life and death. Halliday (1948) summarizes the biologic viewpoint: "1) The human organism, although composed of parts may also be regarded as an integrated unit or living person. 2) Illness represents a vital reaction or mode of behavior of a person to factors in the environment which he meets as he moves in time. 3) The cause of illness is therefore twofold, [viz.] certain characteristics of the person and certain factors of the environment."

Yet, an exclusively biologic viewpoint is too restrictive. First, a focus on pathology persists, and pathology as the sine qua non of illness has obvious limitations. Boyd (1965) insists: "Lesions may explain symptoms but not disease; they may answer the question *how* but not the much more profound question *why*." Second, the biologic approach requires that observations be confirmed by the scientific method; thus, psychical phenomena which cannot be physiologically verified are accepted uneasily, if at all. For example, because one cannot prove which processes are involved, how can one account for the conversion reaction? Or, how do hostility, guilt, and subjective states exert their effects on the metabolism or alter physiology? In biologic terms, there is even greater difficulty explaining the influence of psychosocial events on health and illness along the spectrum ranging from the exotic voodoo death to the ordinary dilemmas of daily life which involve disappointment or frustration.

THE PSYCHOSOMATIC CONCEPT

Psychosomatic concepts supplement the biologic; they assume that mental events are real even if intangible, and they embody a psychologic approach to the study of illness. Halliday (1948) defines a psychosomatic affection as: "A bodily disorder whose nature can be appreciated only when emotional disturbances, that is, psychological happenings, are investigated in addition to physical disturbances, that is, somatic happenings." He then notes shortcomings: "The allocation of a disorder to the psychosomatic category depends fundamentally on quantitative factors."

In discussing concepts of disease, Wolff (1962) reminds us that Claude Bernard perceived disease as the outcome of attempts at adaptation; these attempts produce disease because, although they are appropriate in kind, they are faulty in degree. But Wolff thinks that disease in humans has a more complex meaning because of man's highly developed nervous system; therefore, evoked reactions which are labeled "disease" may be wrong not only in magnitude but also in kind.

An emphasis on the quantitative implies that the psychic and the somatic are separate systems which can be individually weighed for their etiologic value. Attempts to find strict cause and effect relationships are a logical consequence; unfortunately these efforts usually neglect multifactorial etiology and abet the natural inclination to gain understanding by dichotomizing so that the patient is seen as having *either* psychic *or* somatic disease, and not *both*.

FIELD THEORY

Field theory, articulated by Kurt Lewin, provides an integration of etiologic principles requisite to a more comprehensive concept of illness. Lewin (1951) defines a field as "the totality of coexisting facts which are mutually interdependent." This, obviously, is holistic. The organism and the total environment are mutually interdependent. They are a system composed of parts and subsystems which, in reality, never exist in isolation, but continually transact with and influence each other. Therefore, as Hall and Lindsey (1957) state, "Behavior is a function of the field which exists at the time the behavior occurs." And, as Spiegel (Grinker, 1953) explains, "Since the field is a continuum of patterned, transactional processes, the structure-function of any one part of the field affects the structure-function of all the other parts of the field, and, therefore, of the whole field." Spiegel continues, "The structure of functional interdependence of all the parts of the field makes statements describing dominance or hierarchical relations of one part of the field over another essentially meaningless. For example, biological, psychological, and cultural events are considered to be parts of the field; the particular forms one takes will depend upon the reciprocal relations among all three. One cannot be derived from another but must be considered as having spatial and temporal coexistence." In commenting on this psychosomatic-social field,

Grinker adds: "When stressful forces succeed in straining or disintegrating parts of the field, foreboding somatic signs may be observed and, in the human being, the signal of anxiety may be experienced."

Wittkower and Cleghorn (1954) apply field theory to illness. Signs and symptoms of illness are viewed in a field of six components: 1) the field of the individual as he began to react to the disease, 2) the field of the environment: physical, bacterial, cultural, economic, and so on, 3) the field of the observer: his relationship to the field and influence on the form and content of the data he receives, 4) the field of the mechanism, involving the cause and effect relationships and reactions of the human machine (e.g., biochemical or physiological processes), 5) the field of purpose, in which illness is seen as a link in a circular chain of self-regulating events (e.g., the patient became ill so that he could escape the stresses of work) and, 6) the field of methodology (e.g., cardiac catheterization rather than auscultation), in principle and in practice.

Halliday (1948) gives this theory practical form when, in discussing principles of etiology, he states: "The question, What is the cause of the onset of this illness?, is tripartite, namely: 1) What kind of person was this? i.e., which characteristics are relevant and causal? 2) Why did he become ill when he did? i.e., which factors of environment are relevant and causal? and 3) Why did he become ill in the manner that he did? i.e., which part contacted the factor and which bits and pieces by preceding movement and ensuing movement finally made manifest the particular mode of behavior?"

For every patient he sees, the consultant should ask himself these three simple questions: What kind of person is he? Why did he become ill when he did? And why did he become ill in the manner he did? Formulating thoughts about the patient this way brings holistic concepts directly into everyday practice. Moreover, we find that the physicians and surgeons we work with are quite receptive to our teaching from this framework.

THE ECOLOGIC CONCEPT

For the physician, the ecologic approach means that he must always assess the illness in the context of the patient's environment as that environment influences illness and the patient's capacity to deal with it. In his studies of illness and social environment, Hinkle (1961) concludes that there are no discrete psychosomatic diseases, but that all illness is to some extent influenced by the social environment. He describes the ecologic viewpoint: "The ecologist views life as based upon the maintenance of a dynamic steady state in a highly ordered system, and he is concerned

with the interactions that occur between this system—the living organism
—and the environment in which it exists." The ecologic approach "is biological, and . . . (the ecologist's) assumption is that those aspects of
human biology that are 'social' or 'behavioral' are different from the re-
mainder of the natural world only in degree, complexity, and order."

Thus, the comprehensive approach involves much more than eliciting
the medical history and attempting to make it conform to a medical
model. The physician must use the tools of anthropology, sociology, and
psychology as he evaluates each patient. From anthropology he learns that
particular cultures include unique attributes and traits which both define
and influence illness and that a patient from a given cultural experience
may be expected to have acquired characteristic reaction patterns. From
sociology he learns that certain attitudes and values are associated with
special levels in the society and with specific group situations. When this
information is used along with that obtained from the evaluation of the
patient's psychologic status, the physician can then understand how the
patient views his own life situation at a particular time.

The patient's estimate may be crucial. For example, Hinkle (1961)
even correlated patients' opinions of their life situations at given times
with the number of concurrent illnesses; periods in life perceived as
highly satisfactory were also times which included a low incidence of
illness. While stressing that the approach of the ecologist is biological,
Hinkle continues by saying: "The weight of the evidence is that man's
interaction with his social and interpersonal environment is relevant, not
just to his emotional state or to his mental health, but to all of the illness
that he experiences. This relationship is, in the last analysis, a life and
death proposition for him."

SUBJECTIVE CONSIDERATIONS

Concepts of illness include the subjective. A physician's appraisal of a
patient involves his reactions to the patient and his criteria for defining
illness as well as his personal and professional concerns. These range from
his own state of mental health and physical well-being to his clinical
know-how and financial objectives. How he appraises illness is influenced
by his value judgments, ethical standards, and attitudes. For example, an
alcoholic has been defined as one who drinks more than his physician.
Moreover, the physician's social class, background, and aspirations are of
immense importance. Scott (1958) in commenting on Hollingshead and
Redlich's work (1958), notes that rates of neurosis under treatment are
more a function of the therapist's social distance from the patient than of
the patient's financial limitations. Of course, illness may be iatrogenic. The

zealous physician's insistence on repeated diagnostic procedures can transform a patient's worries about his chest into the inexorable conviction that he has heart disease. And, physicians bear the responsibility for many cases of addiction to narcotics.

THE COMPREHENSIVE CONCEPT

The comprehensive approach, grounded on ecologic principles, is a derivative of these various concepts. It adheres to the following propositions:

1. Patients are people under stress; illness and health are on a continuum, embodying various adaptive and maladaptive reactions.
2. The mind and body are merely phases of the same system.
3. Multiple etiologic factors are responsible for all illness.
4. The human organism, his physical and social environment, his past history and present purpose, and his relations with others are all intertwined, not only constituting the cause, but also determining the form, the character, and the degree of the reaction to stress.
5. The constitutional endowment, as well as developed patterns of response (resistance or susceptibility), contribute to the reactions which are termed illness.
6. Finally, the physician's perception of illness and all the facets of his relationship with the patient are intrinsic to the comprehensive approach.

For even the mind depends so much on the temperament and disposition of the bodily organs that if it be possible to find some means by which man might commonly be made wise and able . . . I believe it is in medicine that it ought to be looked for.

(Descartes, *Discours de la Methode*, Part VI)

IS MENTAL ILLNESS A MYTHICAL CONCEPT?

Any discussion of concepts of illness must consider the current controversy: Is mental illness a medical problem or sociocultural one? In his book, *The Myth of Mental Illness*, Szasz (1961) attacks the traditional view of mental illness as an object or a condition which is alien to the afflicted person and thus subject to removal by therapy. He says: "It is customary to define psychiatry as a medical specialty concerned with the study, diagnosis, and treatment of mental illness . . . Mental illness is a myth. Psychiatrists are not concerned with mental illness in their treatment. In actual practice they deal with personal, social, and ethical problems of living."

Physicians discuss mental illness as if it exists in a discrete form like tuberculosis or a fracture. That assumption rests at one extremity of a continuum; at the other pole is Szasz's contention that all mental illness is only sociocultural. Parsons (1964) enters the debate, emphasizing a social definition of mental illness. He describes "sociocultural diseases," stating: "The primary criteria for mental illness must be defined with reference to the social role performance of the individual. . . . It is as an incapacity to meet the expectations of social roles that mental illness becomes a problem in social relationships. . . . Mental health is rather concerned with capacity to enter into such relationships and to fulfill the expectations of such memberships." These expectations vary from culture to culture. Clausen (1959) insists that "cultural definitions of the specific problems involved [mental illness] vary tremendously and bear little resemblance to psychiatric definitions. . . . Psychiatric knowledge and the mental health movement are social products, certainly subject to study." Parsons (1964) adds to this that "in the United States we are more likely to interpret a difficulty in an individual's fulfilling social role expectations as a disturbance in capacity, i.e., as illness, than is true of other types of societies with other types of value systems." And so, this argument concludes, mental illness may be viewed exclusively as a socio-cultural event.

Clausen's and Parsons' thesis has obvious, but only partial, validity. That mental illness involves the interpersonal and the social is clear. But, all illness has social implications; tuberculosis, syphilis, in fact all the contagious diseases, and even heart disease or cancer, are affected by interpersonal and sociocultural forces. These forces influence the definition, the incidence, the cause, and the treatment of the illness. It is reported, for example, that the incidence of psychoneurosis in the Russian Army during World War II was incredibly low. The Russians ascribe this to high morale. But, Western observers are skeptical, believing that, because the label was in political disfavor, the psychoneurotics were diagnosed otherwise or were forced into combat and swelled the already immense casualty rolls.

Attempts to define mental illness as a purely sociocultural phenomenon are subject to all the pitfalls found in discarded notions of single-factor etiology. The comprehensive concept of illness, with its emphasis on ecologic factors, assumes that sociocultural forces are vital and that they must be understood in both the social and medical view for the work between the psychiatrist and the patient to be therapeutic.

In speaking about solutions to the controversy over concepts of illness, Szasz (1961) states: "The task is to redefine the problem of mental illness so that it may be encompassed under the general category of the science of man. Medicine itself contributes to this enterprise, as do numerous other disciplines." This position is not new. Medicine should be the science of man; and to fulfill its commitment, it must embrace and build on sociologic and psychologic theory and practice. Throughout history, medicine has always drawn from a variety of physical, biological, and social sciences; Pasteur, after all, was not a physician.

This controversy is salutary because it emphasizes the psychosocial and the psychosomatic when, for too long, they were neglected in favor of the purely somatic. But holding one belief or emphasizing one extremity of this continuum, e.g., the sociologic, is both narrow and restrictive. Mental illness is primarily a concept concerned with behavior; and behavior is determined not only by sociocultural forces but also by the biological and the psychological. Thus, mental illness cannot be defined only in social terms.

Furthermore, the controversy about the nature of mental illness is superficial because it does not recognize that illness and medical practice are integral aspects of the social history of a society or of an era. This was affirmed by Burton (1927) in the Seventeenth Century, Trotter (1807) in the Eighteenth Century, and particularly by Henry Sigerist (1951) in the last few decades. What is recognized as illness? How is it defined? The frequency, the form in which it is expressed, and especially the care-taking measures are influenced by and in turn reflect the social climate and the prevailing philosophies. What value is placed on an individual's health, or life? What responsibilities for health does the society assume?

REFERENCES

BOYD, W. Pathology for the Physician, 7th ed. Philadelphia, Lea and Febiger, 1965, p. 4.

BURTON, R. The Anatomy of Melancholy. New York, Tudor Publishing Co., 1927.

CLAUSEN, J. A. The sociology of mental illness. In Merton, R. K., Broom, L., and Cottrell, L. S., Jr., eds. Sociology Today: Problems and Prospects. New York, Basic Books, Inc., Publishers, 1959, pp. 485–508.

GREGG, A. What is the meaning of disease? In Challenges to Contemporary Medicine. New York, Columbia University Press, 1956, pp. 25–48.

GRINKER, R. R. Psychosomatic Research, New York, W. W. Norton & Company, Inc., 1953, pp. 159–160, 165.

HALL, C. S., and LINDSEY, G. Theories of Personality. New York, John Wiley & Sons, Inc., 1957, p. 240.

HALLIDAY, J. L. Psychosocial Medicine: A Study of the Sick Society. New York, W. W. Norton & Company, Inc., 1948, pp. 17, 26.

HINKLE, L. E. Ecological observations of the relation of physical illness, mental illness, and the social environment. Psychosom. Med., 23:289, 1961.

HOLLINGSHEAD, A. B., and REDLICH, F. C. Social Class and Mental Illness: a Community Study. New York, John Wiley and Sons, Inc., 1958.

LEWIN, K. Field Theory in Social Science: Selected Theoretical Papers. Cartwright, D., ed. New York, Harper & Row, Publishers, 1951, p. 240.

MEERLOO, J. A. M. Illness and Cure. New York, Grune & Stratton, Inc., 1964, p. 44.

PARSONS, T. Definitions of health and illness in the light of American values and social structure. *In* Social Structure and Personality. New York, The Free Press of Glencoe, 1964, pp. 258–291.

SCOTT, W. A. Social, psychological correlates of mental illness and mental health. Psychol. Bull., 55(2):65, 1958.

SIGERIST, H. E. A History of Medicine. London, Oxford University Press, 1951.

SZASZ, T. S. The Myth of Mental Illness. New York, Paul B. Hoeber, Inc., 1961, p. 297.

TROTTER, T. A View of the Nervous Temperament. London, Longsman, Hurst, Rees, and Orme, 1807.

WITTKOWER, E., and CLEGHORN, R. A. Basic concepts of psychosomatic medicine. *In* MacLeod, A. W., Wittkower, E. D., and Margolin, S. G., eds. Recent Developments in Psychosomatic Medicine. Philadelphia, J. B. Lippincott Co., 1954, pp. 3–28.

WOLFF, H. Concepts of disease. Psychosom. Med., 24(1), 1962.

3 THE NATURE OF CONSULTATION WORK

Utilizing the comprehensive-ecologic concept of illness, the psychiatric consultant stands at the interface bridging psychiatry and medicine. His position is new, and the opportunities are great. As Sandt and Leifer (1964) indicate, psychiatric consultations are viewed within three major frameworks: "1) as a community service to social work agencies, schools, criminal courts and mental health clinics, 2) as an educational device for teaching psychiatry to medical students and house staff, and 3) as a diagnostic and therapeutic tool in general hospitals." Established consultation programs are essential resources which should be available to all physicians. A study of consultation work shows that it has evolved through three phases.

THE PATIENT-ORIENTED APPROACH

First the psychiatrist focused his efforts on proving that he could contribute to the care of general medical and surgical patients. Psychiatric consultations were patient-oriented (Bernstein and Kaufman, 1962; Cushing, 1950; Weisman and Hackett, 1960). They were in the medical tradition, emphasizing diagnosis, evaluating psychopathology, and providing treatment or disposition for the patient. Kaufman (1953) states that this orientation was historically necessary; it enabled the psychiatrist to take his place in the family of physicians. Many psychiatrists still adhere to the patient-oriented consultation because it is an accustomed approach which fits standardized medical practices. However, this approach is limited because the consultant deals primarily with the patient and responds only to the explicit questions raised by the referring physician.

Experience revealed shortcomings: first, level of psychopathology

16

was not a consistent indication for referral, and second, physicians' concerns were usually more complex than their referral requests indicated. Another orientation was called for. Although Balint (1957) insisted for years that working with the referring physician was much more productive than seeing the patient for a brief consultative hour, only recently, the work of Beigler et al. (1959), Schiff and Pilot (1959), Meyer and Mendelson (1961), and others stressed the consultee's role. They studied the types of, and the reasons for, referrals, focusing on the referring physician's role in producing or alleviating disturbed behavior. The consultant, they advocated, must teach the principles of medical psychology to referring physicians.

THE CONSULTEE-ORIENTED APPROACH

With the advent of the consultee-oriented approach, consultants' activities were enlarged in scope; they were no longer limited to diagnostic or treatment services. Schiff and Pilot (1959) state that consultations act as ". . . a lever with which to deal with the resistances of the house staff to psychiatric principles, to extend the house staff's understanding of these principles, and, in some cases, to 'popularize' psychiatry." This orientation acknowledges that the referral request is a plea for help on the part of the referring physician, existing in both overt and covert forms. Schiff and Pilot list four situations particularly appropriate for the consultee-oriented approach: 1) a breakdown in the physician-patient relationship, 2) a lack of consensus between the patient and the medical staff about the severity of the illness, resulting in the patient's leaving the hospital against medical advice, 3) the mismanagement of coexisting medical and psychiatric problems, for example, the doctor's feeling of omnipotence may be destroyed by his inability to cope with the patient's emotional distress, and 4) discord within the staff stemming from divergent points of view regarding patient management.

The consultee orientation calls for interviewing the physician as well as the patient. This interview is designed to elicit the underlying reasons for the request, gauge the physician's knowledge of the problem, expose uncertainties, and assess the capacities of the medical staff for patient care from which suggestions for treatment can be developed.

THE SITUATION-ORIENTED APPROACH

Today, in accord with the comprehensive-ecologic concepts of illness and the current emphasis on community and social psychiatry, consultation activities have moved into a third phase, the situation-oriented.

It extends the consultant's interests and activities to incorporate the total patient milieu. Greenberg (1960) describes this type of consultation at length; he emphasizes a total approach to the patient and the importance of dealing with the consultee's anxiety. This orientation accepts as fact that paramedical personnel, other patients, and visitors, as well as the consultee, contribute to and, indeed, may determine the need for consultation. Also, the milieu is not limited to the patient in his bed, or even to the hospital, but radiates to include the family, place of work, and community. Thus, the consultant is concerned with the influences, intrinsic to the milieu, which produce illness and complicate treatment. This view subscribes to and even goes beyond the concept of the operational group formulated by Meyer and Mendelson (1961); the consultant enlists the help of others.

From our experience at the University of Florida, we found that a rigid adherence to any particular orientation is unwise. Therefore, we developed an eclectic approach derived from traditional concepts, one which varies with each situation. Each orientation may be applied discriminately, individually or in combination with others. However, we use the situational approach most frequently because it possesses the greatest opportunities for effective consultation work.

PSYCHIATRIC CONSULTATION WORK

Psychiatric consultation work differs from consultative activities in the other medical specialties because most physicians believe that referral to a psychiatrist is beset by special difficulties.

First, physicians think that their patients hesitate to accept psychiatric referral because of the stigma attached to mental illness. Both physicians' and patients' opinions about psychiatry influence referral procedures and produce special problems. To a limited extent, more favorable attitudes toward psychiatry are expressed by patients with higher educational and socioeconomic status, although personal contact with mental health workers is the most significant determinant (Schwab et al., 1966; see also Attitude Changes). Brodsky (1965) notes that the growing acceptance of the psychiatric consultation derives from current attitudes which look upon the psychiatrist as an authority on human behavior.

A second difficulty peculiar to the psychiatric consultation is posed by those patients who attempt to avoid the encounter in order to maintain their neuroses. They feel they cannot relinquish established patterns of behavior; they display resistance, an intrinsic part of the neurotic organization, as they try to retain the primary and secondary gains of illness. Affability, compliance, or pseudo-agreement, as well as covert

intimidation and more conventional defensive measures are used to op-
pose the referral. By definition, psychiatric referral involves the whole
person in contrast to more conventional medical referrals which usually
specify that the consultant diagnose or treat only a part of the person.
For example, when the psychiatrist works with his patient, that person's
behavior and values, indeed his whole life are scrutinized. On the other
hand, a cardiologist is primarily concerned with the patient's heart, a
surgeon with the indications for surgery. Therefore, as clinical experience shows, patients unquestionably accept referrals to other specialists
while they may be reluctant about psychiatric referral because it involves
submission of the whole person and threatens to jeopardize the neurosis.

For physicians, as well as patients, elements of mystery still surround
the psychiatrist. Many physicians think they cannot inform their patients,
in explicit terms, how the psychiatrist works or what he will do. Divergent training, differing concepts of illness, and problems with communication cloud understanding between psychiatrists and other physicians.
In training, the psychiatrist is too often deprived of contact with his
medical colleagues, particularly when he works in a removed part of a
general hospital, or when he takes his residency in an institution which
cares only for the mentally ill. Conceptually, the psychiatrist stresses
diagnosis and treatment by the inclusion rather than the exclusion of
illness factors. And psychiatric terminology, with its proliferation of
jargon, obstructs communication.

Lastly, both psychiatrists and other physicians have enlarged the gap
between medicine and psychiatry. Psychiatrists often discard their medical
role and even, at times, flagrantly disavow their medical knowledge.
Other physicians pretend ignorance of human behavior or even, more
irrationally, fear that the psychiatrist will analyze their private neuroses
or evaluate their characterologic disturbances.

Despite its complex nature, consultation work is an appropriate
means for meeting the staggering demands for psychiatric care. When
psychiatrists work closely with their medical colleagues, their skills and
knowledge are made available to many more patients than when they are
practicing in more conventional surroundings. At the same time, the
mutual interest and the cohesion of effort for patient care remove barriers; physicians learn from psychiatrists, and psychiatrists are saved
from remaining isolated members of an esoteric profession (see Beigler
et al., 1959).

THE THEORETICAL BASIS

Theoretical models support the consultant's activities and provide
a basis for the further development of this work.

THE THERAPEUTIC CONSULTATION MODEL

In their article, "The Organization and Function of a Psychiatric Consultation Service," Weisman and Hackett (1960) wrote about the "therapeutic consultation." An essential element was the "change in emphasis from disease orientation, in which the patient is an illustration of pathological processes, to patient orientation, in which individual personal motivation and impaired ego capacity influence the adaptation to illness. The predominant clinical problem for which the consultation was requested became the focal point of investigation, not merely as a symptom of disease or as an indication of the physician-patient relationship, but more as an expression of crisis or conflict with which the patient, as a human being at that instant in time, was confronted."

Weisman and Hackett conceptualize the "therapeutic consultation" by distinguishing among the impersonal, intrapersonal, and interpersonal factors involved. In this schema, the impersonal consists of the crisis imposed on the patient, a situation beyond the patient's control, environmental factors such as mandatory retirement, an accident, or even a natural catastrophe. The intrapersonal or the intrapsychic is primarily concerned with conflict (affecting the illness or produced by the illness) and with the patient's adaptive capacities: ego strengths, defense mechanisms, and fantasies. The interpersonal is the patient's relationships with family and others.

Weisman and Hackett (1960) recognize four fundamental principles of consultation work: 1) a rapid evaluation, 2) the psychodynamic formulation of the major conflict, 3) an effective program for therapy, and 4) the active implementation of that program by the psychiatrist. Their emphasis on the psychodynamic formulation of the major conflict is particularly valuable and is further developed in a special article. They conclude by pointing out that the patient-oriented viewpoint coupled with a psychodynamic formulation of the factors associated with crisis, conflict, and reality testing, provides a basis for the therapeutic consultation.

Their model is sound but limited because the interpersonal focus is viewed almost exclusively from the perspective of the patient. Insufficient consideration is given to the staff's reactivity to, contribution to, or participation in interpersonal processes.

THE OPERATIONAL GROUP MODEL

In an effort to obtain a greater understanding of consultation patterns and processes, Meyer and Mendelson (1961) analyzed referral procedures for 60 medical inpatients at Johns Hopkins. They defined the operational group as involving the physicians, nurses, and other personnel, as well as the hospitalized patient. The request for psychiatric consultation reflects a crisis within the group, usually a disruption of trust and communication between the patient and the "caring-for" people. Two necessary conditions precede the consultation request: 1) staff uncertainty, developing when the patient's behavior defies understanding (in terms of the information available about him); and 2) a continued feeling of responsibility for the patient. It is not the actual level of overt psychopathology which creates uncertainty about the patient. Instead, it is the perception of the patient's behavior as disproportionate, not meeting the physician's expectations for the patient's condition, that engenders uncertainty. Uncertainty arouses the physician's anxiety and this interferes with the doctor-patient relationship; the physician feels alienated and the patient begins to doubt the physician's competence. The effects of uncertainty spread to involve the nurses and paramedical personnel; the entire hospital situation becomes antitherapeutic. At this point, if the staff does not feel an ongoing sense of responsibility, the patient may be discharged abruptly or manipulated into a situation in which he is apt to sign out of the hospital against advice. However, when there is a continued sense of responsibility, the physician calls for consultation. The entrance of the psychiatrist redefines the operational group, thus reducing anxiety and establishing trust and communication. The interactions between the patient and the staff then become therapeutic. Sometimes merely initiating the referral request is sufficient because the staff has taken positive action which they regard as constructive.

This theoretical model accounts for many inconsistencies in referral processes and explains, at least in part, why some patients are referred for consultations while others, with the same or greater degrees of psychopathology, are not. Although this theory is valuable in its general applicability for inpatient consultation work, several questions arise. First, would the same problems be encountered with private medical inpatients? Second, does making the request for consultation always reduce the referring physician's anxiety? It may have the opposite effect; the physician may feel he is losing control over the patient through the referral. Finally, this model does not incorporate Abrahams and Golden's (1963) astute observation, verified by clinical experience, that increased communication and trust between the physician and his patient may lead to requests for referral as the physician obtains greater understanding of the patient and wishes to maximize his therapeutic role.

THE COMMUNICATION MODEL

Sandt and Leifer (1964) propose a communication model and discuss the significance of the language used in referral notes. Consultation requests are often ambiguous, reflecting the physician's attitudes toward, and his expectations of, the consultant. In their schema, the referral event has three components: 1) the sender—patient, physician, or family, 2) the message itself, and 3) the receiver. An analysis of the referral language can reveal: the expected role of the psychiatrist, camouflaged values and feelings held by the patient and staff about psychiatry, and whose agent (patient's or referring physician's) the psychiatric consultant is.

For Sandt and Leifer, consultation requests are phrased in three types of instrumental (calling-for-action) language: communicative, promotive, and suggestive. *Communicative* language refers to the straight transmission of information: "This patient has colitis; please evaluate for ulcerative colitis." *Promotive* language is more persuasive, asking for specific action: "This patient has an anxiety reaction; provide psychiatric treatment, both immediate and long-term." *Suggestive* language is communicative and promotive; it inculcates certain emotions in the receiver: "Please take this hostile man off our hands; he is paranoid, in trouble all the time, and we can't put up with it any longer." All language, the authors say, may be conceptualized as ranging along a continuum from the communicative to the promotive, with the suggestive a form of both. Therefore, the consultant must be prepared to analyze the attitudes of the sender as expressed in the note in order to adopt the suitable approach: patient-oriented, consultee-oriented, or situation-oriented.

The consultant can use this communication model to obtain a greater understanding of the complexities of consultation work, particularly when he recognizes the limitless ramifications, both denotative and connotative, of our language. Sandt and Leifer have begun an exploration of the applicability of communication principles to consultation activities; their endeavors need further development and clinical testing.

Recently, Brosin (1968) has stressed that "the several communication systems in the consultation process are of crucial importance in the relations of psychiatrists with other members of the medical profession and, indeed, with everyone in the health professions." He maintains that after the initial request for consultation is transmitted, both the sender (encoder) and receiver (decoder) enter into a subsequent message system in which each one encodes and decodes. Thus, the nature and the quality of the work performed by the consultant will be influenced by his ongoing communications with the consultee.

SUMMARY

These theoretical models are not mutually exclusive. Weisman and Hackett's (1960) emphasis on viewing the patient from the impersonal, intrapersonal, and interpersonal dimensions can be combined with Meyer and Mendelson's (1961) concept of the operational group to provide the consultant with structure for his work. Sandt's and Leifer's (1964) discussion of referral language aids the consultant in analyzing the complexities of the referral, and Brosin's emphasis on communicative systems points to the process on which improved consultation procedures depend.

REFERENCES

ABRAHAMS, D., and GOLDEN, J. S. Psychiatric consultations on a medical ward. Arch. Intern. Med. (Chicago), 112:766, 1963.

BALINT, M. The Doctor, His Patient, and the Illness. New York, International Universities Press, Inc., 1957.

BEIGLER, J. S., ROBBINS, F. P., LANE, E. W., MILLER, A. A., and SAMELSON, C. Report on liaison psychiatry at Michael Reese Hospital, 1950–58. AMA Arch. Neurol. Psychiat., 81:733, 1959.

BERNSTEIN, S., and KAUFMAN, M. R. The psychiatrist in a general hospital: His functional relationship to the non-psychiatric service. J. Mount Sinai Hosp. N.Y., 29:385, 1962.

BRODSKY, C. A social view of the psychiatric consultation. Psychosomatics, 8(2): 61–68, March/April, 1967.

BROSIN, H.: Communication systems of the consultation process. In The Psychiatric Consultation. W. M. Mendel and P. Solomon, ed. New York, Grune and Stratton, 1968.

CUSHING, J. G. N. The role of the psychiatrist as a consultant. Amer. J. Psychiat., 106:861, 1950.

GREENBERG, I. M. Approaches to psychiatric consultation in a research hospital setting. Arch. Gen. Psychiat. (Chicago), 3:691, 1960.

KAUFMAN, M. R. The role of the psychiatrist in a general hospital. Psychiat. Quart., 27:367, 1953.

MEYER, E., and MENDELSON, M. Psychiatric consultations with patients on medical and surgical wards: Patterns and processes. Psychiatry, 24:197, 1961.

SANDT, J. J., and Leifer, R. Psychiatric consultation. Compr. Psychiat., 5:409, 1964.

SCHIFF, S. K., and PILOT, M. L. An approach to psychiatric consultation in the general hospital. Arch. Gen. Psychiat. (Chicago), 1:349, 1959.

SCHWAB, J. J., CLEMMONS, R. S., VALDER, M. J., and RAULERSON, J. D. Medical inpatient's reactions to psychiatric consultations. J. Nerv. Ment. Dis., 142(3), 1966.

WEISMAN, A., and HACKETT, T. The organization and function of a psychiatric consultation service. Int. Record Med., 173:306, 1960.

SECTION TWO   Fundamentals

4   THE ROLE OF THE CONSULTANT

[Psychiatry's] interests are biographic, and its procedures are those of history. It is essentially humanistic since it deals with man's relations to himself and to others. . . . I believe that the principal contribution of psychiatry . . . lies in its humanizing influence. It has kept man himself at the center . . . rather than his enzymes or the chains of proteins of which he is composed.

Binger (1966)

The role of the psychiatric consultant is not rigidly defined. It involves more than performance; it includes sense of purpose. As a specialist in comprehensive medicine the consultant is a model for other physicians.

Both Cushing (1950) and Beigler et al. (1959) describe the consultant's essential obligation: to provide psychiatric skills and knowledge for general medical and surgical patients. Kaufman (1953) insists on the dynamic qualities vital to this role; the effective consultant is a catalyst, and more, an integrator. To this we add that he is an interpreter. As a consultant, the psychiatrist is catalytic when he uses the information gleaned from his comprehensive evaluation to change an arid, or incompletely understood, case history to one of meaning and interest. When the physician learns why and how the patient's complaints emerge from the stresses of the past, compounded with the problems of the present, even the "crock" loses his dullness, and individualized responsible management replaces stereotyped approaches. To fulfill his role, the consultant has to integrate the conventional data about the patient (medical history and results from examinations and laboratory procedures) with knowledge of personality dynamics and the meaning of the illness to the patient. This synthesis clarifies how and why the patient reacts in his unique manner.

Integrating the data is only the first step. Next, the consultant must interpret the patient's behavior to the staff. Then, their view can change from disease orientation to person orientation. When the staff reinterpret the patient's illness and behavior in the light of their increased understanding, management can become therapeutic.

Further, the consultant must utilize his medical training as fully as possible. Too frequently, psychiatrists reject this background to which they gave a decade of their lives, and in doing so violate the holistic concepts which they espouse. Although the term holistic is overworked, receiving more lip service than practice, both the concept and the approach are fundamental to psychotherapy and mandatory for consultation work. By adhering to holistic concepts, with full regard for the inclusion of medical and psychological facts, the consultant can use his skills interpersonally with the staff to promote patient care.

The consultant is a model for others as he approaches patients and deals with interpersonal problems. These problems are not limited to difficulties between the patient and the staff, such as threats to omnipotence or overidentification. They also exist among the staff members as controversy due to personality differences, competitiveness, and discrepant views of the patient. Berblinger (1968) emphasizes the importance of the psychiatrist's role as a relationship expert. He cautions, "A competing doctor-patient relationship and a feeling of exclusion on the referring physician's side are probably greater obstacles for communication between colleagues than differing theoretical premises or frames of reference." He notes that psychiatrists seldom ask for consultation from other psychiatrists, and we have observed that psychiatrists who overvalue psychogenic concepts are sometimes reluctant to refer their patients to medicine or surgery.

So, the major role of the consulting psychiatrist is to be the specialist in comprehensive medicine. Specifically, this role requires the evaluation and treatment of the patient with a deliberate synthesis of the medical, psychological, and sociocultural processes which combine to produce illness and influence recovery.

Above all, the consultant is a teacher; he has opportunities to convey the principles of medical psychology to his colleagues. Finally, there is a need for documentation, study, and research. Too frequently, anecdote or impression is relied on when clinical research could provide the observations and the data from which principles can be formulated and taught.

THE CONSULTANT'S ROLE IN CONTRIBUTING TO MEDICAL THEORY AND PRACTICE

A discussion of the psychiatric consultant's role leads logically to a consideration of psychiatry's contribution to medical theory and practice.

1) As a basic science, psychiatry focuses on human behavior in health and disease and studies it scientifically. 2) Psychiatrists have confronted the age-old mind-body dilemma directly. Their insistence on the unity of the mind-body has fostered holistic approaches essential for the treatment of any sick person. 3) Psychiatry leads in the research with, and treatment of, patients with psychosomatic diseases. In fact psychosomatic medicine has been largely, but not exclusively, a psychiatric specialty. Psychiatric tenets concerning various psychosomatic illness, such as peptic ulcer, are now accepted; all physicians are cognizant of the effects of conflicts and stress on structural disease. 4) The concept of functional illness has changed from a vague label applied to illness in which organic pathology could not be found to an acceptance that "All human illness is functional since normal functioning is disturbed. The fact that the heaviest impact of the illness may be at the somatic or psychic level is of less moment than the understanding that basically all human illness involves disorder of functioning" (Strecker, 1957). 5) Psychiatry has underscored the importance of multiple factors in the etiology of disease. 6) Psychiatry is encouraging the development of team medicine. Psychiatrists collaborate with their medical colleagues, use milieu therapy, and are bringing together behavioral scientists, such as sociologists and psychologists, as well as ministers and lawyers, to join in a more comprehensive effort to prevent and treat mental illness. 7) Psychiatry is assuming the responsibility for teaching medical psychology.

The consultant's role is to carry these contributions to fruition. A recent editorial in *The Southern Medical Journal* (August 1966) states, "A number of factors are increasing the momentum of the *rapprochement* occurring between psychiatric and nonpsychiatric medicine . . . Fortunately for everyone concerned, the facts of modern society and modern medicine are forcing the psychiatrist and the nonpsychiatric physician to face each other across the hospital bed, or across the examining table in the clinic or emergency room." [The italics are the author's].

Lastly, Binger's (1966) emphasis on psychiatry's humanizing influence should be heeded by the consultant as he ponders his role. Of the medical specialists, he is farthest from the physical sciences and closest to the humanities. But, Kaplan (1967) observes: "In America the (psychiatrist) is trained in the backyards of science and is deprived of intensive training in the humanities. Medical training turns out physicians who are preponderantly pragmatic, scarcely versed in experimental method and the philosophy of science, and practically illiterate about the broad issues of the Western cultural tradition." Physicians are accused of ignorance not only of philosophy and literature, but also of life itself except for the hospital, the office, and the world of the sick.

Of course, this is not uniformly true. American medicine includes in its ranks such distinguished poets as William Carlos Williams. And, the new emphasis on the history and philosophy of medicine is reminding medical professionals that some of the great physicians of the past were Renaissance men who made significant contributions in many fields and brought to medicine a humanistic view. We see this trend reflected in the work of the modern medical student, and we wish to offer an example from our own medical college at the University of Florida.

METAMORPHOSIS: ON BECOMING A DOCTOR

we worked
at learning
over this veda
that torah
in silent cells
in the busy temples built to bones
monks meek and wan
vested in our order
discipled fast to mortal gods
painfully inscribing that symptom this cure
on the wrinkling parchment of our youth
fingering our rote questions and answers
like beads
strung together
to reach the cross of cure

we grew
in work
to feel with hands the withered pulse
to prod the wilting flesh with drugs
seeing bellies break and hearts stop
agonized by caring
we pushed our roots deep in earth
and trimmed away our fruitless limbs
cutting off our thumbs of rage
pruning our fingers of laughter
always eyeing harvest time
we thrust out buds of self-acceptance
our tree was leaved in jargon
words hard as stones
that talk of each petal
of deaths flowers
sprawled in fields around us

we endured
the manyfooted autumn crawl
the fallen leaf
the lean winter
cloistered
in our chrysalis
grown
in our spring change
to emerge in summers ritual way
among the brightly flowered fields

FRED FREVRIER
Class of 1968

Beginning at least with Freud, a humanistic background has been deemed desirable for psychiatrists. Unfortunately, neither medical school nor psychiatric residency often include or even stimulate disciplined inquiry in the letters and arts. The consultant must reach toward logic, ethics, literature, and the fine arts to enrich his knowledge of man and equip himself to play his role wisely and well.

REFERENCES

BEIGLER, J. S. et al. Report on liaison psychiatry at Michael Reese Hospital. AMA Arch. Neurol. Psychiat., 81:733, 1959.

BERBLINGER, K. The teaching of psychiatric consultation techniques. In The Psychiatric Consultation. W. M. Mendel and P. Solomon, eds. New York, Grune and Stratton, 1968.

BINGER, C. The two faces of medicine. N. Eng. J. Med., 275(4), 1966.

CUSHING, J. G. N. Role of the psychiatrist as a consultant. Amer. J. Psychiat., 106:861, 1950.

Editorial. Southern Med. J., 59:979, 1966.

KAPLAN, D. M. Why I am not a psychiatrist. Harpers Magazine, Feb. 1967, p. 45.

KAUFMAN, M. R. The role of the psychiatrist in a general hospital. Psychiat. Quart., 27:367, 1953.

STRECKER, E. A. Contributions of psychiatry to medical theory and practice. Med. Clin. N. Amer., July 1957.

5 THE RELATIONSHIP BETWEEN CONSULTANT AND PATIENT: TRANSFERENCE AND COUNTERTRANSFERENCE

Even though the consultant usually sees the patient for only one or two sessions, the relationship is vital. Angyal (1965) says the therapeutic relationship is ". . . the drama of the struggle for decision . . ." It is structured by the situation, the patient's expectations, and the consultant's obligations to him as well as to the consultee. Because the psychiatrist spends much of his time exploring the patient's personal as well as medical history, the relationship between the patient and the consultant is endowed with a degree of intimacy frequently lacking in the more conventional patient-physician encounters.

The patient visualizes physicians as healers having knowledge and skills which alleviate distress. He expects the consultant to provide assistance to his referring physician. Yet, he has fears as well as hopeful expectations. He is afraid that he may reveal too much of himself, that he will be labeled neurotic, and that this epithet will be attached to him throughout his hospital stay or during his visits to the clinic. Moreover, the patient fears that the personal, and often guilt-ridden, information he discloses will be relayed to his physician who will then hold a lowered opinion of him.

The patient has other fears. He wonders what the psychiatrist expects, and he worries whether he is saying the "right" thing and about which information is *really* important?

The consultant should anticipate these expectations and fears, and unearth them during the early part of the interview with a question such as, "What do you honestly think about seeing a psychiatrist?" Then, the patient feels that his attitudes, expectations, and fears are important and that the psychiatrist will accept him.

TRANSFERENCE

Classically, transference is derived from the unconscious and is rooted in the repetition compulsion; intensive transference usually develops during psychoanalysis or in the course of intensive psychotherapy. The patient endows the psychiatrist with the attributes and roles held by various significant persons in the patient's past, and with characteristics (usually fantasies) which match the patient's idealized image of a therapist who will meet his personal needs. The therapeutic relationship mirrors, in a capsule, the patient's interpersonal and fantasy existence. As Freud explained, a transference *neurosis* develops. Success in treatment coincides and indeed, is synonymous with, the resolution of the transference neurosis, because as the patient is able to objectify this crucial relationship he will also attain the capability for handling other interpersonal relationships satisfactorily.

During consultations, transference develops in only limited forms; it is enmeshed within the patient's expectations, hopes, and fears about his medical illness. A patient may say: "You remind me of my father or mother," or, with more generalized feeling, "You are like a friendly teacher or minister I knew," or, "You are the first doctor who really understands my illness." The concept of transference has been broadened to include all of the patient's attitudes toward, and preceptions of, the psychiatrist (Orr, 1954). Accordingly, very often he will say, "This is the first time I have had an opportunity to talk about all of these things with someone who really listens." Obviously, maintaining a keen awareness of the patient's attitudes toward him helps the consultant.

COUNTERTRANSFERENCE

Countertransference is defined as the psychiatrist's attributing to the patient certain characteristics of persons who were significant in his own life. This concept has also been enlarged to include all the consulting psychiatrist's fantasies, attitudes, perceptions, and feelings about the patient. Thus, the encounter between the consultant and the patient is complicated by feelings and attitudes, held by each, which may undergo further development during the consultative experience.

In their article on the countertransference problems of liaison psychiatrists, Mendelson and Meyer (1961) discuss the potentially disruptive effect of certain kinds of countertransference phenomena. They describe four elements of the consultation situation which produce feelings and responses in the psychiatrist that interfere with his clinical effectiveness. The psychiatrist: 1) works in the medical setting with its incoveniences, 2) sees patients with severe organic disease which may result in death, 3) faces the dilemmas and frustrations posed by patients with severe character disorders in relation to medical illness, and 4) tries to meet his medical and psychiatric responsibility even when there is severe family and social pathology.

These elements vary in importance. There are obvious physical and psychological inconveniences for the consultant, but they are not insurmountable. Frequently the consultant does not have an office in an inpatient unit or in a clinic; he has to see the patient at the bedside or in a borrowed office. Thus, he may lack privacy and comfort. Also, consultations involve urgency. The consultant is under pressure to see the patient immediately and provide a formulation, diagnosis, and treatment plan. Although these difficulties arouse feelings of irritation and frustration, they should not be viewed as serious obstacles. The irritation they engender need not affect the consultant's work adversely. Frequently, the discontent, ostensibly produced by these inconveniences, masks an underlying sense of insecurity. This insecurity stems from fear of rejection by the medical staff, reactions to the patient's physical distress, or lack of knowledge about medicine. Inconveniences can be handled. Flexibility is a primary tool in consultation work.

Working with the seriously ill or dying patient is distressing for all physicians, but for the psychiatric consultant this distress is aggravated by additional factors. The consultant may be more disturbed by these patients because he works with them only occasionally; encountering death is not routine for him. Psychiatric training, with its emphasis on humanistic values, heightens his sensitivity. He does not possess all of the defenses available to other physicians, such as relief through action. Consequently, the consultant may identify too sympathetically with the patient and his attempts to grapple with the actual psychological problem are blocked. In approaching the seriously ill patient, a beginner may easily think, "If I were in that condition, I would react the same way." While such feelings are humane, they reflect anxiety and loss of objectivity. When the consultant becomes so personally involved with the seriousness of the patient's physical condition, his effectiveness is automatically limited by the countertransference. He may even doubt his ability to help and succumb to feelings of hopelessness. At this point he tends to restrict his therapy to superficial reassurance, or he may avoid the patient. As Mendelson and Meyer (1961) point out, it is commonly assumed that the disturbed behavior of seriously ill patients is produced by the present stress of the illness; however, disturbed behavior, they say, is derived from and more critically determined by the patient's previous life experiences. The psychiatrist can work with a patient's views of and attitudes toward his past experiences as these influence his reactions to the present illness.

When the consultant overemphasizes the patient's organic pathology to the extent that his perception of the psychological difficulties is clouded, he is just as much at fault as the medical specialist who splits the soma from the psyche. Or, if he defends against his personal involvement with the severe organic illness by saying it is not his concern and that he should devote his time only to the patient with a controlled, relatively less serious medical illness and a discrete psychological problem, then he is acting like the cardiologist who is interested only in the EKG and not in the patient's anxiety. The psychiatrist's reluctance to work with seriously ill patients stems in part from his feelings of inadequacy in the medical realm; a realm which, too often, he deserted completely. The old jokes which describe the psychiatrist as "a doctor who is afraid of blood and death" are altogether too appropriate. But continued experiences with these patients and the maintenance of ties with general medicine diminish these countertransference problems for the consultant.

Dilemmas and frustrations posed by patients with severe character disorders should create few difficulties with countertransference. These patients are considered notoriously difficult to work with because of their intractability. By their erratic behavior, usually characterized by passive-aggressiveness and hostility, they frustrate all physicians. The psychiatrist is trained to deal with these patients, and he encounters them more frequently. In fact, the psychiatrist has a special opportunity to help the consultee with these cases. Most physicians are less astute in detecting characterologic problems than in diagnosing other psychiatric conditions. The consultee who is anxious and guilty because he dislikes a hostile or clinging patient is reassured when the consultant informs him that he, too, has the same reactions. This labels the problem as the patient's, not the physician's, and such corroboration encourages a more objective approach to the patient on the part of the consultee.

Feelings of pessimism and despair, produced by the consultant's encounter with severe family and social pathology, are common. Yet these feelings need not produce intense countertransference which blocks therapeutic endeavors. The psychiatrist is trained to work with colleagues in other fields; he can call upon them to help when medical illness is compounded by poverty and marked social pathology in the home situation. For example, he knows that he can collaborate with a social worker who is prepared to assist with such problems. Thus, at least partial solutions are available.

In consultation work, there are special aspects to both transference and countertransference. The most important point is that these phenomena arise from the matrix of the medical illness. The patient, because of beginning transference, may try to attach himself to the consultant at the expense of the relationship with his referring physician. Of course, patients with characterologic disturbances are prone to manipulate the staff anyway, but the consultant should be aware that transference may be the underlying force which gives impetus to these disrupting maneuvers. Moreover, all of this will be intertwined with the facts of medical illness: symptoms, diseases, diagnoses, prognoses, and financial considerations.

In contrast to the countertransference situations in which the consultant shrinks from work with the seriously ill, the unwary consultant, or the one who disdains his medical colleagues, may become so entangled by his countertransference that he truly believes he is the only one who can help the patient. The consultant must be alert to these feelings and attitudes. With vigilance, he should bring them to light and scrutinize his own involvement in order to diminish their antitherapeutic effects.

REFERENCES

ANGYAL, A. Neurosis and Treatment. New York, John Wiley & Sons, Inc., 1965, p. 246.
MENDELSON, M., and MEYER, E. Countertransference problems of the liaison psychiatrist. Psychosom. Med., 23:115, 1961.
ORR, D. W. Transference and countertransference: A historical survey. J. Amer. Psychoanal. Ass., 2:621, 1954.

6 HOSPITALIZATION

With the assistance of Judith Benninger Brown, M.A.

In nursing, hospitalization [for the patient] is usually referred to as "distressing." In psychological terms, it might be described as "ego threatening"; in sociological terms, "disorganizing."

Elms and Diers (1963)

The comprehensive approach to patient care, with its emphasis on ecology, requires explicit acknowledgement of the special effects of hospitalization on the patient. Illness pervades the hospital environment, and a sense of urgency and importance characterizes the routine activities of the staff as they engage in diagnosis and treatment in combating disease. The hospitalized patient is a "displaced person." Coser (1962) states: "Illness alters a person's social role and his social relationships, and hospitalization dramatizes this change." Therefore, an understanding of the hospital environment, its social structure, and staff expectations of the patient must be combined with comprehension of the meaning of hospitalization for the individual patient. These processes can be conceptualized as an equation: hospitalization + patient = ongoing system (not always in equilibrium). The system may suffer from disruption to the point that there is staff dissension, alienation of the patient, or even a temporary breakdown in working arrangements. Consequently, hospitalization may contribute to the patient's illness or to the development of manifest psychopathology. Schimmell (1964) states that 20 percent of the patients in his study suffered, at one time or another, from complications produced by hospitalization.

THE SOCIAL ORGANIZATION
WITHIN THE HOSPITAL

The social organization of the hospital is vertically and hierarchically arranged, usually along traditional lines of authority. There are three organizations: the medical, the nursing, and the administrative; within each of the three there is a particular hierarchical grouping. This complex arrangement may be strained because of a failure in the combined operation of the three branches.

Providing patient care is the goal of each of these professional groups. It is assumed that they will combine their efforts, even though their immediate interests or long-term goals may vary. However, differences in their educational backgrounds and interests may deter rather than advance cohesion. For example, the physician may be interested in research activities, the nurses primarily concerned with patient care from shift to shift, and the administrators wrapped up in their problems of economics and smooth management. Thus these structural arrangements may not contribute to functional needs; they may even create problems.

TENSION BETWEEN STRUCTURE AND FUNCTION

Further, there is malalignment between the structurally and the functionally arranged orders of importance. For example, although the attending physician or chief of service is ostensibly at the top of the totem pole, the resident or intern is the functioning person whose immediate hour-by-hour decisions have the greatest influence on patient care.

STAFF EXPECTATIONS OF THE PATIENT

Against this background, the staff has defined expectations for the patient. They expect him to recognize both the overt and subtle aspects of their established lines of authority; he is expected to adjust to them, in all of their complexities, on a moment-by-moment basis. Beyond this the staff expects the patient to conform to the hospital environment with its existing rules and regulations. Failure to conform is interpreted as deviancy or trouble, either potential or actual. Besides conforming, the patient is expected to be grateful and to express this gratitude by recovering satisfactorily from illness, by giving wholehearted cooperation, by containing his fears and worries, and by not disrupting the staff or its routine when recovery is not possible.

INVALIDITY OF COMMON ASSUMPTIONS ABOUT HOSPITALIZATION

It is commonly assumed that the tripartite, hierarchically arranged social organization within the hospital promotes the best possible patient care and that the roles of doctors, nurses, and administrators are defined and mutually adjusted for this same purpose. It is also assumed that the entire staff functions for the benefit of the patient, not the organization.

However, organizations develop protective measures to ensure self-perpetuation, often at the expense of their professed functions and goals.

The effects of these processes become apparent to the consultant. In accord with Meyer and Mendelson's (1961) discussion of the operational group, staff tolerance of a patient's disturbed behavior is variable. When a patient's behavior is perceived as disruptive to the organization, the patient is likely to be referred for psychiatric consultation. Thus, while psychiatric referral may signify a disturbed patient, the *event* of defining the patient as disturbed may reflect staff problems, inadequacies, or basic structural deficiencies in the staff society. The patient may become a scapegoat for staff dissension and be shipped off to a psychiatric ward or referred for consultation solely to protect the staff's established structural patterns.

In his book, *Society as the Patient* (1948), Frank states an axiom of sociologic research: One observes a society and gathers certain data on institutions or people who are perceived as being threatening to the society (criminality, sociopathy, high infant mortality, and so on). These individuals or institutions are seen as marginal; the criminal or sick are recognized as deviant. Society then takes steps to eliminate or cure these offenders. Frank asks us to invert the axiom and interpret the existence of a deviant or disturbed individual as somehow reflecting central disorganization in the core of the society.

General assumptions about traditional roles are also under attack. Jourard (1964) asserts that inherent in the nurse's bedside manner is a proscription of self-disclosure; this is obviously detrimental to both patient and nurse. Bursten (1963) notes that the social structure of the staff may actively suppress self-report; for example, expressions of anxiety by a staff member or of dependency by a patient.

Thus, the patient entering the hospital steps into the middle of a complex and intricately involved, but inconsistently organized, social structure.

HOSPITALIZATION AS CONTRIBUTING TO THE ILLNESS

For most patients, hospitalization imposes an added burden on the disease process. It produces reality-based problems: disruptions of family routines, interruptions of normal living habits, and fears about being a captive in the hospital environment. Also, there is added expense attached to illness and hospitalization. The consultant needs to evaluate the effect of these disruptive factors. By assessing the patient's reaction to these problems he can obtain valuable diagnostic data on the illness, a clearer picture of the quality of the patient's relationships with others, and an appraisal of the additional difficulties which will be encountered with convalescence and the return home.

PHYSICAL AND PSYCHOLOGIC INCONVENIENCES

Most patients suffer from the physical and psychologic inconveniences of hospitalization. There is the annoyance of the fixed hospital routine. For example, diet trays are sent to the patient according to the hospital's particular schedule. There is a lack of privacy resulting from repeated examinations and the necessity to share a room with others who may be severely ill and in distress. The noise is vexatious and the furniture uncomfortable.

Psychologic stresses include the strain of adapting to the routine with its barrage of stimuli coming from hospital personnel, equipment, and other patients; accepting a victim status; and feeling the helplessness which accompanies being in the hands of strangers.

The doctor-thing in his white coat unhesitatingly pushed open the door of the hospital room. The door had no lock or latch so that he needed only to push it and felt no need to knock. It was a "semi-private" room, so that the doctor looked from the one "semi-private" to the other, wondering which was his. Finally, the white-coated doctor asked with a rising inflection, "Mr. _____?" The semi-private sitting on the far bed, as if afraid to muss it, was in a new bathrobe and stiff slippers. The far-bed semi-private replied with a rising inflection, "Yes?" In his white coat, the doctor-thing said, "I'm Doctor _____." The patient knew, really knew, that this doctor-thing was truly a man of science. "His" doctor had sent him to "the" doctor.

The doctor-thing, still standing, surveyed the patient-thing with a practiced eye. The patient-thing quickly, even embarrassingly, crushed out his half-smoked cigarette.

"What's the trouble?" asked the doctor-thing.

"I have a feeling here."

The doctor-thing pulled up a chair and sat.

"Point to it," he directed.

"About here," said the patient-thing.

"How long?" "How often?" "Nature of?" "Radiates to?" "Brought on by?" "Relieved by?" "Pain or ache?" "Previous illness?" "Married?" "Children?" "Smoke?" "Drink?" "Job?" "Lie down, please so I can examine you." "Hmm, need some tests." "We'll do a cholecystogram tomorrow, a barium enema next day."

The doctor-thing got up to go.

"Whaa—what do you think it is?" asked the patient-thing.
"Need the tests to tell."
"But Doctor, what do you—anything serious?"
"We're getting the tests."
The doctor-thing strode out of the *"semi-private"* room, leaving the door, *without a lock or latch, open.* (Steiger, 1964)

ADAPTATION PROBLEMS

In her book *Life in the Ward,* Coser (1962) reports that a number of factors tend to disorient patients on admission to the hospital: anxiety about physical conditions, separation from family and accustomed surroundings, and loss of independence. She believes that many patients are not given sufficient opportunity to understand the meaning of the medical and nursing procedures or the roles played by the personnel. She describes two types of patients and their approaches to hospital adaptation: 1) Those mainly seeking gratification of their primary needs approach the hospital as if it were a refuge (hospital-oriented patients). 2) The others, believing that the hospital offers greater facilities for them and their physicians, approach it with more reality-bound expectations (outside-oriented patients). In accounting for these two types of adaptation, she found that the more hospital-oriented patients were older and had a greater number of previous admissions than the more outside-oriented. Also, medical patients are more hospital-oriented than surgical patients. More importantly, she concludes that the patient's roles outside the hospital (in the past and the present) are related to his present roles within the hospital and influence his adaptive behavior. For example, an excessively dependent person who has unfulfilled needs will not only express this dependency within the hospital, but if the needs are gratified by hospitalization he will adapt his behavior to secure further gratification. The changed behavior will have a consequent effect on his roles both within and outside the hospital.

In their article, "The Psychological Aspects of Hospitalization," Wright and Holmes (1963) state: "The doctor should be aware of the patient's interpersonal relationships within the hospital and should learn to recognize and manage certain psychological adaptive reactions common to acute and chronic illnesses." They emphasize the need for understanding the setting in which the illness developed, the patient's expectations of his new environment (which may be colored by memories from childhood or previous problems with hospitalization), and the financial aspects of hospitalization. They note many of the psychologic adaptations: regression, anxiety about separation from family members, secondary gain, pseudo-independence, delirium, depression, and conversion hysteria. In their discussion of pain, they indicate that when the psychic organization for awareness of pain is already involved, and when the patient is in a situation in which a somatic complaint is expected, continued peripheral painful stimulation may not be necessary to keep the pain cycle going. This discussion bears directly on one of the consultant's main problems—providing management for the patient who requests narcotics for pain relief too frequently, or whose continued complaints of pain disturb the nursing staff. The recognition and management of these patients are described in the section on Pain.

INCREASING PSYCHOPATHOLOGY

The effects of illness, medical procedures, and the strange environment may combine to strain the patient's already damaged capabilities for coping with disease; consequently, manifest psychopathology is increased. This is particularly true for delirious patients. Another example is the person with a severe characterologic disorder who is tolerated only by his immediate family, but not by others. The stress of hospitalization and the lack of family protection aggravates the already serious condition; flagrant conflicts between the patient and the staff occur.

SUSPENSION OF PSYCHOPATHOLOGY

In contrast to these more common reactions, the consultant must be alert to those patients whose psychopathology is suspended by hospitalization. Usually this is the patient who is having severe difficulty at work or with the family. For him the hospital becomes a shelter where limited regression is allowed. He is removed from the stresses and strains of everyday living which promoted his unrest. Frequently, these patients are referred late for psychiatric consultation because their overt psychopathology was diminished by hospitalization. They are referred for one of the following reasons: 1) The referring physician has a clear understanding of this process and realizes that definitive psychiatric evaluation is necessary before the patient returns home; 2) no medical reason for hospitalization turns up on the diagnostic work-up, or 3) the patient becomes so comfortable in the hospital that he resists discharge.

SYMPTOMATOLOGY

In an evaluation of depression in general medical patients (Schwab et al., 1965), we found that 70 percent of all the medical inpatients complained of fatigue and lethargy, 68 percent of insomnia, and 52 percent of upper gastrointestinal disturbances. Also, many of the affective symptoms commonly held to be indicative of depression, such as depressed mood, were found in these patients. The frequency with which these symptoms occur produces obvious difficulties with diagnosis. Significantly, it raises an interesting question: To what extent are these symptoms related solely to hospitalization?

Obviously then, hospitalization has antitherapeutic side effects which may appear as overt symptomatology. The emphasis on pliable conformity and obedience to routine may create a sense of dependency which the patient finds difficult to tolerate. His maladaptive responses may also take symptomatic form. Finally, in the hospital environment, pain has come to be associated with the body which is being treated, and consequently, environmental stresses are somatized.

INTERPERSONAL REACTIONS

Difficulties between the patient and one or more of the staff members frequently result in the patient's being referred for psychiatric consultation. There may be a punitive aspect to the referral insofar as the referring physician, whose action may have been instigated by the nurse, will use the referral to label the patient as emotionally disturbed, thus absolving himself of any responsibility for the patient-staff conflict.

The patient can divide the staff into camps so that a civil war arena exists. Communication breaks down, and the effectiveness of the treatment program is jeopardized. The patient's personality disorder is usually central to the conflict and may contain elements of self-defeat and retaliation. A typical example is the passive-aggressive person who is superficially compliant, at least for the first day or so. Later, his underlying hostilities are expressed through passive-aggressive mechanisms: subtle negativism, lack of real cooperation, delaying, and indirection. These patients speak glibly of cooperation, even while they are subverting the staff's attempts to carry out necessary procedures. Transference is responsible for some of these interpersonal difficulties. The patient may visualize one physician as a benevolent father and another as a stern authoritarian figure. Just as commonly, a patient may visualize the nursing staff in terms of maternal, paternal, or fraternal figures.

IMPLICATIONS FOR THE CONSULTANT

Because the effects of hospitalization are manifold, the consultant must be aware that the patient's expectations and fears of the hospital pervade all of his reactions while he is there. The antitherapeutic effects of hospitalization may even produce symptoms. Consequently, the consultant must evaluate each patient's hospital experience. A brief part of the initial interview should be devoted to probing the patient's expectations of, and reactions to, the hospital. The consultant should discuss the patient's relationships with the medical and nursing staff.

In order to create a more therapeutic climate for the patient, the consultant may have to work with the medical, nursing, and administrative staffs. At these times he usually has to get them to modify their demands on, or alter their expectations of, the patient. The consultant must bear in mind that the structural organization within the hospital shifts from time to time and varies from unit to unit. He must be prepared to assess all of these influences as they pertain to the care of the patient.

REFERENCES

BURSTEN, B. The psychiatric consultant and the nurse. Nurs. Forum, 2:7, 1963.

COSER, R. L. The adjustment of patients. In Life in the Ward. East Lansing, Mich., Michigan State University Press, 1962.

ELMS, R., and DIERS, D. The patient comes to the hospital. Nurs. Forum, 2:89, 1963.

FRANK, L. K. Society as the Patient: Essays on Culture and Personality. New Brunswick, Rutgers University Press, 1948.

JOURARD, S. M. The Transparent Self. Princeton, D. Van Nostrand Co., 1964.

MEYER, E., and MENDELSON, M. Psychiatric consultations with patients on medical and surgical wards: Patterns and processes. Psychiatry, 24:197, 1961.

SCHIMMELL, E. M. The hazards of hospitalization. Ann. Intern. Med., 60:100, 1964.

SCHWAB, J. J., CLEMMONS, R. S., BIALOW, M., DUGGAN, V., and DAVIS, B. A study of the somatic symptomatology of depression in medical inpatients. Psychosomatics, 6:273, 1965.

STEIGER, E. A. Medical science and things. J. Health Hum. Behav., 5(1), Spring 1964.

WRIGHT, R. G., and HOLMES, T. H. Psychological aspects of hospitalization. In Lief, H., Lief, V., and Lief, N., eds. The Psychological Basis of Medical Practice. New York, Harper & Row, Publishers, 1963, pp. 219–231.

7 INDICATIONS FOR
PSYCHIATRIC REFERRAL

Indications for psychiatric referrals are characterized by inconsistency even when there are consultation-liaison programs. Criteria for referral have been described at length by numerous writers. Generally, their articles reflect a disease orientation (Mittelman et al., 1945; Kaufman and Bernstein, 1957; Stewart et al., 1962): threats of suicide, psychotic reactions, traditional psychosomatic illnesses, and so on (Pillersdorf, 1951). Brosin (1968) classifies referrals in three categories: 1) routine requests which arise because a symptom or physical sign triggers referral; reassurance on permission to transfer the patient is sought; 2) administrative and legal needs for which the psychiatrist's opinion is considered necessary, and 3) A "genuine appeal for help," for a greater psychodynamic and human understanding of the patient and the family on the part of the physician.

IS THE LEVEL OF PSYCHOPATHOLOGY AN ACCURATE INDICATOR?

On the surface, manifest psychopathology would seem to be the most obvious indication for referral; when viewed quantitatively, overt psychopathology would seem to determine the frequency and character of referrals. But the experience of most psychiatric consultants shows that the level of psychopathology does not necessarily determine whether or not a patient will be referred.

One reason why psychopathology is not an accurate index of current referral practices is that the physician interprets a patient's disturbed behavior subjectively, that is in terms of how much psycho-

43

pathology he considers "outside normal limits." For example, one patient with severe depression accompanying a serious illness may not be referred for consultation because the physician believes that the degree of depression is a natural response to the medical illness; or destructive behavior may be condoned in the patient who has a diagnosed brain tumor. In contrast, even slightly deviant behavior, involving hostile attitudes or critical remarks on the part of a patient whose diagnosis is unclear, may bring an immediate call for an emergency psychiatric consultation. Also, staff members may disagree in the interpretation of a patient's behavior; some may regard it as pathological, while others do not. If those at the top of the hierarchical ladder do not see the psychopathology or do not accept the other's interpretations, the patient may not be referred.

Further reason is that staff tolerance of patient behavior varies on a day-to-day or even hour-to-hour basis. Frustrations with diagnosis, dissatisfaction with responses to treatment, overwork, and personal conflicts account for variable levels of tolerance and influence referrals.

Another limitation is that hospitalization suspends some patient's neurotic problems; some who display obvious psychopathology prior to hospitalization find that the hospital is a sanctuary and their overt psychopathology diminishes.

Thus, the level of psychopathology is at best a somewhat limited guide for referral. When consultation services are first made available, only the obvious problems are referred; the consultant is asked to evaluate psychotic patients for commitment, to help with emergency management, or to provide disposition. In time, after the consultant has demonstrated his ability to help both consultees and patients, the staff refers subtler and more varied problems: preoperative evaluations, management of patients with mixed medical and psychiatric illnesses, and even the advisability of psychiatric care for a family member instead of the patient.

TIMING OF REFERRAL

Alert clinicians diagnose patients' psychotic disorders (schizophrenia, brain syndromes, depressions) quickly and refer these patients for psychiatric consultations to confirm the diagnosis and obtain care. Patients with psychoneurotic reactions (anxiety, conversion, depression) are much more difficult for consultees to evaluate; some of these patients are referred for evaluation early in hospitalization, but many are referred late, if at all. Patients with psychophysiologic reactions and personality disorders are usually referred for consultations late. Clinicians submit patients with psychophysiologic reactions to exhaustive diagnostic work-ups to determine whether structural disease processes are present; also, patients with personality disorders represent a category of diagnoses difficult to define explicitly (Schwab et al., 1965a).

We observed a tendency toward an inverse relationship between the severity of the medical illness and the early timing of the referral request. Internists are more prone to refer the patients for psychiatric consultations early if the admission physical examinations reveal no significant findings. On the other hand, finding organic disease keeps the patient from receiving psychiatric assistance early in the period of hospitalization when the conditions for assistance are optimal (Rossman, 1963; Abrahams and Golden, 1963; Schwab et al., 1965a).

In another study (Schwab et al., 1966) we found that patients who reacted favorably to consultations regarded the timing of the referrals as appropriate. Of all the patients, only 12 percent felt that the referrals were too early; they expressed fears that their medical work-ups had not been completed and that all organic causes for their illnesses had not been ruled out. Only 9 percent believed consultations were requested too late, saying that if their problems were psychiatric their doctor should have obtained this help earlier. Twenty-four percent of the patients would not give definite opinions about the appropriateness of the timing; they responded passively with statements such as "I don't know, that's up to my doctor."

FACTORS WHICH INFLUENCE REFERRALS

In discussing psychiatric referral procedures, Chodoff (1954) mentions two groups of referral factors: those related primarily to the patient and those related to the physician. As patient factors he lists: 1) the patient's attitudes and wishes about seeing a psychiatrist, 2) the patient's endowments or actual life situation, and 3) the nature and severity of the patient's difficulties. He questions the advisability of forcing a really unwilling patient to consult a psychiatrist. But he emphasizes the desirability of psychiatric referral for patients who hold adverse attitudes toward medical care. When appropriate management does not change these patients' attitudes, continued efforts strain both the physician and the patient, and psychiatric referral is indicated. He implies that psychiatric consultation necessarily means psychotherapy when he asks whether patients who are not good candidates for psychotherapy should be referred for evaluation. Such a view is now unacceptable; consultants have an array of skills which can be utilized flexibly for many patients. Consequently, whether or not the patient is a good candidate for psychotherapy does not bear directly on the consultation problem.

In discussing factors relating to the physician, Chodoff (1954) emphasizes the importance of the physician's background in psychiatry. Physicians who maintain interest in their patients' emotional problems handle referral procedures more effectively than those who are not interested in these aspects of their patients' difficulties. The physician's attitude toward the patient is important; he should refer patients whom he dislikes or does not respect. Chodoff also stresses the importance of the physician's self-knowledge, noting that self-awareness enables him to handle a wide range of psychiatric problems and to recognize his own limitations. He concludes by stating that the question as to whether a particular patient should be referred to a psychiatrist depends not only on what kind of person the patient is and what is the matter with him, but also on what kind of person the physician is.

In an analysis of the reasons for psychiatric referral, Abrahams and Golden (1963) develop these concepts, stipulating three groups of factors which influence requests for consultations:

1. *Factors having to do with the patient in the hospital setting that stimulate a request for psychiatric consultation*
   (a) *Threat of suicide*
   (b) *Heterodox overt sexual behavior*
   (c) *Expression of overt hostility toward the staff*
   (d) *Rapid change in behavior pattern from one which had appeared static*
   (e) *The dying patient and his management*
2. *Factors having to do with the doctor that stimulate psychiatric referral patients*
   (a) *Difficulty in communicating with patients*
   (b) *More effective communication between doctor and patient. (A doctor who develops an unusually good relationship with his patient will learn of his patient's problems and seek the solution. This is also a function of the time the patient spends on the ward.)*
   (c) *Irrational guilt over management of the patient, often conspicuous in the dying patient*
   (d) *Presence of "psychosomatic" illness in the physician similar to an illness in the patient decreases the rates of referral for psychiatric scrutiny*
   (e) *Doctors' tendency to belittle value of brief psychotherapy in a general hospital setting*
3. *Factors having to do with hospital's management which affect the rate of psychiatric referral of patients*

(a) *Rapid diagnostic work-ups in teaching institution to save costs of hospitalization tended to discourage a personal interest in the patient and his emotional problems, thereby decreasing the number of referrals*

(b) *Positive attitudes of important authority figures such as the attending staff man regarding the value of psychiatric referral tended to increase the quality and rate of psychiatric referrals*

(c) *Certain administrative policies with "legalistic" import ("the hospital has to protect itself," as from litigation in case of suicide) affected referral*

PATIENTS' OPINIONS ABOUT THE NEED FOR REFERRAL

When this organization of the factors influencing referral is combined with Chodoff's (1954) emphasis on the referring physician's psychiatric background, as well as with Meyer and Mendelson's (1961) concerns with the consultee's anxiety, uncertainty, and continued responsibility, psychiatric referral processes are given some structure. But patients' opinions about the necessity for referral are not included. In one study we found that 72 percent of the patients referred for consultations believed the consultations were necessary and another 15 percent believed consultations might be indicated. Among medical inpatients not referred for consultation, the same study showed that 16 percent believed they should have received a psychiatric consultation while another 18 percent felt that one might be indicated; only 66 percent believed a consultation was not necessary (Schwab et al., 1966).

CHARACTERISTICS OF PATIENTS RECEIVING REFERRALS

An evaluation (Schwab et al., 1965b) of two groups of medical inpatients, 100 consecutive referrals for psychiatric consultation and a matched nonconsultation group, indicated that the consultation patients had certain group characteristics which differentiated them from the others. These included: an increased number of chief complaints, frequently subjective in character and of little variety, involving few organs and systems, but related to emotional, neurologic, and sensory modalities. These medical patients' complaints were monotonously repetitive. Ninety-two percent of the 17 chief complaints were limited to illnesses involving only four systems: the psychobiologic unit, the musculoskeletal system, the nervous system, and the gastrointestinal system.

The consultation patients were differentiated by a greater number of previous hospitalizations, previous professional contacts with psychiatrists, the use of tranquilizers, the number of significant adverse events and separations in the life history, and the frequency of abdominal and gynecologic surgery. Adverse events included recent deaths or illnesses of near relatives, marital discord, and disturbed family relationships, as well as abortions, injuries, and natural catastrophes.

The consultation patients as a group had significantly fewer positive findings on the physical examination, compared with the controls: 43 percent versus 76 percent. The absence of positive findings in over half of these patients affirms our clinical knowledge that many complaints without demonstrable physical manifestations are psychogenic in origin and represent disguised pleas for help. They are calling cards which provide access to medical care. Emotional liability, a depressed or inappropriate affect, or disproportionate responsiveness during the admission work-up were significant findings distinguishing the consultation group from the others. This study emphasizes that the mental status examination is an important guide for evaluating patients for referral.

In conclusion, indications for referral are comprehensive only when they are derived from holistic concepts, are based on clinical knowledge, and include an awareness of the staff's role, an understanding of the influence of hospitalization, and a feeling for the patient's interactions with his family.

REFERENCES

ABRAHAMS, D., and GOLDEN, J. Psychiatric consultations on a medical ward. Arch. Intern Med. (Chicago), 112:766, 1963.

BROSIN, H. Communication systems of the consultation process. *In* The Psychiatric Consultation. W. M. Mendel and P. Solomon, eds. New York, Grune and Stratton, 1968.

CHODOFF, P. When should the physician refer a patient to a psychiatrist? Med. Ann., 23:313, 1954.

KAUFMAN, M. R., and BERNSTEIN, S. A psychiatric evaluation of the problem patient. J.A.M.A., 163:108, 1957.

MEYER, E., and MENDELSON, M. Psychiatric consultations with patients on medical and surgical wards: Patterns and processes. Psychiatry, 24:197, 1961.

MITTELMAN, B., WEIDER, A., BRODMAN, K., WECHSLER, D., and WOLFF, H. G. Personality and psychosomatic disturbances in patients in medical and surgical wards. Psychosom. Med., 7:220, 1945.

PILLERSDORF, L. The psychiatric referral: When and how? Ohio Med. J., 47:527, 1951.

ROSSMAN, P. L. Organic diseases simulating functional disorders. GP, 28:78, 1963.

SCHWAB, J. J., CLEMMONS, R. S., SCOTT, M. L., and FREEMON, F. R. Problems in psychosomatic diagnosis: II. Severity of medical illness and psychiatric consultations, Psychosomatics, 6:69, 1965 a.
—— Differential characteristics of medical inpatients referred for psychiatric consultation: A controlled study. Psychosom. Med., 27:112, 1965 b.
SCHWAB, J. J., CLEMMONS, R. S., VALDER, M. J., RAULERSON, J. D. Medical inpatients reactions to psychiatric consultations. J. Nerv. Ment. Dis., 14 (3), 1966.
STEWART, M. A., TUASON, V. B., GUZE, S. B., and SATTERFIELD, J. H. A study of psychiatric consultations in a general hospital. J. Chron. Dis., 15:331, 1962.

8 MAKING THE PSYCHIATRIC REFERRAL

Teaching referral techniques is one of the consultant's foremost tasks. Using good referral practices has everyday value for referring physicians and obvious benefit for the consultant.

Binder (1952) conceptualizes difficulties with psychiatric referral as having two bases: 1) objections and resistance on the part of the patient, and 2) inadequate understanding of psychiatry on the part of the general physician. Undoubtedly, certain patients object to psychiatric referral. Jaffee (1963) reports that patients find it difficult to accept psychiatric referral when pain is their chief complaint; many do not understand how pain can be produced by emotional causes. Earlier, Carlson (1958) noted that the most difficult patients to refer were those with a neurosis expressed through disturbed physiological functioning and those with fundamental characterologic problems. For example, the patient with infantile pride and feelings of omnipotence is antagonized by the mere mention of psychiatric referral. The extremely dependent patient resists referral because it poses a threat to his clinging relationship with his personal doctor. This also happens with less pathologically dependent patients who are fond of their physicians. Bartemeier (1957) believes that adverse reactions may be due to the referring physician's failure to estimate the intensity of the patient's attachment to him.

Some stigma still surrounds the psychiatric referral. Watters (1952) states: "Referral to a psychiatrist may be viewed as a triple threat: first to the patient's ego, . . . second, . . . to his family, because mental illness has ramifications reaching into the past, . . . and last, . . . a threat to society, which defends itself by stigmatizing the patient. . . ." Some medical patients whose illnesses are declared "psychogenic," fear that they will be ostracized by family or friends.

There are financial considerations (the consultant's fee and the cost of hospitalization) which not only produce opposition to referral on the part of the patient, but also deter the referring physician. In the past many insurance programs rejected claims for payment when there was only a psychiatric diagnosis. But most insurance programs now furnish some coverage for psychiatric illness.

PATIENTS' REACTIONS TO REFERRING PHYSICIANS

Orland (1960) believes that physicians' concerns about their patients' reactions to consultation are excessive; our research is confirmatory.

Some physicians tend to have a basic mistrust of referral in general. They regard patients as their own property. They fear that referral will mean loss of patients, will reveal inadequacies (at least in the area for which the referral is made), or will endanger established doctor-patient relationships. Some of these general concerns are not so evident when the referral is to a psychiatrist, because many practitioners do not feel they are under any real obligation to have acquired psychiatric skills, or even much knowledge of the field, except for screening and diagnostic purposes (Kaufman and Margolin, 1948). Also, because the psychiatrist's work is thought to be different from that of other practitioners, the physician has fewer worries about his patients being "stolen."

Regardless of these mitigating factors, physicians do have particular concerns about psychiatric referrals. These concerns take the form of disquieting questions: "What will the patient think about the request for psychiatric consultation? Does the patient think that I have regarded him as crazy because I have called in a psychiatrist? Does this mean that the patient will think I cannot understand him? Or, am I trying to drop the patient?"

Consultations can create problems. Brodsky (1967) contends that the very personal relationship between psychiatrist and patient quickly displaces that which existed between the referring physician and his patient. He says, "Following the consultation, the old relationship between referring physician and patient seems pallid to both."

Because referral processes are frequently discussed but rarely studied, we (Schwab et al., 1966) obtained data about patients' reactions to their referring physicians. We interviewed 30 consecutive medical inpatients for whom psychiatric consultations were requested. We asked: "What did you think of his decision to refer? Did it change your opinion of him? If so, how?" Of the 30 patients, 20 (66 percent) evinced accepting and positive attitudes towards their physicians after the consultations, 5 (17 percent) revealed mixed and ambivalent reactions, and 5 (17 percent) were hostile and derogatory. These differential reactions to referring physicians were not related to age, sex, marital status, or duration of illness. Nor were these reactions related to patients' attitudes toward the medical profession in general.

The patients who reacted positively to the psychiatric consultations likewise regarded their referring physicians favorably. But hostility towards the referring physician does not necessarily mean that the patient will not work with the psychiatrist, even though he has mixed feelings about the advisability of doing so. The majority of those who were hostile to their referring physician were ambivalent, not hostile, towards the consultation.

Most of the patients (70 percent) did not change their opinions of their referring physician as a result of the referral. Of the six who did change, the direction of the change is important: four revealed that the referrals increased their respect and heightened their regard for their referring physicians, while only two indicated that their opinions of the referring physician were lowered. Of the five patients reporting unfavorable reactions to their referring physicians, four said that the consultations did not change their opinions. These unfavorable reactions seem rigid. Such "fixed" adverse reactions may reflect the quality of the patient-doctor relationship, may be a consequence of the patient's previous experience with physicians or psychiatrists or both, or may be manifestations of defense mechanisms related to illness and resistance to psychiatric work. These patients should be referred for psychiatric consultations.

The physician's attitude about referral influences the patient (Jaffee, 1963). Referrals should be made in a positive tone. The physician should make it clear that referral does not mean that the case is hopeless or that the patient will be deserted. Orland (1960) insists that the referring physician can perform valuable educative functions for patients by explaining what the psychiatrist will do and how the psychiatrist works. He adds: "Specifying the purpose of the referral, whether for evaluation or therapy, facilitates a rapid approach to the consultative problem with a particular patient."

Binder (1952) urges the consultee to answer patients' objections to psychiatric referrals directly and truthfully. He emphasizes that the referring physician's empathy with the patient is decisive.

Watters (1952) notes that referral opens many opportunities for the consultee to lend hope to the patient and to work constructively with him after the consultation. He stresses that the physician should take an active role in making the referral.

The consultant should teach physicians how to prepare their patients for referral. We estimate that about 10 percent of the patients at the University of Florida Teaching Hospital do not receive adequate information about the consultation from the consultee, or this is conveyed to them so quickly, or so euphemistically, that they find it easy to forget that the consultee has mentioned a consultation. Of course, forgetting may be a defensive maneuver revealing the patient's ambivalence about the consultation.

GUIDELINES FOR REFERRAL

The consultant can supply referring physicians with the following guidelines:

1. An open, forthright discussion. This discussion must be candid and should explain in simple terms why the referral is necessary. The referring physician should not rely on diagnosis by exclusion, telling the patient: "You ought to see a psychiatrist because we can find nothing wrong with you." Instead, he can say: "The evidence indicates that there may be an emotional problem which accounts for your symptoms. The consultant can help us determine whether this is so."

2. Recognition of the patient's feelings. The physician should encourage the patient to ventilate his feelings about the impending consultation. In itself, ventilation is salutary, and it alerts the physician to distortions. When the fears are out in the open and the distortions are dealt with, the patient is better able to accept the consultation (Bartemeier, 1957).

3. Clarification of the psychiatrist's role: no prejudgment. The consultee should state that the psychiatrist is being called in only to ascertain the extent and meaning of the patient's emotional distress, and that the consultant will not attempt to make a case for psychogenic etiology.

4. Not a last resort measure. Very importantly, the consultee should not load the dice against the psychiatrist. Frequently a physician informs the patient, implicitly or explicitly, that the consultation is a last-resort measure. In doing so, he injures the referral procedure, increasing the patient's anxiety and the possibility of distortion.

5. Realistic expectations of the psychiatrist. The consultee should not oversell psychiatry, or promise miracles, so that the patient's expectations reach magical proportions and disappointment follows. This disap-

pointment will be reflected not only toward the psychiatrist, but also toward the referring physician.

REFERENCES

BARTEMEIER, L. H. On referring patients to other physicians. Northwest Med., 56:312, 1957.

BINDER, H. J. Helping your patient accept psychiatric referral. J. Okla. Med. Ass., 45:279, 1952.

BRODSKY, C. A social view of the psychiatric consultation. Psychosomatics, 8(2): 61, March/April, 1967.

CARLSON, C. C. How to refer a psychosomatic patient to a psychiatric specialist. GP, 18(6):105, 1958.

JAFFEE, M. Psychiatric referral. Rocky Mountain Med. J., 60:26, 1963.

KAUFMAN, M. R., and MARGOLIN, S. C. Theory and practice of psychosomatic medicine in a general hospital. Med. Clin. N. Amer., 32:611, 1948.

ORLAND, F. The general practitioner and the psychiatric referral. Med. Times, 88:1426, 1960.

SCHWAB, J. J., CLEMMONS, R. S., VALDER, M. J., RAULERSON, J. D., Patients' reactions to referring physicians. J.A.M.A., 195:1120, 1966.

WATTERS, T. A. Certain pitfalls and perils in psychiatric referral. Amer. Practit., 3:198, 1952.

9 REACTIONS TO CONSULTATIONS

How the patient will react to him, with cooperation or hostility, worries the resident beginning consultation activities and interests the experienced consultant striving to improve working relationships with patients and consultees. The importance of medical patients' reactions was recognized as early as 1948 by Kaufman and Margolin (1948). Theoretically, patients' reactions should be determined by attitudes toward psychiatry, developed through life, and now modified by the immediate realities of the medical situation. Brady and his co-workers (1959), Gynther et al. (1963), Nunnally and Kittross (1958), and others, investigated attitudes toward psychiatry. In general, more favorable attitudes were observed in patients with more education, in those from higher socioeconomic classes, and in those having professional contacts with psychiatrists and mental health workers. Most of these studies, however, sampled only the opinions held by psychiatric patients, hospital personnel, selected student groups, or the general public. Until recently, few data have been available concerning medical patients' attitudes.

The hospitalized patient would be expected to react more favorably to psychiatric intervention; he has already declared his patient status, and he logically expects to be helped in the hospital. Lipsitt (Zinberg, 1964) states: "The extensive experience of psychiatric consultants to the major hospital services has demonstrated repeatedly that patients who otherwise are not receptive to psychiatric treatment or referral usually accept willingly (and often gratefully) a psychiatric assessment which is proffered in the more familiar traditional medical or surgical ward setting."

We (Schwab et al. 1966) studied reactions to psychiatric consultations in two groups of medical inpatients: one group of 50 consecutive patients for whom the medical staff requested consultations, and a matched group of 50 nonreferred patients. At the beginning of the consultation, favorable or mixed reactions to the resident consultants were expressed by more than 80 percent of the referred patients. At the end of the consultation, acceptance was even greater. The shift, however, lacked stability and probably reflected the impact of the immediate encounter with the psychiatrist; most of these patients reverted to previously held attitudes when interviewed 24 hours later by an independent researcher. A one-year follow-up study supported the latter findings.

These data are helpful to the resident; when first consulting, he is uncertain of his ability to function in this new role. He is afraid that he will be rejected or not even given a fair chance during the brief consultative period. Knowing that more than 80 percent of the patients accepted their referrals cooperatively, or at least weighed the consultations with healthy skepticism and mixed opinions, should diminish the resident's sense of insecurity.

We searched for factors related to patients' differential reactions to consultations. Sociocultural factors were not significant, although unmarried patients tended to react less favorably. Age, sex, educational level, and annual income were not significant. The extent of the patient's knowledge about psychiatry was also not significant. However, we found that patients who obtained their knowledge of psychiatry from professional sources, such as advanced reading or intensive therapy, reacted more favorably than those who obtained knowledge only from the popular news media. Neither a previous brief encounter with a psychiatrist nor, surprisingly, the experience of a close family member with psychiatric care correlated with the patient's differential reactions.

The duration of the illness for which the patient was hospitalized was not significant; patients with illnesses of short duration reacted as favorably as patients with illnesses of longer duration. Referring physicians frequently delay consultation requests for patients with acute illnesses because they fear that these patients will not accept referral. However, postponing requests for indicated psychiatric consultations leads to chronicity with its consequent adjustment to illness. Family and working relationships crystallize into distorted patterns which, in themselves, increase resistance to change. Elements of secondary gain multiply with time so that the patient becomes more refractory to psychotherapeutic intervention.

Patients who believed that their total life situations were either adversely affected by their illness or were associated with their illnesses without obvious cause and effect relationships tended to react more favorably to consultations than those who saw no such associations. Obviously, those who believed they needed psychiatric consultations reacted more favorably. Because patients' illness-related factors are more directly related to their reactions to consultations than the non-illness related factors (age, sex, and so on), it follows that the staff's attitudes toward the consultation, particularly as transmitted to the patient through preparation for referral, are crucial to the patient's reception of the psychiatrist. Therefore, orientation of the hospital personnel is extremely important. When they are accepting and favorable toward psychiatry, patients incline in that direction; unfortunately, the converse is also true. The physicians and nurses may reveal their own doubts or communicate derogatory opinions of psychiatrists by informing patients that consultation is a last-resort measure; the patients are then placed in a double bind. If the medical staff's frustration, anxiety, and hostility emerge in naked or only slightly camouflaged forms, the cards are stacked against the psychiatrist.

In the control group of 50 patients not referred for psychiatric consultation, one third of them stated that a consultation either was indicated, or, might have been. These patients, none of whom received consultations, were asked how they would respond to referral. About 80 percent answered that they would cooperate (26 percent with complete acceptance); the one-year follow-up study showed that these percentages remained constant.

Two points of clinical value emerge from these studies. First, the overwhelming majority of the medical patients (those referred and those not referred) either reacted favorably, indicated they would accept, or at least held mixed opinions about a psychiatric consultation. Less than 20 percent had rejecting attitudes. This 20 percent appears to be a hard core group that maintains these rigid and unyielding attitudes toward psychiatry. Second, many medical patients not referred for psychiatric consultations believed that they should have been referred while they were hospitalized.

Although the findings provide important information about patients' reactions to psychiatric consultations, such data have certain limitations. First, it is hazardous to apply facts about groups to specific individuals. Also, how a patient reacts to a consultant does not necessarily predict the ultimate effect of the consultation for the patient. Further, the data do not take into account the value of the consultant's work to the consultee and other staff members.

We find that a patient's hostile, rejecting attitudes toward the psychiatrist at the beginning of the consultation certainly do not mean the consultation will be unsatisfactory. Anger and rejection are usually superficial defenses, veiling a fear of disclosure, a sense of helplessness, or an anticipated rejection. When the consultant identifies the roots of these fears and works with the concealed feelings, these patients are usually responsive. In fact, we encourage such a patient to express his anger toward the referring physician or the psychiatrist to let him know we can accept such feelings.

For the consultant, working with hostile patients is usually more satisfactory than working with those who react to the consultation over-enthusiastically. Extreme enthusiasm is indicative of a patient's unrealistic expectations of the psychiatrist or of utter dependency and a fragile ego. In general, the overenthusiastic patients have greater psychopathology than the hostile ones; they quickly become management problems and frequently require intensive psychotherapy because they have less ego strength than those who react with defenses characterized by anger and rejection.

REFERENCES

BRADY, J. P. Attitudinal factors influencing outcome of treatment of hospitalized psychiatric patients. J. Clin. Exp. Psychopath., 20:326, 1959.

——— REZNIKOFF, M., and ZELLER, W. W. The psychiatric attitudes battery: A procedure for assessing attitudes toward psychiatric treatment and hospitals. J. Clin. Psychol., 15:260, 1959.

GYNTHER, M. D., REZNIKOFF, M., and FISHMAN, M. Attitudes of psychiatric patients toward treatment, psychiatrists, and mental hospitals. J. Nerv. Ment. Dis., 136:68, 1963.

KAUFMAN, M. R., and MARGOLIN, S. G. Theory and practice of psychosomatic medicine in a general hospital. Med. Clin. N. Amer., 32:611, 1948.

LIPSITT, D. R. Integration clinic: An approach to the teaching and practice of medical psychology in an outpatient setting. In Zinberg, N. E., ed. Psychiatry and Medical Practice in a General Hospital. New York, International Universities Press, Inc., 1964.

NUNNALLY, J., and KITTROSS, J. M. Public attitudes toward mental health professions. Amer. J. Psychol., 13:589, 1958.

SCHWAB, J. J., CLEMMONS, R. S., VALDER, M. J., and RAULERSON, J. D. Medical inpatients' reactions to psychiatric consultations. J. Nerv. Ment. Dis., 142(3), 1966.

SECTION THREE   Procedures: Techniques and Practices

10   RESPONSIBILITIES

From the lore of clinical medicine, there is a timeworn aphoristic definition of a consultant as the one who does the rectal. It is offered as a preachment to the young for thoroughness and against squeamishness.
(Mallott and Earley, 1968)

By definition the consultation is interpersonal—minimally, a triangulated situation involving the consultee, the patient, and the consultant. For the psychiatrist, obligations exist in many directions. His fundamental responsibility, of course, is to provide improved patient care; however, there are other obligations.

First, the consultant is obliged to respond promptly to the call for service. Frequently, psychiatrists handle consultation requests in too routine a manner; physicians complain of tardy responses. Delay provokes increased anxiety in the staff and the patient. Psychiatrists are accused of failing to participate as actively as other physicians in general medical activities. A surgeon hastens to answer requests for his service, e.g., to evaluate a patient's abdominal pain for appendicitis. He rightfully regards his skills as important, and the alacrity with which he responds is tangible evidence of the premium he places on his efforts. When the psychiatrist delays, he derogates the importance of the consultation for both the consultee and the patient. With such rationalizations as "not having enough time" or "preferring to work with a definite schedule," many psychiatrists reveal implicit doubts about the value of their specialty.

The consultant should respond promptly to consultation requests, answering every one within 24 hours. When this is not possible, and particularly for inpatient consultations, the consultant should notify the medical and nursing staff of the exact time when he will see the patient.

By establishing a definite time, he allays the staff's anxiety. Occasionally, action of this sort is therapeutic in itself; the staff knows that something will be done at an appointed time. When time is limited, another alternative is to see the patient briefly for a five to ten minute introduction and then inform both the patient and the staff that he will return the next day at a certain time. The consultant should note on the chart: "Patient was seen briefly for an introductory session, and consultation will be completed at the specified time tomorrow."

Second, the consultant should obtain a complete understanding of the reasons for the consultation—the unstated as well as the overt. A discussion with the consultee prior to seeing the patient is imperative. At that time, the consultant can obtain a brief review of the case and learn the reasons for the request. Thus he is able to grasp the nature of the relationship between the staff and the patient. The time spent with the consultee decreases the amount of time needed with the patient. The consultant elicits significant information by asking how the consultee views the patient. Just verbalizing this question helps the consultee clarify his own attitudes toward the patient and makes the consultant's later discussion of the patient more meaningful to him.

Prior to the consultation the consultant can glean valuable information from the nursing staff and other personnel. This increases their involvement in the case and enlists their aid for the treatment program to be developed.

Complete familiarity with the medical record is also essential. A brief but comprehensive review of the medical history, physical examination, and findings from diagnostic procedures consolidates the consultant's view of the patient as a total human being, one whose psyche is not split from his soma. Reviewing the record educates the psychiatrist; it keeps him in touch with general medicine and provides him with a common ground for his activities with the staff.

Third, the consultant must observe medical ethics. He has a fundamental obligation not to "take over" the patient; the consultee is the primary physician. Occasionally there are exceptions; the consultee may indicate beforehand that he wants the psychiatrist to implement any program he deems necessary and to discuss it with the patient. However, unless there has been explicit agreement on this point, the consultant must review his findings with the consultee before he informs the patient of plans for therapy. In addition, treatment programs are more successful when the psychiatrist discusses his findings and his plans with the nursing staff.

Fourth, the consultant should attach a copy of his written report to the chart so that it will become part of the permanent record to be utilized by the staff on future admissions.

Fifth, every consultation ought to be a learning situation for the consultee. Through a greater understanding of the case material, he learns medical psychology with a clinical orientation. Also, he learns from the interactions among the patient, consultant, and himself. The consultee gains insight into *how* he reacted to the patient and *why* he reacted in a specific manner. The consultant describes the patient's behavior and clarifies the reasons for it; the case history, psychodynamics, formulation, and outlined plans for treatment enlarge the consultee's knowledge of psychiatry. He also learns about medications prescribed for emotional disorders. Obviously, he becomes more familiar with psychiatrists.

REFERENCES

MALLOTT, I. F., and EARLEY, L. W. The consultation situation and program content. *In* The Psychiatric Consultation. W. M. Mendel and P. Solomon, eds. New York, Grune and Stratton, 1968.

11 THE CONSULTATION

READING THE REQUEST

The request for psychiatric consultation is a plea for help from the consultee. Because the consultee is not always able to specify why he needs help, the consultant must be aware that the request embodies both explicit and implicit components. Weisman and Hackett (1960) call these the overt and covert reasons for referral.

The explicit request for consultation may take several forms. It may be vague and merely ask, "Please evaluate," or "For diagnosis and treatment." Sometimes, specific questions appear on the request. These vary from asking for opinions about diagnosis to asking for an evaluation of the suicidal risk or the need for commitment.

Implicit factors lurk: the staff's concerns about the patient, their difficulties with him, and their personal dilemmas which involve attitudes toward psychiatry. Both consultee-oriented and situation-oriented approaches acknowledge that these implicit factors exist in every case and must be coped with.

The request for consultation may be made by telephone, by a personal meeting between the consultee and the consultant, or by a written note. The telephone call and the personal meeting give the consultant an opportunity to evaluate the referring physician's concern. Following any verbal request, the consultant should ask the referring physician to fill out a routine consultation form. This is necessary so that the request and the consultant's reply can become part of the patient's record. When the request is in writing, the consultant must arrange a meeting with the consultee prior to seeing the patient. The importance of this meeting is discussed under RESPONSIBILITIES.

The consultant extracts valuable information by scrutinizing the written request; its language hints at the consultee's real feelings about the patient or about the psychiatrist. For example, scanty information may indicate lack of knowledge about the patient or little involvement with him. A quality of rejection appearing in the note usually indicates a derogatory opinion of the patient, of psychiatry, or both. On the other hand, a written request which asks specific questions, outlines pertinent medical data, and describes feelings, signals a sophisticated and interested consultee.

REVIEWING THE MEDICAL RECORD

A brief review of the patient's chart is essential. Although this perusal need not take more than a few minutes, it offers the consultant important data and significant clues. He should ask himself:

1. Is the medical history complete? Is it meaningful? Is it sketchy, perhaps revealing the consultee's incomplete understanding? Or is it exhaustive and perhaps filled with so many details that there is no distinct clinical picture?

2. What were the physical findings on admission? Have they changed? Do they confirm or contradict the complaints?

3. Has the diagnostic work-up been completed? Was consultation sought only because all laboratory tests were within normal limits?

4. What is the quality of the medical and nursing staff's progress notes? Do they portray what is taking place with the patient or are they merely routine notations? Does only one shift of nurses have difficulty with the patient? Are the staff's views of the patient in agreement?

5. What medications have been given? Are they contributing to psychopathology (e.g., steroids affecting an acute brain syndrome)? Are they for staff convenience (e.g., how often is the patient receiving narcotics or sedatives)?

BASIC MEDICAL WORK-UP

Besides diagnostic procedures and laboratory tests which are specifically indicated by the nature of the presenting symptom, Palerea (1965) recommends that the medical work-up of every patient with psychiatric symptomatology should include a detailed medical history, a careful physical examination, and a laboratory routine consisting of a complete blood count, urine analysis, a VDRL test for syphilis, a determination of blood sugar, urea nitrogen, and cholestoral levels, chest x-ray, and an electrocardiogram. To this list I would add that an electroencephalogram should be obtained for a great majority of the patients.

THE SETTING

When seeing inpatients, the consultant may have difficulty obtaining privacy for his interview. If an ambulatory patient is in a two- or four-bed unit, the consultant should find an open room on the medical floor or escort the patient to his own office. If the patient is not ambulatory, bedside consultations, with curtains drawn, are necessary. The experienced consultant is successful in this setting, and the beginner will have little difficulty when he overcomes his own discomfort.

In every case, the consultant should go to the patient's room as a matter of courtesy. Additionally, he gains information by observing the patient's appearance and his bedside effects. For example, the consultant can see whether the patient has books, flowers, or pictures of the family; the patient's social class, educational level, and the family's interest in him may be evident. Although the hospital is only a temporary home for the patient, many bring personal possessions. And every scrap of information that the psychiatrist accumulates, through observation or otherwise, is helpful.

APPROACHING THE PATIENT

Through experience, each consultant eventually develops his own techniques for approaching the patient. Some consultants do not state explicitly in their introduction, or even during the later phases of the consultation, that they are psychiatrists. In working on certain services such as neurosurgery, some say they are "neuropsychiatrists." But we have found that a simple, forthright statement of fact is the best introduction. The consultant entering the patient's room can say, "Hello Mr. Smith, I am Dr. Jones, a psychiatrist. Your doctor asked me to see you for consultation." When this is done openly and without embarrassment, it explains the consultant's presence and initiates a style for the interview, a style characterized by a spirit of inquiry, lack of prejudgment, and mutual respect. This approach is effective, probably because it clears the air at once, without leaving room for deception or misinterpretation.

Then the psychiatrist should ask the patient what his physician said about the consultation. Although most referring physicians discuss the referral with their patients, a few find it difficult to do so and leave this task of breaking the ice to the psychiatrist. When necessary, the psychiatrist should be willing to accept this responsibility because he is the expert in human relations and has skills for handling adverse reactions. However, the consultee's failure to prepare the patient for referral is usually telling evidence of his uncomfortable relationship with the patient.

Next, asking the patient simply "How do you feel about seeing a psychiatrist?" is an extremely useful technique. This permits the patient to express feelings at the beginning of the interview and lets him know that feelings are important and that they will be accepted. The patient may disclose hidden fears, asking, "Does my doctor think I am crazy?" Or, he may ask openly or indirectly, "Hasn't my doctor found what is wrong?"

As the consultation progesses, the patient also worries: "What does the psychiatrist want me to say?" "Will I be able to tell him what he wishes to know?" "Will the information I give him be used against me?" "Will the staff hold a changed opinion of me?" At this point the consultant should help the patient come to grips with his expectations of the consultation and its meaning. The psychiatrist must not rely on glib statements of reassurance; attitude is more important. We say, "Neither your doctor nor I is sure that there is a psychiatric problem; we are working together, and I am here only to see whether there are emotional problems contributing to your illness."

THE INTERVIEW

The consultant should proceed with the interview in his own style as comfortably as possible. The openness of his introduction has already set the tone for the entire interview. Asking the patient how he feels and what he thinks about his illness is the next step. This is essential; it brings to light the patient's view of his illness (obvious distortions may be revealed), and it enables the consultant to order his thoughts about the illness. This interest in the patient's medical complaints is appropriate. But the patient should not be allowed to give a detailed medical history at this point; a long recital might serve as resistance to the psychiatric interview. As the patient is discussing his illness, the consultant should inquire about feelings and events associated with the onset of the illness or the development of new symptomatology. How the patient responded to previous illnesses, hospitalizations, or surgery, is germane.

The personal and family history must be explored, focusing on the quality of the patient's relationships with parents, siblings, and spouse. The consultant should inquire about: needs, happiness, values, and meaning. This discussion should evolve in such a way that the patient sees his life in sharp perspective and can evaluate how he reacts not only to its exigencies, but also to the broad contours.

Then the consultant should devote five or ten minutes to a formal mental status examination. Inexperienced consultants may be embarrassed to ask obviously intelligent patients to do serial sevens or to interpret a proverb such as "People who live in glass houses should not throw stones." However, when the consultant becomes accustomed to doing a mental status examination on every patient and discovers its importance, he loses his reluctance to engage in this routine part of the evaluation. The patient accepts this examination as openly and honestly as the consultant presents it; it is no more out of place than some of the simple physical examination procedures, such as asking a healthy-looking young person to move a joint in which there is no evidence of illness and about which there is no complaint.

WHEN TO TERMINATE THE INTERVIEW

Sometimes the conventional hour is insufficient; the consultant may receive too little or too much information, and he may be unable to crystallize his impressions of the patient. When more time is needed, it is best to break off the interview after an hour and return the following day, usually for a shorter period. In our experience, prolonging a single interview increases confusion. Only rarely can the consultant achieve a more effective formulation after an hour and a half than after an hour.

When terminating such an interview, the consultant can inform the patient that he wishes to think about their discussion, that he would like the patient to give it more thought, and that he will return the next day at an appointed time. Repeatedly, we have found that the patient begins the second interview by giving the consultant additional information. Being away from the patient for a day mulling over the interview increases the consultant's objectivity, uncovers gaps, and enables him to detect areas of resistance. A brief interview, often as little as 20 minutes, on the second day suffices to complete the case formulation, diagnosis, and treatment plan. When a second interview is necessary, the consultant should inform the consultee and write a short progress note.

HOW TO TERMINATE THE INTERVIEW

Terminating the interview requires certain skills. The consultant is under an obligation not to inform the patient of the results before meeting with the consultee. He should tell the patient frankly that he wishes to discuss his findings with the consultee, and he should reassure the patient that the consultee, the consultant, or both will meet with him later.

Occasionally, a problem arises when, at the end of the interview, the patient tells the consultant that he does not wish to have certain personal matters divulged to anyone else: the referring physician, nurses, or particularly his family. This puts the consultant in a bind, especially if the information is essential for case formulation. How secret information will be used should be discussed freely with the patient. Obviously, every detail need not be revealed to others. An element of trust must be maintained; the psychiatrist should secure the patient's permission to give at least a guarded description of personal material to the consultee, with the provision that this is confidential and that the consultation note will not contain embarrassing details.

THE DISCUSSION WITH THE CONSULTEE

After seeing the patient, the consultant should meet with the consultee to inform him of the findings and obtain his reactions. Of course, when there is an emergency, the consultant must immediately outline a treatment plan and enlist the aid of the consultee and nursing personnel. Usually, a short conference with all concerned expedites treatment.

In the discussion with the referring physician, there should be mutual agreement about what the patient should be told and who will speak to the patient. In most cases, the referring physician gives the psychiatrist permission to see the patient again for this purpose. At this point, interpersonal difficulties may arise between the patient and the consultee, between the patient and the consultant, or between the consultee and consultant. In general, these difficulties involve lack of trust on the part of the patient toward the consultee or consultant, dislike extending in either direction, or controversy about the diagnosis and treatment plan. Such problems must be dealt with directly and worked through to a satisfactory conclusion. Following the interview with the consultee and the nursing staff, the consultant should write his note and place it on the patient's chart.

CASE FORMULATION

The demands of consultation work, seeing patients quickly and supplying recommendations promptly, place a premium on the consultant's skills in case formulation. By definition, to formulate is "to reduce to or express in a formula," or "to put into a systematized statement . . ." (Webster). For the consultant, all these definitions are important; he must reduce the mass of accumulated data from the medical work-up and the psychiatric examination to a succinct, organized group of statements which cohere. These statements must be selective and meaningful, expressing pertinent facts which give the consultee a schema for understanding the patient and providing treatment.

According to Masserman (1955), the psychiatric examination should yield four categories of data: a description of the present illness, a personality evaluation, the mental status results, and a dynamic formulation. The dynamic formulation, he states, consists of "valid deductions from the anamnestic data as to: a) the patient's physical and intellectual endowments, b) his acquired tendencies and behavior, including special capacities and vulnerabilities, and c) the weight of other factors relevant to prognosis and therapy."

Weisman (1959) notes that formulation has been confused with case description and diagnostic impressions. To him, formulation is directed toward evaluating conflict. He lists three requirements basic to this formulation: the *explanatory* (indicating the source of conflict), the *logical* (appraising the conflict systematically), and the *operational* (using methods by which conflict may be revealed and expressed). Weisman proposes a quadrilateral formulation whereby conflict may be understood from the following viewpoints: 1) the regulatory functions of the ego, 2) the predominant emotional problems at hand, 3) the quality and the quantity of the object relationship, and 4) the nuclear elements of the conflict itself.

Noyes and Kolb (1963) emphasize the importance of constructing a diagnostic formulation, stating: "An effort is made to coordinate and correlate the various symptoms and behavior manifestations and to articulate them one with the other, with the result that a comprehensive, consistent, meaningful, natural-history picture of the personality is obtained, a dynamic formulation that avoids speculative assumption and makes sensible the patient's life history."

We conceive of the case formulation as a summary statement of the data gathered from the patient's past history and present illness, explaining not only what is happening, but how, and why. Personal, constitutional, and environmental influences must be evaluated in this light; the patient's resources must be assessed. From the formulation, the consultant derives a diagnostic classification. The diagnosis is viewed only as a hypothesis, to be supported or rejected by the data. The formulation and the diagnosis lead logically to recommendations for treatment and a statement concerning prognosis.

THE CONSULTANT'S REPLY

The consultant's note becomes a permanent part of the patient's record to be read not only by the consultee, but also by physicians and nurses on future hospital and clinic admissions. Obviously, its main purpose is to communicate the consultant's findings to the consultee. The note should be focused to: 1) answer specific questions raised by the consultee, 2) present, in precise terms, factual data about the patient which support the psychiatrist's formulation and his diagnostic impressions, 3) respond to unstated, implicit concerns of the consultee and the staff, and 4) indicate how the consultation helps both the patient and the consultee.

The consultant should analyze his written note for style and content. With respect to style, clarity and brevity are important. A one-page note is usually sufficient. In the past, consultants drafted four to five type-written pages about each patient. Significant data were mixed with in-consequential details. This verbiage was usually ignored by the busy consultee who had neither the time nor the interest for it; he would search frantically for the summary. Thus, much of the consultant's work was not communicated clearly, and a teaching opportunity was lost. Therefore, the note should be concise, emphasizing the significant findings and offering a coherent portrayal of the patient.

Adhering to a consistent format is recommended. First, there should be a brief statement of the reasons for consultation, the chief complaint, and the highlights of the present illness. The past history should point out the number and types of previous illnesses and, more importantly, the patient's reactions to them. The next section, the personal history, should contain essential data: childhood development, schooling, relationships with parents and siblings, adolescence, sexual and marital history, and occupational history. Correlations between significant events and illnesses should be unearthed and the life style displayed. The physical examination should be mentioned, at least by writing the word, "reviewed," indicating that the consultant is familiar with the data accumulated by the work-up, x-ray reports, and other laboratory findings. The psychiatric examination should be given a separate heading and the consultant should describe the reactions to the consultation as well as the more traditional subjects such as: orientation, memory, affect, mood, and thought content.

Then the case formulation should be stated succinctly, emphasizing the logic which led to the clinical impression. Frequently, two clinical impressions are necessary: the patient's reactive disorder and his personality diagnosis (e.g., conversion reaction; hysterical personality). Diagnostic terms should fit those found in the APA *Diagnostic and Statistical Manual of Mental Disorders*.

The last section includes the consultant's outline for treatment and disposition. These recommendations should be phrased specifically. Finally, the consultant should conclude with a thank you and sign his name.

OUTLINE FOR THE CONSULTANT'S NOTE

1. A short statement of the reasons for the referral.
2. The Chief Complaint and Present Illness. May be covered by a brief statement under the heading *Presenting Problem*.

3. Past Medical History. Interpret its significance instead of listing illnesses.
4. Personal History. Outline pertinent events and sketch the family history, including attitudes.
5. Physical Examination and Laboratory Findings. Summarize. The words, "reviewed" or "negative," may suffice.
6. Psychiatric Examination. Be concise and to the point.
7. Formulation. Make it brief but telling.
8. Clinical Impressions.
9. Recommendations. Be definite and specific.
10. "Thanks" and signature.

Three sample requests and the consultant's replies follow.

FOLLOW-UP

The consultant will have to make follow-up visits to most of his patients while they remain in the hospital. Obviously, his advice is needed by the staff on a day-to-day basis for severe management problems. Also, the consultant's willingness to see such patients briefly, every day, encourages the staff to intensify their efforts to help. Their anxiety is reduced when the consultant shares their burdens.

For patients without psychiatric problems or those for whom arrangements have been made for psychotherapy after discharge, the follow-up may be brief. The consultant need spend only a few minutes, or just say, Hello. Making regular rounds is a suitable means for seeing these patients expeditiously.

Patients regard these follow-up visits as expressions of interest and tangible evidence of the psychiatrist's role as a specialist in comprehensive medicine. They contribute much in influencing patients' attitudes toward psychiatry, changing the ambivalent or unfavorable toward the more positive.

THE FEE

In the past, some psychiatrists avoided consultations because they had difficulty obtaining adequate fees for their services. Now, expanded private and government insurance plans provide fees for psychiatric consultations. Newer mental health programs, with their emphasis on community psychiatry and psychiatry in the general hospital, are making funds available for psychiatrists to pursue consultation activities on a part-time basis. Many experienced psychiatrists, and even beginners, find that consultation

CONSULTATION REQUEST
HOSPITAL AND CLINICS
UNIVERSITY OF FLORIDA

Name
Address
Hospital #
Other Identification

Consultation Requested:	Psychiatry
Requested By:	Medicine
Date of Previous Consultation	Walk _____ Stretcher _____ Wheelchair _____ Bedside ___X___

Pertinent History and Findings: 18 yr. old W.M. student	Provisional Diagnosis:
and clothing salesman. Bloody	This patient has
diarrhea. Divorced parents.	Reason for Consultation and Specific Questions: colitis; please
Poor male identification.	evaluate for ulcerative colitis.
Medications Influencing Findings:	

CONSULTANT'S REPLY:

CC: Diarrhea

FH: Patient's mother had diarrhea two days before.

PH: Patient's early life was filled with familial trauma. At age 13 he witnessed his father being shot by his mother, and at age 16 his parents divorced. Subsequently, his mother was "taken up" by a man whom the patient does not like and who, the patient says, abuses her. The patient has been shifted back and forth between the parents during the last few years. He has one younger brother, and an older one, age 21, who was married at 16, went AWOL from the Air Force, and is now serving a prison term for car theft. The patient is close only to his mother, and turns to female figures for aid and advice. However, he has realistic goals and tries to earn enough money to finance his college education by working during the day and taking courses only at night.

PE: The patient appears to be ill. Sigmoidoscopy and biopsy support impression of acute inflammatory, ulcerative disease of the colonic mucosa. Shigella found on culture.

Psychiatric Examination: Mental status within normal limits. Patient does present a somewhat effeminate appearance, but by history, he has formed several heterosexual relationships.

Formulation: The patient has severe family pathology, but he is trying to work his way through this in a healthy manner. He lacks adequate masculine identification, and needs guidance as well as an opportunity to express his previously repressed anger toward his parents. With evidence of diarrhea in the community, the finding of shigella, the absence of previous attacks, and the lack of significant psychopathology, the diagnosis of ulcerative colitis cannot be made at this time. Also, no reactive psychiatric diagnosis can be made. Should the symptoms persist, or recur with repeated psychic trauma, further evaluation should be undertaken.

CHART COPY

71

Impression: Acute Colitis, probably due to Shigella. Adult situation reaction--
extreme family pathology.
Recommendation: Evaluation of resources available to help patient. Arrangements
have been made for social worker to consult with him. She will check
financial resources and interview family members in an attempt to locate
patient in a more healthful setting.

Thanks,

CONSULTATION REQUEST
HOSPITAL AND CLINICS
UNIVERSITY OF FLORIDA

Name
Address
Hospital #
Other Identification

Consultation Requested:	Psychiatry
Requested By:	Medicine
Date of Previous Consultation	Walk _____ Stretcher _____ Wheelchair ___X___ Bedside _____

Pertinent History and Findings: 27 yr. old W.F.	Provisional Diagnosis:
Acute intermittent porphyria; angina;	This patient has an
MI 2 yrs. ago.	Reason for Consultation and Specific Questions: anxiety reaction and
Familial hypercholesterolemia	is passive-aggressive;
Medications Influencing Findings:	provide psychiatric
Meprobamate 400 mg tid	treatment, both imme-
	diate and long-term.

CONSULTANT'S REPLY:

CC: Pain in chest

PI: Good health until 1960 when she developed post-partum dyspnea and persisting fatigue. In 1962, she awoke with crushing substernal pain radiating down both arms. EKG & SGOT confirmed a myocardial infarction; serum cholesterol 675 mg%. During 1962-3 numerous hospitalizations for anginal syndrome and anxiety attacks with chest pain. Also, diagnosis of duodenal ulcer 1963. Evaluation here in 1963 showed cholesterol 786 mg% which decreased to 450 mg% on diet and bedrest symptomatically improved. Coronary angiography Sept 1963 demonstrated complete obstruction of the right coronary artery with collateralization. Glucose tolerance curve 132 mg% at 2 hours. UF Hospital admission 1964 for evaluation of abdominal pain--diagnosis of intermittent porphyria. Now, patient re-enters complaining of frequent attacks of burning chest pain associated with emotion or exertion and not well relieved by nitroglycerine or narcotics. Patient has orthopnea, dyspnea, ankle edema, "nerves," and inability to carry on routine household functions.

FH: Porphyria and diabetes in mother. Father, brother and daughter all have hypercholesterolemia. No history of mental illness.

PH: Born and reared in central Florida. Father an engineer, mother a housewife. Birth, early development, play life, school life, all appear normal. Patient is the eldest of three. High school education with better than average grades. Married age 18, three children, no trouble reported in marriage until present illness.

PE: Reviewed.

Psychiatric Examination: Oriented X3, alert, cooperative, anxious-appearing patient. Stream of talk normal. No evidence of hallucinations or thought disorder. Memory intact in recent and remote spheres. Math adequate, abstracts interpreted in a popular vein. 7's adequate. Affect appropriate. Mood lowered. Patient obviously anxious. Insight and judgement fair; perception and grasp good.

CHART COPY

Formulation: Patient was told by another physician not to do anything, or she
would have another MI. She was unable to comply. Consequently, she would
overwork but then anxiously await attacks of chest pain. She is
discouraged; illness and hospitalizations have interferred with plans and
daily activities. Husband has been taking Maalox for 2 years, and her
8-year old daughter is doing poorly in school. The disturbed daily life,
fear of death, frustrations of goals, fear of a breakup in her family, and
the need for multiple medical procedures has produces a great deal of
anxiety which the patient has expressed with both somatic complaints
(anxiety attacks, hyperventilation) and worries. In addition, the patient
has porphyria, which may produce mild anxiety attacks or even acute psychosis.
Impression: Adult situational reaction with anxiety in a patient with multiple
organic disease (coronary artery disease, porphyria, hypercholesterolemia).
Recommend: On-ward psychotherapy aimed at: 1) support and reassurance from
immediate management, 2) develop insight into the etiology of the anxiety,
and 3) help the patient accept a life with limitations. Visits three times
a week planned.

Thanks,

CONSULTATION REQUEST
HOSPITAL AND CLINICS
UNIVERSITY OF FLORIDA

Name
Address
Hospital #
Other Identification

Consultation Requested:	Psychiatry
Requested By:	Surgery
Date of Previous Consultation	Walk ____X____ Stretcher _____
	Wheelchair _____ Bedside _____

Pertinent History and Findings:	Provisional Diagnosis: Paranoid
25 yr. old W.M. with perforated D.U.	
Surgery 10 days ago.	Reason for Consultation and Specific Questions: Please
Convalescing	take this hostile man off our hands--he
Medications Influencing Findings:	is paranoid, in trouble all the time,
None	and we can't put up with it any longer.

CONSULTANT'S REPLY:

CC: Recovering from surgery for stomach ulcer.

PI: The patient has had both intermittent and chronic indigestion, and abdominal pain for over one year. About three weeks ago became much worse. He was admitted to this hospital as an emergency ten days ago, diagnosis--perforated peptic ulcer. Now convalescing satisfactorily from surgery. After surgery, he was combative and hostile. At this time, he appeared depressed but states that he is actively seeking help. He admits he is suspicious about everything but is trying to control his feelings.

FH: The patient is loathe to talk about his mother, but describes her as a kindly, overworked woman for whom he has always wanted to do something, but his efforts are unappreciated. His father is an extremely aggressive, combative, angry man who has had little to do with him now and never played with him when he was a child. No siblings. Patient states that mother and father are not close.

PH: Parents had little interest in him, although his mother was kinder toward him than his father. He tried to stay out of the house as much as possible during his developing years. He was an average student through grade school and high school, but on numerous occasions since childhood he has been in many fights. He fears that he will inflict a mortal wound on his opponent. Now, he expresses concern about his ability to control these aggressive feelings. However, he cannot identify the source of his anger. Since graduation from high school, he has worked at a number of odd jobs and has been an "automobile mechanic" for four years. He admits that he did not follow the diet and medication program which physicians had prescribed for ulcer. Recently depressed and has actively contemplated suicide.

PE: Reviewed. Patient is convalescing satisfactorily from surgery and is now ambulatory.

Psychiatric Examination: Orientation, memory, and attention normal. His affect is inappropriate, more in degree than in kind. In recounting his personal history he showed some loosening of associations by interrupting his discourse

CHART COPY

75

to tell of his many adversaries in the world. He described "gangs" which are
out to "get him," "bosses who never gave him a fair deal," and he hints of
plots arranged by acquaintances and strangers to "get him." It should be noted
that he thinks he has felt this way about others since he was a child. There
are no hallucinations but the patient does describe a paranoid delusional
system concerning plots by adversaries. Mood is obviously depressed.
Calculations are within normal limits for his educational level. He interprets
proverbs poorly; for example, to the proverb, "people who live in glass houses
shouldn't throw stones," he muttered, "People are always throwing things and
are out to get you." This means "that if someone is trying to break you then
you are going to have to break them." Judgment and insight are poor, but
patient does express concern about his inability to control his feelings.

Formulation: This patient's life story is one of unfulfilled dependency needs with
some compensation in doing for others (particularly his mother), who are
unappreciative. Poor identification with an extremely aggressive, combative,
hostile father. The patient is "mad at the world" for not meeting his needs
and has some direct anger toward his father. His inability to follow medical
advice may be related to guilt feelings in many areas, especially in regard to
mother. Patient appears to have been decompensating during the last 10 years.
At times has been overtly paranoidal and aggressive, then developed a peptic
ulcer, and now depression. At present, his compensation is tenuous.

Impression: Paranoid personality, borderline psychotic reaction. Possible
schizophrenia, paranoid type.

Recommend: Chlorpromazine--give a 25 mg test dose at once, then if tolerated, give
patient 50 mg Q6H for 2 days and then 75 mg Q6H. Will follow to work
specifically with his hostility which is disruptive. Have discussed this with
nurses. I feel that the management difficulties are lessening. Arrangements
will be made for follow-up medical care and psychotherapy in outpatient clinic
after discharge. Psychological testing will be requested.

Thanks,

work is an excellent means for maintaining or building up a referral practice. In fact, they derive a substantial portion of their total income from
consulting.

The amount of the fee should be consonant with the psychiatrist's
regular charges for his time and the patient's ability to pay. Every patient
should be billed by the consultant, either directly or through the hospital
or clinic business office, after arrangements for billing procedures are
established with the administration.

REFERENCES

MASSERMAN, J. The Practice of Dynamic Psychiatry. Philadelphia, W. B.
Saunders Co., 1955.
NOYES, A., and KOLB, L. Modern Clinical Psychiatry, 6th ed. Philadelphia,
W. B. Saunders Co., 1963, p. 135.
PALEREA, E. P. Medical evaluation of the psychiatric patient. J. Amer.
Geriat. Soc., 13:14, 1965.
WEISMAN, A. D. Psychodynamic formulation of conflict. Arch. Gen. Psy-
chiat. (Chicago), 1:288, 1959.
―――― Hackett, T. The organization and function of a psychiatric consulta-
tion service. Int. Record. Med., 173:306, 1960.

12 WORKING WITH THE STAFF

THE NURSE

Emphasis on the situational approach, the ward milieu, and the small group (Meyer and Mendelson, 1961) has finally drawn attention to the hitherto neglected role of the nurse in psychiatric consultation work. Physicians recognize the decisive role played by the nurse in caring for patients. But, as Bursten (1963) states: "What is less evident is the role of the nurse in initiating the referral to the psychiatrist."

THE NURSE AND THE REFERRAL

The nurse, in her daily activities, has an excellent opportunity to detect patients' emotional distress and observe psychopathology in its early stages; indeed, she may have the best and often the only opportunity. She is aware, perhaps more than any other member of the medical team, that no patient's hospital course is static. She sees variable behavior and diverse responses to procedures, illness, and treatment, as they fluctuate on an hour-to-hour basis. Management problems are usually reflected, at least in the beginning, in the nurse-patient relationship. As she engages in routine tasks, she may be the first to observe lack of cooperation, hostility, mild confusion, or anxiety about diagnosis and prognosis. Although formal mechanisms usually require that a physician make the referral request, it is frequently the nurse who prompts the consultee to ask for consultation. Bursten (1963) points out, "The formal organizational structure of the hospital serves to conceal the real source of the referral."

Before seeing the patient, the consultant should talk to the nurse for a few minutes. In actuality, the nurse, who may be overlooked, serves as both a communicator and a source of communication. Her notes should convey information, although too often they are scanty and stereotyped.

The nurse's participation in treatment programs is vital. She becomes easily involved, especially if she is included in the small group discussion

78

which follows the consultation. In all cases, the consultant should interpret the patient's behavior to the nurse.

THE CHANGING ROLE OF THE PROFESSION

1. Traditional nurse-physician relationships are changing. The nursing profession is striving for increased status. Indeed, many nurses now act as administrators and delegate the direct patient care to nursing assistants or other auxiliary personnel.

2. The nurse's traditional bedside manner is under scrutiny. Jourard, in his book *The Transparent Self* (1964), avers that the nurse's approach to the patient is usually too rigid, serving a defensive purpose which precludes self-disclosure by the patient. He says: "The bedside manner can actually obstruct . . . attempts to 'integrate psychiatric and mental health concepts into programs of nursing education and nursing care.'" A hidden function of the bedside manner, he believes, is to foster increasing self-alienation in the nurse, desensitizing her to her own experiences and handicapping her attempts to know the patient.

These factors (the changing role of the profession and the reevaluation of traditional nursing approaches to patients) must be kept in mind by the consultant. To obtain smooth working relationships, he should treat the nurse, as a professional colleague, with dignity and respect. It is rewarding to invite the nurse to attend conferences between consultants and consultees and to accompany them on ward rounds. The consultant who values the team approach and rightfully regards the nurse as an important member has little difficulty securing her cooperation and enthusiastic participation.

DEALING WITH ANTITHERAPEUTIC RESPONSES

In view of the changing role of the nurse, in which she may be an administrator who has little personal contact with patients, the consultant must identify the key personnel involved. In many cases, the licensed practical nurse, nurse's aide, nursing assistant, or other subordinates are the ones who maintain the ongoing contacts with patients. The consultant should include them in his small group discussions of ward problems and treatment plans.

The nurse's emotional response to patients may contribute to, or even precipitate, management difficulties. An alert consultant is usually able to detect instances of unusual identification, excessive sympathy, or projected anger. The consultant should be cautious, not interpreting her behavior until he has weighed the unconscious determinants which are present. He should discuss such reactions with the nurse privately; in these discussions, the primary focus should remain on the patient. The consultant may decide to prescribe a change of assignments in order to avoid further clashes between specific nurses and patients.

The nurse's antitherapeutic reactions may in reality be retaliations against the attending physician or other staff members; she may be denying the patient rational and adequate care because of her antagonism toward them. Patient care may also be hindered by the nurse's sense of inadequacy, frustration, and anxiety. At these times, support by the consultant is usually sufficient to enable her to retrench and then function in accord with the patient's needs. Generally, staff nurses are eager to receive guidance, increased understanding, and even specific instructions from a consultant.

NURSE CONSULTANT PROGRAM
AT THE UNIVERSITY OF FLORIDA

As noted by Johnson (1963), a nurse consultant is in the best position to translate and transmit pertinent data about the patient and the situation to the nursing staff and to report their reactions, as well as the basic information, back to the consultant. This is particularly effective when mechanisms for transmitting this information are established.

For about two years we had a coordinated consultation program in which a psychiatric nurse consultant and two or three nursing students worked on the consultation service (Holstein and Schwab, 1965). This operational alliance enhanced the development of our total consultation program. The nurses attended case conferences and work rounds. Besides assisting the psychiatric consultants directly, they contributed information concerning patients' illnesses and characteristics of the patient-nurse relationship. The nurse consultants helped the staff nurses implement the psychiatrist's recommendations.

This coordinated program had specific strengths: communication between psychiatrists and nursing consultants was increased by frequent contact and joint involvement with particular patients. There was a cohesion of effort and a sense of unified mission. The staff learned the multidisciplinary team approach. Barriers between consultants and staff nurses were broken down. Finally, with such a coordinated consultation program, patient care was improved and greater opportunities for teaching and training resulted.

THE SOCIAL WORKER

Social structure influences mental illness; social disability can be crippling for individuals; and emotional distress, in turn, compounds social difficulties. Collaborating closely with a social worker is the consultant's best means for overcoming some patients' specific social impediments.

Social workers are vital links between the patient and the community; they have a tradition of more than 60 years of service. Their responsibilities increased through the years as the profession expanded and developed new ways of applying skills. A GAP Report (1948) states: "The social case worker deals with a wide range of social and personal problems. To enumerate them would be to name the whole gamut of human ills, failure and frustration, such as unemployment, poor housing, need for money, need for medical care, need for help in planning care of children and need for help with disturbed interpersonal relationships." Thus, social workers render services which meet practical reality needs.

Social workers contribute specific strengths to a consultation program. Because their education includes a background in psychology, sociology, economics, and medical problems as well as social case work, they have a necessary psychosocial orientation. They are accustomed to dealing directly with patients' financial needs (obtaining expensive medications for the indigent patient); providing community resources (finding help for the unwed mother or needed welfare assistance during convalescence); and dealing with family problems (arranging for foster home care for children or nursing homes for the aged). The social worker on a consultation service has an opportunity to utilize fresh approaches in meeting the exigencies of the service. Halloran (1965) says: "We encourage variations and innovations appropriate to the particular service."

Social case work is a term applied to a modified form of psychoanalytically oriented psychotherapy which has defined goals; it is considered to be the province of the social worker. Bibring (1964) says that psychotherapy by the case worker should utilize abreaction, clarification, and manipulation rather than the conveying of insight. She imbues the concept of manipulation with special meaning by calling it *redirective manipulation*. Redirective manipulation involves altering attitudes toward surrounding persons and mobilizing the patient's emotional system for the purpose of adjustment, with little or no interpretation.

Bibring's emphasis on these particulars is not uniformly accepted. Kaplan (1963) argues that there is little difference between the psychotherapeutic techniques used by psychiatrists and social workers. He says, "It seems evident that both psychiatrists and social workers treat the basic psychopathology as well as the clinical disorder. . . . In many instances, patients receive the greatest benefit from social case work therapy carried out under medical supervision."

ROLE OF THE SOCIAL WORKER ON A CONSULTATION-LIAISON SERVICE

1. Dealing directly with social pathology. Poverty, ignorance, or circumstance not only produce illness, but also deprive the patient of an

opportunity to regain health. Psychiatric social workers are familiar with community resources; the consultant's despair about coping with overwhelming social pathology and adverse environmental circumstances diminishes when he sees the social worker tackle these problems and provide at least partial solutions.

2. Assisting with diagnosis. The social worker's interviews, with the patient's spouse or other family members, gather information about psychosocial factors which may be necessary for definitive diagnosis. On many occasions our understanding of a particular case was imperfect until the social worker interviewed the family, or visited the home, and then joined in the clinical conferences. The GAP Report (1948) continues: "It is vital that the social history be considered as a constantly reformulated body of information. It consists of material revealed as an outgrowth of a purposeful relationship. . . . This dynamically developed social history provides the foundation for a continuing relationship of the psychiatric social worker to the patient and the family and community."

3. Providing psychotherapy. With supervision, psychiatric social workers can conduct psychotherapy with many medical and surgical patients in the hospital, during convalescence, or after discharge. Also, the social worker can act as a co-therapist with the consultant in family therapy, in coordinated interviews with a spouse or significant family member while the consultant is seeing the patient separately, and in group therapy. Multiproblem families can present so much psychopathology that any single therapist is easily overwhelmed. When the consultant teams up with a psychiatric social worker, his efforts are reinforced, and their discussions provide needed objectivity for each.

4. Interacting with the community. The psychiatric social worker should be the liaison person between the general hospital and community agencies (especially mental hygiene clinics). In this capacity, the social worker is a valuable advisor to the consultant. He can make arrangements for the patient's follow-up care in a mental hygiene clinic or assist family members in obtaining needed psychotherapy. The social worker also can: 1) explain hospital facilities and programs to the patient and the family; 2) assist families with problems arising from the patient's admission; and 3) establish relationships with the family which encourage them to maintain a positive, nonrejecting attitude toward the patient (see GAP Report).

5. Education. The psychiatric social worker on a consultation-liaison service can contribute to the education of students, house staff, and physicians by broadening their knowledge of the following areas: family relationships, the impact of socioeconomic stresses on family life, the avail-

ability and utilization of community resources (educational, vocational, legal, recreational, and so on). Importantly, the social worker's psychosocial orientation remedies deficiencies which exist because of the physician's greater emphasis on biologic processes at the expense of the social.

6. Participating in research. The social worker is in a particularly favorable position to undertake research which is specifically directed toward the psychosocial aspects of illness. By gathering data about patients after discharge from the hospital, and with follow-up studies, the social worker can complement the consultant's endeavors.

The following case illustrates how a social worker can help with some of the problems encountered by a consultant.

The medical staff referred a 47-year-old white widow for psychiatric consultation because she appeared anxious and labile. She was undergoing a diagnostic work-up for weight loss (35 pounds in four months). They asked, "Is this patient depressed? Please evaluate."

The consultant replied that the patient's life history has been a long ordeal of poverty and misery. She was one of 15 children; she left school in the sixth grade to help her mother take care of the children. At 22 she married a man who could barely support a family; since, she has worked as a maid earning $120 per month. Her husband died three years ago after a long illness. Her small house is crammed; her 18-year-old daughter and 22-year-old son, with his wife and two small children, also live with her. The son seems content to share the mother's poverty; he works only occasionally. He and his family moved in with the mother only six months before. The patient felt that she was caught in a bind—she would like the son to obtain work and move away; on the other hand, when she thought of "throwing him out," she felt guilty. She has ruminated about what she should do, has felt "blue," and is filled with remorse and guilt. In the past weeks she has been preoccupied with her weight loss and vague bodily aches and pains.

The consultant diagnosed an acute psychoneurotic reaction with elements of anxiety and depression. He recommended sedation and asked the psychiatric social worker to see the patient's son and daughter. After two interviews with them and one with the patient, the social worker accomplished the following: The son realized the futility of the present living arrangement and, with the help of the social worker and an employment agency, obtained a job and agreed to move. The patient received limited financial support from an agency for one month in order to tide her through convalescence.

When seen for follow-up one month later, she was greatly improved; she had returned to work, had regained 12 pounds, and her depression was obviously lifting. The son had moved and was working, but there were some doubts as to how long he would continue this independent existence. The social worker supported the patient in her efforts to keep the son and his family at some distance and help them at a distance, rather than merely sharing poverty with them.

THE CLINICAL PSYCHOLOGIST

The consultant's effectiveness can be enriched by a good working relationship with a clinical psychologist. Dickel (1966) compared the training of physicians and clinical psychologists, emphasizing the necessity for the two fields to recognize, respect, and offer their services to each other. He notes that there are obvious differences in orientation between psychiatrists and psychologists; at times, they even disagree about who should rightfully evaluate and treat the mentally ill. Dickel pleads for mutual consideration and combined efforts: "That clinical psychology has a place beside and within medicine in the diagnosis, therapy, and research of many human disorders is accepted and encouraged."

An editorial in the *Annals of Internal Medicine* (1962) called attention to the value of simple, self-administered psychological tests which can be scored by objective criteria. Fitts' Self-Concept Scale (the TSCS), the well-known MMPI, the Cornell Medical Index, Eysenck's Personality Inventory, the Beck Depression Inventory, and other instruments are now widely used in general medicine. They provide precisely the kind of data and the kind of reasoning used by clinicians, and they can be applied in a systematic manner. The editorial concludes that these instruments carry "promise for both the research worker and the clinician. . . . these tests provide so much information so cheaply that they may well become routine parts of any ongoing epidemiologic study. . . . For the clinician . . . it means that simple and reliable tools will for the first time become available to assist him in the most critical of functions, the psychologic assessment of his patients."

Thus, the consultant should take advantage of the psychologist's special abilities for: diagnosis, evaluation of patients' responses to self-administered psychological tests, assistance with treatment programs, and development of research for a consultation-liaison program.

ROLE OF THE CLINICAL PSYCHOLOGIST

1. Testing. The clinical psychologist's primary contribution to consultation activities is testing patients to clarify diagnostic problems. For example, organic brain disease can be diagnosed early by refined psychological test procedures, and well-developed projective instruments

like the Rorschach aid in differentiating schizophrenia from certain character disorders or depressive illnesses.

2. Psychotherapy. The clinical psychologist can also conduct individual or group psychotherapy with many consultation patients. When there is close cooperation between the psychologist and the consultant, and particularly when the consultant as the team leader provides supervision, these psychotherapeutic endeavors are unusually successful.

3. Research. A clinical psychologist's contributions to the entire field of consultation-liaison psychiatry can be substantial. Systematized research is lacking; concepts, procedures, and clinical problems require objective study. The psychologist can assist with research design and data analysis.

INDICATIONS FOR PSYCHOLOGICAL TESTING

These indications for referral can also be phrased as specific questions to the psychological consultant (see also Wortis and Halpern, 1958).

1. Differential Diagnosis
    (a) Brain damage vs. schizophrenia or depression
    (b) Neurosis vs. psychosis
    (c) Personality disorder vs. psychosis
    (d) Malingering vs. posttraumatic neurosis
2. Assessment of Mental Functions
    (a) To determine whether the patient is mentally retarded
    (b) Borderline intelligence (the inadequate personality)
    (c) Is there a marked discrepancy between verbal and performance skills (the sociopath)?
    (d) Degree of intellectual impairment (organic brain disease)
3. Conflicts and Mental Mechanisms
    (a) What are the major areas of disturbance (anxiety?)
    (b) Sexual identification
    (c) What are the major defense mechanisms (denial? repression? projection?)
4. Formulation
    (a) Explicate dynamics
    (b) Confirmatory evidence (thought disorder?)
5. Convalescence and Prognosis
    (a) What intellectual tasks can the patient perform?
    (b) What are the patient's personality strengths or special abilities?
    (c) Serial testing
6. In all cases in which the consultant may have to testify as an expert witness
    (a) Posttraumatic or compensation neurosis

(b) Competency, particularly for patients with organic brain syndromes

(c) Divorce, custody, wills

(d) As a court-appointed witness in criminal cases.

REFERRAL TO THE PSYCHOLOGIST FOR TESTING

When the patient is referred for testing, the consultant must supply the psychologist with the reasons for his request and the facts about the medical illness and psychosocial stresses. He should also have a brief discussion with the psychologist, both before and after the testing. The written referral request should always pose specific questions.

The following case history illustrates the value of a referral for psychological testing, particularly when specific questions are posed:

The psychiatric consultant referred Mr. C., a 41-year-old white male for psychological testing because he was unsure about the diagnosis. Since an automobile accident two months before, the patient had been hospitalized three times for the treatment of persistent headaches and severe pain in the neck and arms. The consultant asked: 1) comment on differential diagnosis between a psychophysiologic and a conversion reaction; 2) please evaluate personality for type; and 3) what are the main defenses?

The Psychologist's Reply: The MMPI, TAT, Rorschach, HTP, and the Bender-Gestalt were administered. Mr. C. was superficially cooperative, but was irritated by this further investigation into his symptoms. The patient was resistant, insisting that his headaches were real — but that he was not worried about his condition. During testing, he had a more severe headache, and his irritation became obvious. A review of the patient's life shows that his existence is barren and routine; he has no interests or hobbies except hunting; and, he regards his job as a "drag."

Interpretation: The data indicate that the patient is a socially oriented, passive person who develops symptoms under stress and uses somatization to achieve neurotic ends. Further, he is a bland, repressive person who has little insight into his feelings. He receives much love and attention while sick; this is important because he has severe dependency problems. His underlying hostility broke through during testing and was evidenced by his Rorschach responses: "animals were cut open, gnawing, eating, etc." His interpersonal relationships have little depth or warmth; he denies his sexual impulses; and he relates primarily in a dependent, immature fashion. His intellectual resources for dealing with the world are accurate but limited.

Conclusion: Mr. C. has the personal history, past medical history, and psychopathology which fit the pattern for the diagnosis: conversion reaction. Personality diagnosis: passive, immature, dependent male. His main defenses are denial and repression; they are used to conceal his hostility and his awareness of his own needs and inadequacies. He probably will not be responsive to intensive psychotherapy.

The psychologist's report both supplemented and confirmed the psychiatrist's impressions about the patient. General supportive therapy was instituted (physical therapy, analgesics—consisting only of aspirin to avoid possible addiction, and progressive activity). Little attempt was made to probe into the patient's basic personality problems, but with minimal prodding and slight direction, the psychiatrist encouraged the patient to ventilate his feelings 15 to 30 minutes per session. No attempt was made to "rush" the patient out of the hospital; instead, a gradual return to activity was effected, and the patient is now being seen weekly for brief visits in the outpatient clinic. Although he still complains of headaches, these complaints are more moderate, and he has returned to work part-time.

Thus, psychologic tests can be used to support clinical impressions, aid in the diagnostic appraisal, and complete the work-up, particularly where some litigation may be involved. Data obtained from psychologic testing achieve their grestest value when they are incorporated into the consultant's comprehensive understanding of the patient and the illness.

REFERENCES

BIBRING, G. L. *In* Zinberg, N. E., ed. Psychiatry and Medical Practice in a General Hospital. New York, International Universities Press, Inc., 1964.

BURSTEN, B. The psychiatric consultant and the nurse. Nurs. Forum, 2(4):7, 1963.

DICKEL, H. A. The physician and the clinical psychologist. J.A.M.A., 195(5):365, 1966.

Editorial. Psychological tests and medical prognosis. Ann. Intern. Med., 56(3):524, 1962.

GAP Report No. 2, p. 1, Jan. 1948.

HALLORAN, H. M. The role of the caseworker. *In* Kaufman, M. R., ed. The Psychiatric Unit in a General Hospital. New York, International Universities Press, Inc., 1965.

HOLSTEIN, S., and SCHWAB, J. J. A coordinated consultation program for nurses and psychiatrists. J.A.M.A., 194:491, 1965.

JOHNSON, B. S. Psychiatric nurse consult in a general hospital, Nursing Outlook Forum, 11:728, 1963.

JOURARD, S. M. The Transparent Self. Princeton, D. Van Nostrand Co., Inc., 1964.

KAPLAN, A. H. Social work therapy and psychiatric psychotherapy. Arch. Gen. Psychiat., (Chicago), 9:497, 1963.

MEYER, E., and MENDELSON, M. Psychiatric consultation with patients on medical and surgical wards: Patterns and processes. Psychiatry, 24:197, 1961.

WORTIS, S. B., and HALPERN, F. Psychological tests and indications for their use. Med. Clin. N. Amer., May:741, 1958.

13 CONSULTATIONS IN THE CLINIC AND IN PRIVATE PRACTICE

With the assistance of Roy S. Clemmons, M.D.

Many of the principles and techniques which have been described for consultations with inpatients are equally applicable to clinic work or private practice. The purpose of this chapter is to note some of the differences produced by the particular arrangements of clinic or office practice.

CONSULTATIONS IN THE CLINIC

Kaufman (1953), Fox (1963), Lipsitt (1964) and others (Grinker, 1953; Bibring, 1956; Schiff and Pilot, 1959; Overley, 1963) have discussed the psychiatrist's contribution to patient care in the general medical clinic. Based on the 1957 work of Grotjahn and Treusch (discussed below), we developed the psychiatric cross-consultation technique for our general medical clinic. This cross-consultation is not radically new, but it is distinguished from the more traditional clinic consultation because it maximizes the consultant's opportunities for teaching.

UNIVERSITY OF FLORIDA CROSS-CONSULTATION CLINIC: DESIGN AND OPERATION

Patient eligibility for these cross-consultations is determined primarily by the willingness of the referring physician to present the patient, share the interview, and discuss the findings with the consulting psychiatrist. These consultations take place in the general medical clinic; arrangements for them are made through the clinic secretary. Patients are seen on the same day that the requests for consultation are received.

Two psychiatrists participate; one of them devotes three hours, three afternoons a week, and the other provides the same amount of time on the remaining two days. To obtain a consultation, the referring physician, usually a member of the medical or surgical staff, contacts the clinic secretary who sets up the consultant's schedule for the afternoon. By noon, she can tell him how many consultations have been arranged, thus enabling him to use his time to best advantage.

The referring physician, in addition to filling out the standard consultation request, meets with the psychiatrist at the designated time to discuss the case. One or two members of the house staff and several medical students usually complete the group. After a 10 to 15 minute discussion, the consultant, the consultee, and frequently one or more of the students meet with the patient in a clinic office. In this medical setting, the consultant interviews the patient for about 30 minutes. He and the rest of the staff then retire to discuss the case and formulate recommendations for a treatment program. The consultant writes the consultation note.

When appropriate, the referring physician is encouraged to undertake the psychotherapy, with the consultant offering supervision. Thus, indicated psychotherapy is carried out concurrently with the medical work-up and treatment. In this way, psychotherapy loses its mysterious aura and becomes a form of medical treatment.

ACHIEVEMENTS

1. Communication among those involved in patient care is remarkably improved. Ideas are exchanged; the consultation becomes a two-way process, with both the consultant and the consultee benefiting from each other's specialized knowledge.

2. Educational opportunities are increased. For example, the consultee or medical student may even spend a few minutes at the end of the hour asking the consultant for his opinion about another case.

3. The number of requests for these consultations is growing. One reason for this success is that there is little or no lapse of time between the request and the consultant's intervention.

4. Much of the burden of routine evaluation is removed from the psychiatric outpatient clinic. Also, the need for referring clinic patients to the emergency room for consultation is practically eliminated.

5. Keeping the consultations in the general medical clinic, away from the psychiatric clinic or the emergency room, reinforces the holistic approach and diminishes the tendency to shuttle patients from one specialty clinic to another. As a result, the so-called "crock" is accepted in the general medical clinic.

6. Physicians and students are encouraged to undertake psycho-

therapy with their patients. Also as the psychiatrist works in the medical milieu, he comes to understand physicians' problems and his recommendations become more realistic.

7. The psychiatrist is accessible; emergencies are handled promptly.

CONSULTATIONS IN PRIVATE PRACTICE

For private practice, Grotjahn and Treusch (1957) proffer an unusual model of the consultation; the psychiatrist goes to the consultee's office. The psychiatrist is a guest, invited by both the consultee and the patient; his guest status emphasizes his secondary, but important, role. The consultation is located in a medical context. And in this familiar setting, the patient need not erect a new set of defenses.

TECHNIQUE

Grotjahn and Treusch (1957) discuss the technique of this type of consultation. The consultee briefs the psychiatrist for about ten minutes. Then, the patient joins them in the office. The consultee retains his usual seat; the patient sits in such a way that he is not between the two specialists, and so he can see them both at the same time. This arrangement reduces the likelihood that the patient will feel torn between his psyche and soma. Both the consultant and the consultee participate in the interview. After the patient leaves the office, the psychiatrist voices his recommendations. In certain cases, however, the patient remains in the office for the summation; then, the psychiatrist addresses himself to the physician, while the patient only listens to his remarks. In all cases, after the psychiatrist leaves, the consultee concludes the interview with the patient.

Treusch's and Grotjahn's (1967) consultation procedure has now evolved as "family consultations," in which the psychiatrist, internist, patient, and close family members participate in the interview. Because the interview takes place in the internist's office, the family members are able to develop the theme of the consultation. Treusch and Grotjahn emphasize that "psychiatric family consultations offer a technique for better diagnosis and understanding in many conditions confronting the physician in family practice. Neither the patient, his family, nor the physician should expect anything more. . . . In a way, it is a partial return to the values of the old-fashioned family physician, with present-day psychiatric sophistication."

ALTERNATIVE PROCEDURES IN PRIVATE PRACTICE

Only rarely, unfortunately, can the consultant take advantage of the procedures described by Grotjahn and Treusch (1957). Usually, the referring physician calls to make an appointment or has the patient do so himself. A written request may not be provided; thus, it is necessary for the consultant to gather most of the pertinent information by telephone. The psychiatrist should set up a system to take telephone referrals personally because a discussion with the consultee is mandatory. The psychiatrist must gather information about the reasons for referral, the quality of the patient's relationship with his physician, the medical procedures, and the treatment programs. This discussion also serves to maintain rapport with the referring physician. After seeing the patient in his office, the consultant should discuss the findings with the consultee by telephone.

THE NOTE

For all consultations, the psychiatrist should complete a written note.

REFERENCES

BIBRING, G. L. Psychiatry and medical practice in a general hospital. New Eng. J. Med., 254:366, 1956.

FOX, H. M. Psychiatric consultation in general medical clinic. An experiment in post-graduate training. J.A.M.A., 185:999, 1963.

GRINKER, R. R. Psychotherapy in medical and surgical hospitals. Dis. Nerv. Syst., 13:269, 1953.

GROTJAHN, M., and TREUSCH, J. V. A new technique of psychosomatic consultations: Some illustrations of team work between an internist and a psychiatrist. Psychoanal. Rev., 44:176, 1957.

KAUFMAN, M. The role of the psychiatrist in a general hospital. Psychiat. Quart., 27:367, 1953.

LIPSITT, D. R. Integration clinic: An approach to the teaching and practice of medical psychology in an outpatient setting. In Zinberg, N. E., ed. Psychiatry and Medical Practice in a General Hospital. New York, International Universities Press, Inc., 1964.

OVERLEY, T. M. Discovering the functional illness in interview. J.A.M.A., 186(8):776, 1963.

SCHIFF, S. K., and PILOT, M. L. An approach to psychiatric consultation in the general hospital. Arch. Gen. Psychiat. (Chicago), 1:349, 1959.

TREUSCH, J. V., and GROTJAHN, M. Psychiatric family consultations. Ann. Intern. Med., 66(2): 295, February, 1967.

14 ROUNDS

Attending medical or surgical ward rounds is an important activity for the consultant. Daily rounds are not necessary; rounding with the staff once or twice a week usually suffices. When there is an established liaison program, or a university hospital setting, making such rounds is essential. However, any psychiatrist who wishes to maintain a close liaison with his fellow physicians should devote one or two hours a week to rounding on a service of his choice.

Making rounds on a service from which the consultant is receiving many referrals offers him an opportunity to survey all the patients on that service. He understands how his patients are relating to the other patients, medical staff, nurses, and attending physicians. He sees his patients in a situation less structured than the conventional psychiatric interview. He gains an appreciation of the milieu as it changes, from week to week, in patient composition, personnel, and ward relationships.

Further, he can assess the effectiveness of referral procedures. Some patients are referred promptly, while others are referred too late, if at all. The consultee's blind spots become apparent.

On services from which the consultant receives few referrals, he learns why consultations are not requested and how the staff is managing patients who should receive consultations.

The consultant usually may choose either to accompany attending physicians or to make regular morning work rounds with the house staff. Rounding with the attending physician frequently turns out to be a high-level conference between two professionals; the psychiatrist's contributions may not filter down to the house staff, nursing staff, or students. Therefore, we found that attending the house staff's work rounds, prior to their rounds with the chief of service, has distinct advantages. The psychiatrist's teaching efforts can be concentrated on the students and house staff who are still in training. He is working directly with the personnel who have the closest contacts with patients. Also, the house staff appreciates the psychiatrist's interest; their willingness to learn increases. In fact, they use the information derived from these rounds to supplement their presentations to the attending physicians.

ATTAINING CONSULTATION WORK OBJECTIVES

Some of the objectives of the consultant's work are more easily realized on rounds than elsewhere. 1) The holistic approach: When the psychiatrist mingles freely with the rounding staff, he is identified by them and the patients as part of the treatment team. Joint efforts lead to patient orientation rather than disease orientation. 2) A working liaison: When the consultant shares the staff's routine, as well as their concerns about particular patients, a growing familiarity develops. The staff's fear of criticism is dispelled, and distorted views of psychiatry are diminished. Also, the presence of the psychiatrist is supportive; the staff is less fearful of patient psychopathology. 3) The teaching of medical psychology: Opportunities for bedside teaching in the medical tradition are plentiful. For example, the staff can watch the psychiatrist question a patient briefly. The importance of multiple etiology emerges.

GUIDELINES FOR MAKING ROUNDS

1. Do not interfere with essential activities. On work rounds the staff is under pressure to see each patient briefly. They must evaluate his daily progress, review diagnostic procedures, and make plans for treatment. If the consultant obstructs these necessary activities, he will be unwelcome. The staff will make this known by disregarding his presence or derogating his contributions.

2. Blend with the staff. This usually requires wearing a white coat and carrying a stethoscope or reflex hammer, not to disguise his identity as a psychiatrist, but to put both the staff and the patients at ease. Also, the consultant should mix with all the individuals on the rounding team, not devote his attention exclusively to the resident in charge.

3. Participate in examinations and share concern. When the psychiatrist is interested in learning from the staff by asking why they request certain laboratory procedures, he will be kept up-to-date on changes in medicine, and the staff will appreciate this chance to teach. The consultant should evince an interest when unusual physical findings

are displayed, and he should share the staff's concern about the critically ill patients or those with complex medical problems.

4. Limit teaching activities. Do not attempt to make every case "psychiatric" and do not monopolize the staff's attention. Teaching on rounds is most effective when the consultant responds directly to the staff's questions about a particular patient, and when he interjects his comments only occasionally. Discussing the obvious psychopathology or a particular management problem of only one or two patients on any given day is probably the maximum teaching that can be achieved. Although this may not seem to be much on one occasion, when it is done over a number of months, the consultant will find that he has actually imparted a great deal of knowledge to the staff.

15 CONSULTATIONS WITH SURGERY

Against the perils of surgery the patient will either defend himself or react.

Beaton (1965)

Although the consultation principles and practices that have been presented are generally applicable to most inpatient situations, the consultant's work with surgeons and surgical patients has some special features.

First, a surprisingly high incidence of mental illness, predominantly psychoneurotic or characterologic, has been found in surgical patients (Titchener, 1956); some form of important psychiatric disorder was present in 86 percent of 200 patients. In another study, about 10 percent of those admitted to a surgical service were seeking relief for psychological problems as the primary reason for surgery (Zwerling et al., 1955). A report of the National Committee against Mental Illness (1964) revealed that one out of every ten surgical patients was suffering from definitive mental illness. Thus, a surgical service should be a fertile source of referrals for the consultant; his efforts with these patients should be gratifying because he is working at a critical juncture with those who have definite and often serious afflictions.

Second, some patients are addicted to surgery, while others procrastinate, delaying needed surgery until their chances for recovery are jeopardized. This delay is a serious problem. Wahl and Golden (1966) report that about 43 percent of the patients they studied delayed surgery until their disease processes were severely advanced. Ignorance about symptomatology was not an important cause of this pathological delay; it accounted for only 5 percent. The significant psychological reasons for delay were fear of punishment, fear of death, and suicidal wishes. On

96

this same subject, Titchener and Levine (1960) state: "Delayers feared illness and the need for treatment too much; delayers feared something else more than the consequences of sickness; or delayers were too proud." Because these patients delay surgery, or even seeking medical assistance of any sort, the consultant must attempt to ameliorate the psychologic consequences of delay. Further, when these patients are in the hospital, consultation may be sought because manifestations of their psychopathology, other than delay, appear preoperatively and postoperatively. And of course, the consultant will have to deal with some of these patients because they will remain severely ill inasmuch as needed surgery could not be performed in time.

Third, both the working situation and the atmosphere on surgical inpatient units differ from those present on medical or pediatric wards. The surgeon spends much of his time in the operating room; thus, the consultant has less opportunity to develop a close relationship with him. The consultant usually finds that he spends a greater part of his time with the nurses than with the surgical staff who are on the unit only when making ward rounds or when a patient's critical condition necessitates their presence.

Fourth, the surgeon-patient relationship has its own unique characteristics. The surgeon's interest is focused on the operation; he is generally less involved with long-term patient care and total management than his medical colleagues. Also, the operation is usually the patient's chief concern. Consequently, the surgeon, more than other physicians, is dependent upon the consultant for instituting comprehensive care.

POLYSURGERY

The problem of the polysurgical patient, who not only submits to, but even seeks repeated operative procedures, is challenging. These patients are interesting; they display many of the fundaments of psychiatric theory. In working with them, the power of the unconscious, rich fantasies, and vivid symbolization emerge with striking clarity. Moreover, one must deal with the surgery, the decisive action, as well as the more ordinary worries and events of the neurotic's life. Only suicide approximates polysurgery as an event in which the unconscious determinants and the action are so overtly joined. But, when a patient commits suicide, the psychiatrist's further work is limited; he can only speculate about the causes. With the polysurgical patient, however, the psychiatrist has an opportunity for continued therapy, albeit difficult, as well as study.

In a definitive discussion of polysurgical addiction, Menninger (1934) states: "Frequently the neurotic patient forces himself upon the surgeon, demanding the operation either verbally, or as is more often the case, demanding it in some physiological way." Menninger distinguishes between the gains for these patients: the *primary* or paranosic gain (relief of anxiety) and the *secondary* or epinosic gain (solicitude of friends, relatives, and staff; dependency and so on). The polysurgical patient is dominated by the repetition-compulsion. Menninger emphasizes the patient's unconscious motives for polysurgery: 1) To avoid facing something else which he fears more. In some cases, the surgical procedure is the lesser of two evils; for example, surgery to postpone a wedding. Or, in others, surgery may be sacrificial, providing a focus which staves off psychosis. 2) To obtain a transference relationship with a father figure. The underlying dynamic is that the patient seeks a "father" and, to accept this relationship, he must receive pain. 3) To fulfill an ungratified wish for a child. This is particularly true of cases in which either the patient or her mother has had a Caesarean section. 4) To be symbolically castrated. Menninger reinterprets this symbolism more specifically as "the wish to be relieved of anxiety by submitting to castration." The symbolic castration (any surgery) fulfills the wish to avoid death, and may be conceptualized as *saving the whole by sacrificing a part*.

In his analysis of the psychological motivation which prompts patients to seek surgery, Hollender (1958) says that it is a price some patients feel they must pay to obtain gratification. This is dramatically illustrated by a case in our recent experience. An intelligent married woman in her late twenties could enjoy sexual relations only during the first few postoperative weeks when her wounds were still healing and the scars were fresh; she had had 18 "surgeries" in seven years. Also, the surgery is an atonement which aids in relieving guilt. Some of these patients punish themselves with accidents or illnesses and then turn to surgeons, asking them to inflict the further punishment which is unconsciously demanded by a harsh superego.

Other patients seek surgery in the hope that it will uncover evidence of structural disease which will justify their symptoms, thus allowing them to maintain their neuroses, their warped attitudes, and their distorted interpersonal situations. Surgery also expunges the guilt springing from hostility toward others.

Wahl and Golden (1966) emphasize that surgery gives the patient permission to regress, that guilt is assuaged by the shedding of blood, and that the surgery fulfills a primary process need for symbolic sexual gratification. They note that in seeking surgery the patient handles unresolved fears of death by a counterphobic mechanism; the polysurgery enables the patient to demonstrate to himself repeatedly that he has "mastered death." They describe the typical patient as a woman who is unhappy and lonely, and who has a long history of sexual unresponsiveness. As a child, she was deprived of affection and, instead, the parental relationship was characterized by sadistic and seductive qualities. While in the hospital, the patient has a strong need for attention. She derogates the efforts of previous physicians. Finally, after many operations, the resultant anatomical and physiological changes produce further problems which in turn necessitate continued medical care and surgery.

Titchener and Levine (1960) discuss clinical signs, other than the obvious scars of previous surgeries, which identify these patients. First, many polysurgical patients are depressed and apathetic prior to surgery; their depression is associated with somatic complaints. Hostility, bitterness in the patient's interpersonal relations, self-depreciation, and self-revulsion are indicative of "operation-suicide." Second, dramatization (bizarre behavior or casual indifference in the face of surgery) reflects the neurotic need for the operation. In our experience, many of these patients are hysterical. They display classical characteristics of hysteria: histrionics, seductiveness, rapid fluctuations from the "little girl" to the "strong woman," sophisticated manipulations of staff and relatives, and a dilettante's knowledge of medicine and surgery. Third, some of these patients have a persecutory ideation with strong masochistic and paranoid traits.

The number of polysurgical addicts is not known. Although the psychodynamics of polysurgery have been studied, there is little clinical research addressed to frequency, family determinants, symptoms, signs, and identification. We (Schwab et al., 1965) found that a group of 100 medical inpatients referred for psychiatric consultations had had a total of 226 surgical procedures; the nonconsultation control group had had 180. This difference between the two groups was not statistically significant. However, significant differences came to light when only intra-abdominal and genitourinary procedures were counted. This study points out that the frequency of intra-abdominal and genitourinary surgery is a better index of neurosis than the total number of procedures. More work is necessary to obtain diagnostic profiles which can be used to detect these patients before polysurgery becomes an obvious way of life.

Wahl and Golden (1966) recommend: "In almost all cases it is valuable and appropriate for the surgeon to obtain a psychiatric consultation [for these patients]." Working with polysurgical patients is a formidable task for the consultant, particularly after they have had very many surgical procedures. Long-term psychotherapy, as well as continued medical management, is necessary for these cases. Excellent communication between the psychotherapist and the patient's personal physician is essential. The surgical procedures will have produced structural and physiologic changes which give rise to symptoms that need medical treatment and which the patient can use as massive resistance to therapy.

THE MEANING OF SURGERY

Many patients come to surgery presenting an outward appearance of equanimity. This is evidence of the courage and faith of the human being and is quiet testimony of the confidence the patient places in the medical profession. However, there is almost always some degree of apprehension; the patient knows that he is placing his life in the hands of another individual.

A cloud of fantasy surrounds the idea of surgery. Although most of the fantasies are unconscious, they include common, even normal, ideas such as: "They will hurt me and I can't endure it. What if the anesthetic won't work? I will crack up and go crazy under the pain and never get back to normal." Or, "Perhaps under the anesthetic I will reveal secrets that I couldn't bear to have known." Some fantasies which represent neurotic solutions to problems are: "I insist upon this operation to solve all my problems. The operation will bring me attention and sympathy. The operation will vindicate me and show me that I am not neurotic." In addition, many people seeking gynecologic or genitourinary surgery feel that the operation will alter their sexual roles in life (Hollender, 1958).

The surgical patient is *submitting* to a procedure. He must cope with his feelings of helplessness. He may feel gratified in his sense of helplessness and experience guilt because of this sense of gratification or because of his abandonment of responsibility (Meyer, 1958). Guilt may pervasively color his attitudes toward surgery so that he conceives of the operation as punishment.

Further, his body image is jeopardized. Anxiety about diagnosis, prognosis, and loss of function are always present. In addition, there are terrors related to anesthesia: of death, of complete helplessness, and of the "unknown sleep."

CONSULTATIONS

The surgeon's request for consultation poses questions related to immediate psychiatric problems: the advisability of surgery in view of existing mental illness, the need for assistance in obtaining the patient's cooperation for a required procedure, or the management of a discrete preoperative or postoperative difficulty. The patient who refuses surgery or the one who speaks openly about premonitions of death is almost always referred for psychiatric consultation. The surgeon expects the consultant to convince the refusing patient to cooperate so that the operation need not be postponed. But for the one who believes he will not survive, the surgeon gladly defers the operation until the consultant has sufficient time to evaluate and help the patient.

When a patient has any emotional illness, the decision to proceed with surgery must be a judicious one. Psychiatric consultation can estimate the emotional consequences of surgery, although it does not eliminate all risk.

Beaton (1965) notes that the obsessive-compulsive usually handles surgery more comfortably than the anxiety reactor, and that the hysteric will temporarily abandon his conversion symptomatology before surgery, only to resume it later. Persons with character disorders present problems during convalescence; they lack needed self-discipline and suffer from poor impulse control. The schizophrenic may go into complete remission after serious injury, only to have the psychosis reemerge with recovery. Severe depression and extreme hypochondriasis are contraindications to elective procedures. In any clear-cut case of emotional illness, planning for postoperatvie psychiatric care is essential.

In all cases, patients' attitudes toward, and expectations of, surgery must be brought to light by the consultant. Every consultant should read Titchener and Levine's book, *Surgery as a Human Experience* (1960), which presents a comprehensive view of the meaning of surgery to patients.

PREOPERATIVE CONDITIONS

The range of problems confronting the surgeon preoperatively covers the spectrum of psychological disorders, but anxiety, denial, and depression are the most common. Surgeons recognize anxiety and are accustomed to handling it when the operative procedure is the focus; they deal with moderate or severe anxiety states without becoming excessively involved with the patient. Routinely, the surgeon uses an authoritative, supportive approach to the highly anxious patient, assuring him that professional skills, facilities, and statistics are in his favor. Sometimes, he even reschedules surgery, moving the severely anxious patient ahead of others, thus reducing time for the build-up of anxiety. Anxiety arising from basic psychopathology and not specifically related to the operative procedure is more serious and, when detected, is an indication for psychiatric consultation.

Janis' work (1958) is important: Patients with no overt preoperative anxiety tended to have more serious postoperative reactions than those with moderate or severe forms of anxiety before surgery. However, those with severe, disorganizing anxiety are poor surgical risks.

Extreme denial is another danger sign. It is prima facie evidence that the patient is not considering the consequences of impending surgery. In these cases, the postoperative reaction is likely to be stormy, particularly when the patient finally has to come to grips with the effects of the surgery and accept the results.

Depression is probably the psychiatric syndrome most commonly missed by surgeons preoperatively. Also, it is predictive of serious psychiatric illness postoperatively, usually continued depression.

Beaton (1965) notes that against the perils of surgery the patient defends himself by three major defense patterns; denial, projection, and reaction formation. He says that denial is a primitive escape; projection is the unconscious placing of the patient's fears and guilts onto those who are caring for him (surgeon or staff); and reaction formation is a type of behavior, the opposite of which the patient would unconsciously like to express (for example, the excessively compliant, almost self-sacrificial patient is often exhibiting a reaction formation against his own hostility toward the staff; further, this patient may not report personal anguish when he should).

POSTOPERATIVE CONDITIONS

Postoperative problems fall into overlapping categories: those carried over, and those resulting from, the procedure. Awakening in an unfamiliar recovery room, surrounded by semianesthetized people is traumatic and may set the stage for psychosis. Refusing to acknowledge amputation, denying a colostomy, or ignoring other anatomical changes are psychological phenomena of consequence. In fact, they may be the first signs that the entire reality-testing system is strained.

Depression and delirium are the two most common postoperative conditions. The depression may be acute, a reaction to the surgical procedure, in which case it is usually self-limited; or, more often, it is a continuation of a long-standing condition which was not clearly recognized before. Postoperative depression has deleterious effects on convalescence: the patient recovers slowly, suffers more complications, and may be suicidal.

Depressive reactions occur as a result of the loss of bodily parts, removal of organs, and disfigurement. Depression represents mourning for the loss, and is also a reaction to exaggerated fears of rejection by, and separation from, those on whom the patient is dependent. Cancer patients tend to feel a sense of abandonment which may be reinforced by realistic factors in their environment. They need closeness, support, and continuity of contact with others.

Delirium, the acute brain syndrome, is a frequent complication of surgery. The effects of anesthesia, the procedure, disturbed physiologic functioning, and electrolyte imbalance may be superimposed on other etiologic factors such as circulatory impairment, infection, or preoperative addiction to alcohol or drugs.

The following case history illustrates a problem with postoperative delirium and describes how the consultant gives his assistance:

A 71-year-old white male was referred for psychiatric evaluation three days after eye surgery for a retinal detachment. The request stated that he was disoriented, hostile, and paranoid; provisional diagnosis was delirium, acute, postoperative. The consultee asked, "Please make recommendations for treatment."

THE CONSULTANT'S REPLY

The presenting problem is acute delirium in an elderly white male who had eye surgery three days ago. The patient admits that he was very confused last night "after he took his medicine"; he wandered around the room because he did not know where he was. He tells, somewhat angrily, that the nurses and doctors "ordered him around like a boy." His past medical history is uneventful, except for mild hypertension for 3–4 years. His personal history is stable; after many years as a steady, skilled worker he retired six years ago and now lives alone with his wife. Their marriage is happy, and although he worries about his blood pressure, he enjoys life and was active and busy until he had trouble with his eye last week. There is no evidence of mental illness, undue reactions to stress, or of psychopathology in his past history.

Physical examination—Reviewed. It should be emphasized to all staff members that this man has diminished vision in his unoperated eye.

Mental status: The patient is now rational and is oriented as to time, place, and person. He admits to disorientation last night and to anxiety about whether his operation will be successful. Except for the anxiety, his affect is now appropriate. His mood is one of concern but he is not depressed. He tells that last night he thought the shadows in the room were strange people. Memory, ability to calculate, intelligence, and ability to abstract are all within normal limits.

He has received excessive amounts of medication: 50 mg Sparine, 100 mg Nembutal; and 50 mg Thorazine at 2200 and again at 2400 hours last night.

Formulation: This elderly white male, who has always been in good health, became disoriented last night following the administration of excessive medication. The failure to recognize that he was almost blind in the unoperated eye and the lack of a structured environment produced black patch delirium.

Diagnosis: Acute brain syndrome, black patch delirium.

Suggest: 1. Improved doctor-patient and nurse-patient relationship by announcing who you are and what you plan to do. Be specific and concrete in approach.

2. Keep personnel contact down to minimum—let a few staff members get to know him well. Treat him with respect.

3. Show interest in the patient's condition. Make comments as to what room looks like—flowers, coloring, what the weather is like, and so on. Comment on the food and how it tastes and smells. Encourage use of other senses—hearing, touch. Keep patient ambulatory but aid him in walking about and finding chairs, bathroom, and hallway.

4. Talk about pleasant successful periods in his life, i.e., references to his hobbies and previous work.

5. Allow wife to stay with patient beyond visiting hours.

6. Keep light on at all times.

7. Have someone read newspaper aloud in morning and at night.

8. Avoid barbiturates; use Thorazine 50 mg q 6h. After 2 days, reduce medicine gradually.

9. Will follow with you. Recommend: Weisman, A. D. and Hackett, T. P., "Psychosis After Eye Surgery." New Eng. J. Med., 258:1284, 1958.

Paranoid reactions are sometimes expressed, particularly by the patient whose libido is heavily invested in his body image. He may focus hostile feelings on the surgeon, other staff members, and those upon whom he is dependent.

Other psychiatric problems result from the discovery of an unexpected malignancy, the necessity for further surgery, a disruption of body image, diminished self-esteem, and difficulties with sexual identification. In addition, there are practical problems concerned with convalescence, restoration of function, and the resumption of family and work activities.

GUIDELINES FOR THE CONSULTANT

1. Evaluate the meaning of surgery. Question the patient concerning expectations, fears, and guilt. Also, elicit fantasies.

2. Resolve fears about anesthesia. A joint conference between the psychiatrist, the anesthesiologist, and the patient is helpful. Explain that

the preoperative medication will make induction of the anesthetic a simple matter. Describe the recovery room in detail and emphasize that an experienced staff is in attendance.

3. Make recommendations for convalescent management. Intractable pain, persistent demands for narcotics, sleeplessness, and interpersonal difficulties are the most common problems. The consultant can deal with all of these. For example, he can advise that visitors or occupational therapy be substituted for narcotics.

4. In conclusion, all consultants should study Hackett and Weisman's excellent two-part paper (1960), "The Management of Operative Syndromes," which provides guidelines for managing specific psychiatric reactions to surgery.

. . . .

In looking back over his many years of experience, Ochsner (1950) deplores the premium placed on the surgeon's scientific skills at the expense of the art of medicine. He emphasizes the need for more psychiatric consultations preoperatively.

REFERENCES

BEATON, L. E. Psychiatric necessities in surgical education. Amer. J. Surg., 110:28, 1965.

HACKETT, T. P., and WEISMAN, A. D. Psychiatric management of operative syndromes. I., Psychosom. Med., 22:2671, 1960. II., Psychosom. Med., 22:356, 1960.

HOLLENDER, M. H. The Psychology of Medical Practice. Philadelphia, W. B. Saunders Co., 1958.

JANIS, I. R. Psychological Stress: Psychoanalytic and Behavioral Studies of Surgical Patients. New York, John Wiley & Sons, Inc., 1958.

MENNINGER, K. A. Polysurgery and polysurgical addiction, Psychoanal. Quart., 3:183, 1934.

MEYER, B. C. Some psychiatric aspects of surgical practice. Psychosom. Med., 20(3):203, 1958.

OCHSNER, A. The importance of psychiatry in surgery. Digest Neurol. Psychiat., 18:91, 1950.

SCHWAB, J. J., CLEMMONS, R. S., FREEMON, F. R., and SCOTT, M. L. Differential characteristics of medical inpatients referred for psychiatric consultation: A controlled study. Psychosom. Med., 27:112, 1965.

TITCHENER, J. L. Problems of delay in seeking surgical care. J.A.M.A., 160:1187, 1956.

——— LEVINE, M. Surgery as a Human Experience. New York, Oxford University Press, Inc., 1960.

WAHL, C. W., and Golden, J. S. The psychodynamics of the polysurgical patient: Report of 16 patients. Psychosom. Med., 7(2), 1966.

WEISMAN, A. D., and HACKETT, T. P. Psychosis after eye surgery. New Eng. J. Med., 258:1284, 1958.

What are the Facts About Mental Illness. Washington, The National Committee Against Mental Illness, Inc., 1, 1964.

ZWERLING, I., TITCHENER, et al. Personality disorder and the relationships of emotion to surgical illness in 200 surgical patients. Amer. J. Psychiat., 112:270, 1955.

SECTION FOUR The Pediatric Consultation

16 TECHNIQUES FOR PEDIATRIC CONSULTATION

by Paul L. Adams, M.D.

TWO METHODS OF CONSULTING

As a psychiatric consultant with pediatricians you may spend considerable time with either the pediatrician or the child patient. Traditionally professionals consulted by seeing patients and then communicating with the referring doctor. This casts the psychiatric consultant into the role of assisting his pediatrician-colleague through a primary orientation toward making a psychiatric diagnosis of pediatric patients, and toward making management suggestions. That is a convenient as well as conventional mode of functioning; for beginners in consultation work it is probably the preferred way. Some pediatricians initially will be puzzled at the new way. So it is better to plan to do the traditional way well; then you can add to it as you improve in skillfulness, and you can carry the more sophisticated pediatricians along with you into new paths.

This traditional pattern of consulting has given way in many settings to the consultation conducted primarily, or solely, with the consultee. This latter consultation mechanism places emphasis on doctor-doctor relations, for the child patient may not even be seen by the psychiatrist. In general medicine this consultation method is new, but not in the specialty of child psychiatry. Child psychiatrists originated teamwork before medical teams and health teams were popular devices; they worked in welfare, health, and education agencies before community consultation became widely adopted. Child psychiatrists long have valued their desire to "work with and through others."

This chapter is concerned with the consultant's relations with pediatricians and with children, and how you can interact artfully and fruitfully with these two groups. It will present suggestions on seeing child patients and on seeing pediatricians, the two modes of consulting. We will deal first with your relations with the pediatrician—the new consultation focus—and then will take up your role with the child directly.

As a psychiatric consultant you will function, as you relate to the pediatrician-consultee, in three challenging roles: collaborator, educator, and supportive resource or helper.

Also, by working with the child patient directly, you will serve in two roles that are among the most exciting and rewarding given to the physician to play: diagnostician and healer or helper.

The most fruitful techniques for dealing with child and pediatrician will concern us. It is wise to know what you are doing in a child psychiatric consultation; and, knowing that, it will become an easier task to explain the meaning of your behavior to the pediatric consultee and to the pediatric patient. Being aware of your roles is a precondition for effectively consulting on a pediatric service.

TECHNIQUES WITH CONSULTEES

LEARN THE WARD STRUCTURE OR SETTING

Since the behavior of a hospitalized child, and likewise the behavior of a pediatrician who is requesting a psychiatric consultation, occurs in a pediatric ward setting, it behooves the resident who answers the call for a psychiatric consultation to get to know the ward structure. This is even a joyous task if your hospital has a medical sociologist or similar behavioral scientist who has studied the pediatric ward and who will brief you about the kinds of human-relations processes operative on the ward.

Does the ward look informal and child-oriented or is there a sterile atmosphere of drab uniformity? Are there signs of humane caring for children? Are there more signs that children must adjust to hospital than there are indications that the hospital exists to serve sick children and their families? Is rooming-in a physical possibility? Or are children largely severed from the tie to family when they enter the pediatric ward? Are there near each child's bed a toy gun and a doll family, or are toys lacking, or centralized in location?

Finding out these things will assist your comprehension of the reality, for the child and his family, of hospitalization here. Unfortunately, this reality is sometimes harsh. Is the turnover of nurses rapid or slow? What do nurses do on the ward? Do the nurses wear uniforms or individually selected clothing? Are they nurses, even the word derives from something hinting at a mothering function, or are they solely administrators, planners, and organizers? Are there among the aides and practical nurses some motherly types who possess intuition about child care? Are the parents of the child patients really welcomed, or held at bay by the ward personnel? What are the policies concerning visitors?

Who on the ward is the manager, the apparent boss, the real boss? Is there a competent chief resident who might regard children's emotional conflicts as of interest? Who writes the orders? Does the attending staff operate with a light or heavy hand? Do the residents, interns, and medical students have any unscheduled time during which you can meet with them for a living consultation? The foregoing are some things to know about the ward setting if you are to consult knowingly on pediatrics.

BE A COLLABORATOR WITH PEDIATRICIANS

You are a fellow physician whose judgements and opinions are called for. You are not in a superrole as the psychiatric consultant. You are not an evangelist bringing a messianic gospel (often in incomprehensible jargon) to pediatricians. You are a psychiatric consultant. You are only different and valuable because of your specialized perspectives and skills, not "super." You are another cobbler with a different kind of last. You stand within a long tradition of close cooperation between pediatricians and child psychiatrists. These two specialists are different nowadays but zones of overlap do exist. Both are concerned with the well-being of children. Moreover, child psychiatry residents and pediatric residents can learn many things from each other, in a collaboration that can be mutually enriching and gratifying.

There are many sound ways of looking at pediatrics as a medical speciality, but as psychiatrists we can select the following way of viewing the field: Pediatricians are divided (at least for our consultation purposes) into 1) those who insist that a pediatrician is himself a superspecialist consultant and 2) those who see themselves as comprehensive caretakers of children in sickness and especially in health. The adherents to the "superspecialist" view usually prefer to locate themselves in a regional center, perhaps a university medical school, where they can put down even stronger and more specialized roots in the basic biomedical sciences. These are the pediatric neurologists, pathologists, psychiatrists, hematologists, and so on. Contrariwise, proponents of the comprehensive view may prefer to engage in the practice of clinical pediatrics or to engage themselves heavily in clinical teaching and clinical research. Incidentally, excellent service, teaching and research come from both camps. Neither has an edge on the excellent market. Also, congeniality to psychiatry and psychiatric sophistication are to be found in both superspecialists and comprehensivists. Their differences are mainly in their views of how their field should develop, and also lie in their distinct professional self-concepts. It is well to know which kind of consultee you are to collaborate with. They will ask different things of you, hold different expectations, and have different styles that may seem inexplicable until you have them "pegged." At times it is easier to serve as a hit-and-run consultant with the superspecialist, for the comprehensive pediatrician may expect to ask more questions, answer more questions, and engage in more give-and-take collaborative work. Almost invariably the superspecialist will want to let you deal with the emotional problems. He may want to divide the labor and let you alone, which is better than adverse intrusion. But the comprehensive pediatrician is more likely to team up with you on ongoing case management.

Equally as important as pegging or typing the pediatrician is identifying the person or persons who really initiated the consultation request. The person who signed the consultation request is often no more than the apparent consultee; the real consultee is the man to see. The real consultee is the pediatrician who wants to talk with you to see what you observe, elicit, and deduce. He has not impersonally fired off a request for your consultation; he desires genuine communication. Only with him can you as a psychiatrist overcome the barriers of bureaucracy, specialization, and dehumanization that seem characteristic of more and more hospital settings. Only with the real consultee can you work together to help the real child. At times the fullest communication should occur with a pediatric nurse, not with one of the physicians, if it is the nurse who is most eager to get your opinions about helping the child who is hospitalized.

Once you have found the person who asked for consultation, proceed to communicate amply, not stingily. Promptness and clarity of feedback are virtues to be possessed by the psychiatrist who consults with pediatricians. Often this informative feedback can be given most effectively by having the pediatrician-consultee present when you interview the patient. In this way, he is prepared to understand how you work: how you collect evidence, how you evaluate it, and finally how you transmit it to a medical colleague. Some of your techniques can be adopted by the collaborative pediatrician. If he tries doing an interview your way, you can be fairly certain that he has developed some confidence in your manner of operating, and has been in a genuine collaborative relationship with you. If you have taught him some psychiatric skills your relationship of collaboration has shaded over naturally into an educational relationship. This will be considered in the next section.

This is a summary of your role as a collaborator with pediatricians:
1. Offer and expect respect and cooperativeness.
2. Determine if the consultee is comprehensive or superspecialist, or mixed.
3. Ascertain exactly who wanted the psychiatric consultation.
4. Give full confidential feedback.

APPROACH CONSULTATION IN YOUR ROLE AS AN EDUCATOR

Ideally, each consultation involves teaching and learning on the part of the consultant and consultee.

The knowledge that you can teach falls into the fields of sociology, anthropology, social work, and psychology, as well as psychiatry. Psychiatry is so infused with the science and arts of human behavior, fields often unfamiliar to pediatricians, that a psychiatric consultant can teach much concerning human development, especially biosocial and psychosocial development. This is information broader than child psychiatry alone, but which is known to child psychiatrists, and it is information that pediatricians still do not hold uniformly as a result of their medical and speciality training. When the psychiatrist transmits a crosscultural perspective on child-rearing practices, symptom formation, psychopathology, definitions of illness, and patterns of sick-child care, he is furnishing some pertinent anthropology for the liberal education of his pediatrician-colleague. When you talk about race, class, status, and reference-groups as these affect children, or about demographic considerations of family size, life expectancy, broken homes, male-female ratios, and so on, you are teaching some basic sociology that may be novel but illuminating to the pediatrician-consultee. When you teach the skills of home visitation, interviewing, hearing and advising parents, or when you stress the balance of assets and liabilities in the family, or tell the consultee of nonmedical community resources from which children and families can obtain help, you are teaching some fundamentals of the child psychiatrist's co-field of social work. Usually these social work affairs are little known by pediatricians. Again, when as a psychiatrist you teach about the testing of intelligence, or of projective testing, or of testing for brain damage or sociopathic trends or psychosis, you impart one very fundamental aspect of that other traditional co-field, clinical child psychology, a profession rarely familiar to pediatricians.

As a psychiatric consultant you are indeed an educator: a teacher of interviewing techniques, of doctor-family relationships, of the principles of psychophysiology and psychopathology, of anticipatory guidance or prevention, of individual differences, of psychotherapy, and of diagnostic assessment in order to select children who are likely to be treatable by pediatricians. Child psychiatrists often seek to work through others. This educational process in conjunction with pediatricians leads you, the psychiatrist, to be clearer, to explain esoteric terminology or even to shun its usage, and in the process to become a more effective teacher and practitioner of your own psychiatric speciality. As an effective educator and consultant you will do a lot to "sell" child psychiatry as represented through you. Selling is hardly called for, and it is certainly not your most important objective, but it would be foolish to tell you that it is not pleasurable.

All does not go smoothly for an educator-consultant. At times you will feel abused, maligned, spurned, and rejected. At times you will be aghast at how unready the pediatrician-consultee is for meaningful dialogue. At such times, discretion, and even curbing your expressions of scorn, would be wise policies to adopt. If, however, the situation is clearly one of inadequate social, affective, and behavioral data collected by the would-be consultee, then offer to return when investigations acquire such data. Frustration is compounded if you are reduced to guesswork and aimless speculation. As Huxley said, an assertion that goes beyond the evidence is more than a blunder; it is a crime. You will be a happier and better educator if you suggest the kinds of additional data that are needed, let the consultee gather these, and then return to consult with him.

There are many to educate: yourself, the consultee-physicians, the medical students, the nurses, the aides, and others. There are many things to teach: human personality development, knowledge and viewpoints from sociology, anthropology, social work, and clinical child psychology and psychiatry, the meaning of illness and hospitalization to child and family, physician-family relationships, how to refer, interview, diagnose, treat and prevent, psychophysiology, psychopharmacology, psychopathology, and psychodynamics, team work, the history of pediatric psychiatry, and more.

HELP AND SUPPORT THE PEDIATRICIAN

Several quasi-therapeutic activities initiated by you can be made available to the pediatrician. Some of these include: 1) Identify his problem clearly. 2) Respect his call for psychiatric help. 3) Probe with kindness his relation to the child patient. 4) Probe transference and countertransference as they operate in the doctor-child/family relationship. 5) Advise him about resources to assist children and families. 6) When appropriate, take over the patient for psychiatric care.

Begin by finding out what the pediatrician's problem is. As psychiatrists we have to understand that people (we, parents of young children, medical and surgical patients, and pediatricians who make consultation requests) ask for help under a variety of circumstances. People—even pediatricians—call for help notoriously when they experience an intolerable burden of pain, anxiety, and loneliness. They call for help when they cannot do it alone. Courageous people call for help more often than do lazy, dependent, or parasitical people. We must let pediatricians garner our support and help, and not be withholding toward them. It is our role to find out the nature of the pediatrician's problem before deciding whether we can be of use to him.

Is he operating only under a compulsion to be thorough? or to round out the hospital chart? You can tell if his consultation request is the genuine article when it seems well-planned, sensible, and justifiable. You can tell if something sticky is going on if he requests the consultation only on the day of discharge, or when the child is literally on the way out of the hospital. Those afterthought consultations are often pointless, and are better omitted if your supervisor will condone your acting in this hardheaded fashion. Sometimes however, the welfare of the patient, if not the welfare of the doctors, is served even when you do an on-the-way-out-the-door consultation. Better late than never.

Is the pediatrician frustrated, feeling helpless and angry because x rays and multiple laboratory tests turned up "nothing rewarding"? That is, nothing that he likes or values? Does he say, "Everything was noncontributory" or "All the findings were negative"? Note that the very terminology connotes a snarl.

Has he seen *the patient*, or has he seen a unique human child who dwells in an interpersonal and symbolic setting? Has he weighed the evidence and come forth with a positive diagnosis of interpersonal and intrapsychic problems? Or is his diagnosis a diagnosis of exclusion, scraped from the bottom of the barrel? A psychiatric diagnosis, even tentatively enunciated by a pediatrician, when it is a diagnosis derived from positive evidence, is like paradise for the consulting psychiatrist.

Is the pediatrician-consultee, following an involved circuit of denial, avoidance, and mounting contempt for the child's problems, trying to ditch the child patient by seeking a psychiatric takeover? Is the assumption of major responsibility by the psychiatrist a warranted turn of events? What inappropriate trends would your takeover tend to reinforce in the pediatrician's conduct as a professional helper of children and families? If he will not squirm too much, you will do psychiatry and pediatrics a good turn by remaining the pediatrician's consultant and helper, not a receptacle for his rejects.

It is a good policy to insist that, even when you take his patient, he agree to keep on providing overall health care for the child. Children are not lucky enough to possess emotional troubles in pure culture isolated and protected from infections and metabolic diseases. Hence, in civilized society, children with emotional conflicts also require ongoing pediatric care.

You can help the pediatrician inestimably as a doctor of children by being so "spooky" as to talk about transference and countertransference that have arisen in his relation with his patients and their parents. Some interrogative ways by which you can sneak into this are now presented. Ask the pediatrician: How does the child feel about doctors? What does he say about the last doctor he saw before seeing you? Does he regard you as being different from other doctors? From other adults? And you, do you like this child? Does he remind you of anyone else you have known? Do you have the feeling that you can be his pediatrician without too many rubs? What do you expect of this Negro child and family (or slum child, or Jewish, or gentile, or tenant farmer, or low-class, or spoiled rich, or female)? What attitudes do you automatically bring, pro and anti, for the people whom you include in your positive and negative reference groups?

If the pediatrician can swallow all this questioning, he will probably be more willing than the average psychiatric resident to talk honestly and openly of transference and countertransference! If he can take the psychiatric exploration of his and the child's distortions, he will be helped by you in a way that borders on experiencing psychotherapy. It is psychotherapy, precisely in a sector of high relevance professionally for the pediatrician-consultee.

Still another way in which you can be helper and supporter of the pediatrician is to help him find appropriate help for the child. This requires you to know community resources: voluntary and professional child care agencies, both medical and nonmedical. From your close association with social workers you sometimes know better than the pediatrician how to locate these child care agencies: welfare departments, special education people, family service agencies, crippled children agencies, child guidance clinics, and so on. Sharing what you have learned can support and help the pediatrician-consultee in his desire to find nonhospital helpers for his child patient. Share with the pediatrician your knowledge of community resources, and propound to him the diversities of the helping mechanism throughout the surrounding community. Show him especially your tactics for beating the waiting list in community child guidance clinics, your stratagems for circumventing their delaying tactics. Where the community clinics are genuinely serviceable, you can explain to him that there is a manpower shortage in all of the professions pertaining to child psychiatry. All of this will help to allay the pediatrician's anxiety, doubt, shame, guilt, anger, and depression; at least at the level of awareness and reality.

The point remains that at times you can help both consultee and patient if you and the consultee decide that you should take the child over as your psychiatric patient. Indeed, a felicitous outcome often results, as you might be the ideal helping resource for the child, family, and pediatrician. Some consultation techniques for working directly with children will be discussed in the section immediately following.

TECHNIQUES WITH CHILDREN

As you see the child patient in consultation you should be aware of: 1) the doctor-patient relationship; in pediatric work this is very often the doctor-child/parent relationship, 2) your role as a diagnostician or identifier of problems, and 3) your role as a helper or healer. For these three aspects of you-in-action, here are some practical considerations of tactics, strategies, and gimmicks.

HAVE A PSYCHIATRIST'S IDENTITY

Declare who you are and what you are doing. Don't play "secret agent," pretending you are just "another doctor that will talk with you a bit." The child deserves to know, and his parents in particular have a right to know, that a psychiatric exploration is the natural next step in the pediatrician's efforts to help. Let everyone know that you are representing psychiatry here.

I have an aversion to psychiatric residents playing "double agent" also. Double agent is a game that evolves from secret agent. Double agent is played in two ways: 1) The psychiatrist poses as someone who does the same things as, and is a mere extension of, pediatrics; while obviously, if he is any good, he is also a loyal agent for psychiatry. Pediatricians themselves, incidentally, often prefer "the outright spook" approach to "the warmed-over pediatric" approach. Better a psychiatrist's identity all the way than a halfhearted double agent's duality. 2) The psychiatric consultant passes confidences back and forth between the child and the child's parents. This is often justified in the name of "confrontation" or of getting to the heart of the matter. The psychiatric heart of the matter is something that ordinarily one is not privileged to know fully in the first hour or two. It takes more time than a blitzkrieg, and is usually calmer than a stampede. A consultation that is totally unlike your treatment procedures is a poor example of psychiatric being-of-assistance. A rule of thumb might be: Consult in keeping with your therapy style. The stampede is neither a model of technique nor is it a goal of psychiatry. For this reason, some mellowness and restraint are indicated when you see the child and his parents. If haste is called for, it might be better to rush in with a competent psychiatric caseworker at your side. The caseworker is expert in working with parents, so also are fellow residents in child psychiatry. A good two-man team is infinitely superior, in child consultation, to a bumbling double agent confronting parents and child, and betraying confidences on both sides.

Tell the child, initially and often, "I am a psychiatrist and something I want to know is . . ." Ask the child what he thinks about you, about your talk, about your being a psychiatrist and so on. This is a little like dirty pool and certainly will not endear you to pediatricians, but occasionally it is well to say, "I will not give you any shots or draw any blood," leaving unstated that you are in some ways a nicer guy than other physicians whom the child has encountered! Explain to him that you try to help out when a child is unhappy, bothered, lonely, worried, scared, can't learn, and has problems. Tell the child in suitable words that your job as a psychiatrist is: to help the child be happier now and grow up to become a good parent when that time comes; to identify his life-problems and have hope within limits that these problems can be solved; to view his troubles (symptoms) as meaning a lot of things to him and his parents that he, you, and they do not yet understand; to have the child come to understand, accept, and enjoy his self-concept, his body, and his dealings with others; to bring into awareness his affects, attitudes, overt behavior; to look closely at fantasies and symbols (dreams, play, early memories, and other waking fantasies are all grist for this mill). This is a big order to achieve and to get across to a child. Nonetheless, it is what child psychiatry does. It is easier to do if you have firmly enlisted the child's cooperation. An explanation of what you are up to has its place in consulting.

INTERVIEW SKILLFULLY IN ORDER TO DIAGNOSE AND TO UNDERSTAND FULLY

Your personal style is important in interviewing children who are hospitalized on a pediatric ward. Your imaginativeness, your intuition, and your spontaneous naturalness will be your greatest assets. If you can content yourself with being just yourself—not a peer, not a parent, but a psychiatrist—you will "be given what to say and do" as the moment occurs. Skills in interviewing can be taught and learned, but too often they boil down only to ways of eliciting content. Hence, the flavor of each consultants practical interviewing skills is highly idiosyncratic. Interview skill is more something evoked than something imposed in an ideal training program. For a psychiatrist the flavor deserves careful study, experimentation, and self-awareness. All of these should be done under continuing supervision, by a teaching psychiatrist, not from reading a prescription such as the present one. However, let us again resort to some guidelines.

Whether you see the child on the pediatrics ward or in a child psychiatry room matters a lot, as does the child's age. So in our prescription (that must be individualized by you) we are thinking of an eight-year-old child whom you are seeing in a room equipped suitably for child psychiatry sessions. At times you may work as a psychiatric consultant in a place designated by pediatricians or even your supervisors. For whatever reasons (but usually relating to shortages of psychiatric space), you may have to interview children at their bedside. Some of what follows might be useful after it is adapted for such on-the-ward consultation interviews. You might ask if the radiologist has to consult at the bedside. If he does, then you can too, of course.

Our guidelines for interviewing the child will include these topics in the order given: 1) Needed equipment, 2) How to get the interview on the road, 3) How to focus on meaningful symptoms, 4) How to confront discrepant histories, 5) How to find out what the child thinks about your psychiatric consultation, 6) How to show that you help families, 7) How to take a history from a child, 8) How to diagnose, 9) How to go after fantasies, and 10) How to organize your consultation report.

1. Certain basic supplies are needed. I prefer a simply equipped room with a table and two low chairs that are easily movable, and within handy reach a gun, a doll family, pencils and paper. The gun is used as an instrument for playing out violence and hostility, the doll family for both hostility and tenderness, and the pencils and paper for drawings. One other piece of equipment that can be useful is a bounceable soft-rubber ball, for this is occasionally the only vehicle for give-and-take between you and the child. A dollhouse (the toilet in it need not actually flush), sandbox, source of water, finger-painting supplies, clay, and many other play media may be utilized, but don't attribute your success or failure to these paraphernalia. The psychotherapeutic and psychodiagnostic encounter is between persons, not things.

Do you need a stethoscope, otoscope, or sphygmomanometer in your basic equipment? Alas, comments on this question lead into impassioned territory where religion, politics, dogmatism, and spleen hold sway. So be careful to learn your supervisor's opinions. You are indeed a physician, and having a medical identity you should be able to carry out a physical examination on children as needed. Always appealing to pediatricians for the necessary physical examinations (especially neurologic or pre-camp) on child patients is cumbersome, nonfunctional, ritualistic, and even silly in child psychiatry general practice. Perhaps, though, if you are a resident doing psychiatric consultations, it would be equally silly, ritualistic, and so on, for you to insist on doing physical examinations routinely. On a consultation service you can make better use of your time if you stick primarily to being a "talking doctor." A good rule of thumb is to look within and inquire, "Am I doing this for the child or for me?" Then try to do what will be best for the child.

2. When the child enters your properly equipped consultation room, you could say, "See what you can find in here that interests you" or "Maybe you'd like to look at some of the toys that are here." This can serve as a springboard to talking about his solitary play; his play with adults, if any, and play with his age-mates.

All the while you are a behavioral observer and through your awareness there are silent questions or hypotheses concerning this child. What is it like to see the world from inside his skin? What does his reticence mean? Why is he fearful, or disinterested, or driven, in appearance? Why does he compulsively touch everything in the room? Why does he ignore me, or seem overly conscious of my approval and disapproval?

If as a psychiatrist you can understand the child through his play, you may not need to talk with him or question him. Even so, with an eight-year-old child, some encouragement of verbal communication is desirable. There is evidence that reality-oriented talk is of value during psychotherapy. Nor is it difficult to stimulate, ordinarily.

3. Elicit the child's story of his troubles. "I am a psychiatrist. I want to help you. What sort of troubles of yours do I need to hear about?" If he pleads ignorance, or says that he has no problems, tell him why children come to psychiatrists, including some of the problems described for you by the pediatrician-consultee. "Children see psychiatrists because they have problems, worries, things that bother them, things that make them unhappy in some way." If he still disclaims having problems: "It is hard to talk to a strange doctor about some of these things. Perhaps it will be easier after a bit. Why did you come into the hospital? What hurt? What is the problem?" You know how the parents and the pediatrician perceive the child's problems. It is impossible that he has no troubles; you know that. Therefore, you might say, "Somebody is worried about your schoolwork (or asthma or stealing or nightmares or bedwetting). Who worries about that?" This ordinarily prompts a child to tell you some things that bother the parents but do not bother him and vice versa.

His problem as he sees it may be a fear of failure; as his parents see it, his problem may be stealing. He may feel accursed by loneliness, while his parents feel accursed by his soiling. Whereas the parents complain of her poor school achievement, she may complain of obesity and its attendant shame. The thing is: Identify the child's meaningful symptoms. Address your interview to "where the child lives" and not to the topics that from hearsay might have seemed intriguing to you. Where he lives is where psychiatry begins to help a child; or it is of no help. Where he lives there are urges, cravings, misunderstandings, perfect understanding, spontaneity, constriction, pain, distorted body image, anxiety, and loneliness. Your job is to learn where he lives and to know his world.

4. Let the child know that you know what the discrepant parental complaints are. Do it simply, not accusingly. A confrontation is not a legal allegation. Encourage him to "talk this over" or "straighten this out" with his parents. Much improved communication within families has resulted from just such easily dispensed advice to child patients. It is helping advice that can be given in the first consultation hour that you spend with a child.

5. Find out, but try not to be a repetitive bore about it, why the child is "coming to see me, a psychiatrist." This often entails finding out what the parents or the pediatrician or both told the child about the psychiatric consultation. Find it out if you can from the child. This will give you a picture of how well and in what terms the child reports what is explained to him by his parents. It will, moreover, provide you with a clue about child-parent interaction, that is a clue to some basic psychiatric data.

6. Explain to the child that your job is to help families. Early in the game tell him that he, and his parents too, have problems, and that your job is to help the whole family with their problems. Since your role in its broad conception is that of professional family-helper, encourage the child to ask his parents about the problems, the things for which the family members are seeking help. One dramatic way to implement your role with the whole family is to hold family group sessions during which problems and their possible solutions can be identified. Sometimes this group approach can be conducted only awkwardly on a pediatrics ward. Also, at times, it lets the resident dodge intimate and confidential talk with a young child. This is a pity, so the learner in child psychiatry might more safely aim to see child and parents separately. Family group evaluations seem to be done best by real "pro's" in individual assessment and interviewing.

A child is never too young to learn that his parents need help. I advocate, but check this with your supervisor, selectively telling the child of some of the parents' problems, while reassuring him that you will not squeal to the parents on what he says. This admittedly dual standard works well for many psychiatrists: Parents can be quoted to the child, but children are never quoted to their parents. It is a sensible way to preserve confidentiality and trust with the child patient, and to enhance the helping process within the entire family.

7. Let the child be your historical informant. All of your accomplishments in medical history-taking are of relevance and utility in child psychiatry. Now you are adding on skills, but hopefully you are not losing any. Chief complaint and its meaning, family history, a drawing of the family, social history, previous illness, and so on, should be elicited (by you or the pediatrician or both) from each child early in his hospitalization. Certainly, you must do an adequate psychiatric work-up.

You could choose to get the historical reports the easy way, namely, from the parents. But if you choose that course, you must forego some of the fun (and value) of hearing about these from the child's standpoint. Most children do not have the extreme ignorance and insensitivity that we as adults impute to them; if they are asked, children can supply useful, valid, and amusing anamnestic materials.

8. Aim toward diagnosis. As in all of medical practice, in child psychiatry diagnoses are made in order to plan and conduct treatment and in order to conceptualize some guesses about outcome. This last is prognosis, of course. When prognosis is given and the conditions spelled out, the prognostication underlines and strengthens the diagnosis. This makes sense and gives more palpable help to the pediatrician-consultee.

True, child psychiatrists often hedge by stressing the difficulties in diagnosis of children; they wax eloquent in testifying to the ease of estimating the "fixed" psychopathology of "fixed" adults as compared to that of children. Nevertheless, the diagnostic process is as essential in child psychiatry as anywhere else. This can be stated in full recognizance of the contemporary vogue for berating "the medical model."

Diagnosis is not a way of life. It is a necessary, but not sufficient, condition for the practice of child psychiatry. Your diagnostic maneuvers can be therapeutic, or they can be unhelpful, from the outset of contact with the child. A lot depends on your intent and skillfulness as the consulting psychiatrist. In this profession it helps to have a heart of gold and the soul of a poet, but lesser resources can be deployed in achieving what matters: full, clear, rich, and natural communication between you and the child.

A child can be keenly responsive to his doctor's warmth of concern and interest for him. The doctor's sincere determination to unravel the child's problems can engage an aloof child, calm a fearful one, and win over a negativistic one. The child senses the offer of help and decides that he'll work with this doctor. This is how it evolves that a clearly unwilling patient, the kind seen recurrently in child psychiatry and pediatrics, can change his tune and radically abandon his uncooperative stand.

When the child cooperates, diagnosis is made firmer, and therapy is enhanced directly. This preparation for therapy should be an omnipresent objective in pediatric consultation even if therapy does not come about. No sharp line demarcates where consultation ends and psychiatric treatment begins. That is why a diagnostic consultation should be helpful to the child.

9. Try to elicit fantasies during the consultation. You learn most and help most when you do not shy away from a child's fantasy, from his primary process materials, or from the severest psychopathology. Verbalizing his inner life and sharing these things with a shrewd-looking adult is the solace and liberation that disturbed children find in child psychiatry. The doctor who hears out the "bizarre fantasies," and who refrains from "shutting up the kid with that psychotic talk" is infinitely more supportive than the back-patting doctor. Do not avoid the symbols of the child, for it is in symbols (some general and some idiosyncratic) that the child lives, moves, and has his being.

The standard tactics for evoking the child's report on fantasies, arranged in the writer's order of decreasing preference, are these:

(a) Dreams. "I want to know a lot about you, and so I'd like you to tell me about your dreams. Let's begin with the dream you had last night . . . the most recent one." Then proceed asking for his recurrent dreams "dreaming the same kind of dream more than once" and his "most scary" dream.

(b) His heart's three deepest wishes. "Make each wish something different from what you have, something you really crave."

(c) Earliest memories. These reflect, as Alfred Adler contended, not so much veridicality of recall as a portrayal in miniature of the current self-concept. This self-concept of the child is a fundamental psychiatric datum.

(d) Daydreams or conscious fantasies. Both act and demonstrate this way, "Let's be silent for a second and you make a picture came to mind. . . . Will you tell me about it?"

(e) "Identifications." These include his favorite color, favorite animal, favorite famous person, and so on.

In addition to all of the foregoing techniques, drawings made by the child, along with his associated narration, help to elucidate the child's fantasy even further.

10. Organize your consultation report. Even if its organization tends toward stereotype or compulsiveness, never mind. You can be fresh and free in content, but put the content into a framework like the following:

Identifying Data. Age, sex, economic class, referring doctor, health status, growth status.

Presenting Problem. What it is. Its meaning to child and family. Duration. Precipitants. Why now?

Associated Problems and Circumstances.

Developmental or Past History.

Family and Subculture. Description. Child's place therein.

Suggestions. a) Housekeeping or custodial: re sleeping, eating, rooming in, location on ward, and the like. b) Diagnostic: include consultants needed. c) Therapeutic: actual maneuvers recommended as intervention into the child's developmental pattern.

A schema of this sort will provide the framework for the full confidential feedback that was referred to earlier, and will now be amplified.

GIVE FULL INFORMATION TO THE CONSULTEE

A consultation report is not a document for evasion, nor is it an occasion for pussyfooting. Let the pediatrician know all that you have learned: assets, liabilities, anguish, incest, even things that are not "nice." Some psychiatrists treat their medical colleagues as if the latter were irresponsible laymen; this makes for trouble. All medical communications have to occur in an atmosphere that presumes honesty and confidentiality to an extreme degree. Alas, you must be certain that the pediatrician will not misuse your consultation report by forwarding it to nonmedical persons or otherwise being indiscreet or unethical. If you are so unlucky as to live with "nonconfidential" doctors, then of course you must edit and withhold facts, as your colleagues deserve that you do. But ideally there are no holds barred, and as a rule of thumb, nothing is to be held back from the pediatrician-consultee.

An effort has been made to give an informal introduction to the techniques found useful in consulting with pediatricians, and in coexisting psychiatrically with hospitalized children. The pediatric consultation can be laborious, but it can be gratifying as well. Hopefully, some flavor of how attractive this aspect of child psychiatry can be has been conveyed.

SUGGESTED READINGS

BRENNEMAN, J. The menace of psychiatry. *Amer. J. Dis. Child.*, 42:376, 1931. A classic statement of the reaches of a pediatrician's antagonism to psychiatry. [Read it and feel lucky to be where and when you are.]

Group for Advancement of Psychiatry: Committee on Child Psychiatry. Contribution of child psychiatry to pediatric training and practice, Report # 21 1952. Delineates areas where pediatrics can be enriched through psychiatric liaison.

KRUG, O. M. exec. ed. *Career Training in Child Psychiatry*. Washington, D.C., Amer. Psychiat. Assoc., 1964. A good definition of the profession, child psychiatry, and of the necessary ingredients for education of a member of the profession.

LOURIE, R. S. The teaching of child psychiatry in pediatrics, *J. Amer. Acad. Child Psychiat.*, 1:477, 1962. A balanced view of what can be taught and ways of teaching effectively.

LUSTMAN, S. L. and RICHMOND, J. B. On the acceptance of realistic goals in medicine. *In* Solnit, A. J., and Provence, S. A. eds. Modern Perspectives in Child Development. New York, International Universities Press, Inc. 1963, pp. 558–574. Deals with the frustrations inherent in medical training and in the ultimate practice of medicine in whatever speciality.

SECTION FIVE   Community Consultation

Community consultation is becoming one of the rapidly expanding areas of clinical psychiatry. Many residencies are now incorporating a community psychiatry rotation into their standard program. And, there are abundant opportunities for advanced training.

In *The Psychiatric Consultation*, edited by Mendel and Solomon (1968), six excellent chapters deal with consultation to schools, universities, government agencies, the clergy, the courts, and industry. Different community consultation settings require specialized approaches.

Hollister (1968) emphasizes that the trend in modern schools to deal with the "whole child" has encouraged the development of both patient-centered and agency-centered consultations in these institutions. Whittington (1968) tells how consultants in colleges and universities can meet special problems by 1) relating to the established college student health service, 2) curbing feelings of omniscience or evangelism, and 3) dealing diplomatically with administrative personnel. English (1968) discusses his work with the Peace Corps as a model for consultations with governmental agencies. He emphasizes that the primary concern is confidentiality and that, initially, the consultant may be in the peculiar position of serving his own colleagues on the staff. This governmental agency required of the consultant that he work with personnel over a long period in many areas other than the strictly psychologic; he was responsible for screening of trainees, morale, trainees' adaptation to their new countries, "re-entry" adjustment, and research evaluation of overseas stress, as well as conventional psychotherapy.

In "Consultations with the Clergy," McWhirter (1968) says the psychiatrist deals not only with the problems of the client as described by the clergyman-consultee, but he may often have to assiduously avoid giving therapy to the clergyman. The consultant will have to familiarize himself with the religious institution involved in order to appreciate the impact of changing religious forms and philosophy on the mental health of both the clergy and the congregation. Pollack (1968) states that the psychiatrist needs special training for consultation with the court. He must preserve confidentiality, inform clients whom exactly he represents (the client or his legal adversary), and he must keep his reports relevant to the legal issues of the case. Levinson (1968) discusses the consultant's work with industry. He offers the interesting observation that the agency itself may be a subject for psychiatric consultation. He views the organization of an industry as a functioning system and searches for its weaknesses and strengths. He cautions that when the consultant deals with individuals from both labor and management, he should not give undue attention to the more powerful figures in the organization.

The chapters in *The Psychiatric Consultation*, written by authorities who are also pioneers in the various areas, are highly recommended for study.

REFERENCES

HOLLISTER, W. G. The psychiatrist as a consultant to the school. *In* The Psychiatric Consultation, W. M. Mendel and P. Solomon, eds. New York, Grune and Stratton, 1968.

WHITTINGTON, H. G. Consultation practice in colleges and universities. *In* The Psychiatric Consultation, W. M. Mendel and P. Solomon, eds. New York, Grune and Stratton, 1968.

ENGLISH, J. Mental Health consultation with a government agency. *In* The Psychiatric Consultation, W. M. Mendel and P. Solomon, eds. New York, Grune and Stratton, 1968.

McWHIRTER, D. P. Consultation with the clergy. *In* The Psychiatric Consultation, W. M. Mendel and P. Solomon, eds. New York, Grune and Stratton, 1968.

POLLACK, S. Consultation with the courts. *In* The Psychiatric Consultation, W. M. Mendel and P. Solomon, eds. New York, Grune and Stratton, 1968.

LEVINSON, H. Psychiatric consultation in industry. *In* The Psychiatric Consultation, W. M. Mendel and P. Solomon, eds. New York, Grune and Stratton, 1968.

17 COMMUNITY CONSULTATION BY THE PSYCHIATRIST

Rufus M. Vaughn, M.D.

Literature dealing with community consultation generally focuses on the consultant as part of a comprehensive community mental health program. In contrast, I would like to emphasize the role of the individual psychiatrist. Some of the principles involved will apply to both individual and group consultations whether the psychiatrist works as a member of a clinic or in private practice.

The psychiatrist's contribution to communities through consultation with agencies is not of recent origin. Such activity has gone on for many years in a number of settings, particularly with social workers in family service agencies. Routinely, members of agencies meet with psychiatrists to present and discuss client problems. The demand for such consultations has grown considerably. Psychiatrists respond positively since the impact of such consultations may extend beyond a single client or patient. Since 1962 particular efforts have been made to include special training during psychiatric residency to assist the trainee in acquiring skills appropriate to this activity.

The psychiatrist is not alone in showing interest in this area. Many health-related professionals, particularly psychologists and social workers, are utilizing techniques of mental health consultation. Unfortunately, there is no systematized or replicable evidence that such consultation activity is useful. Research in this area is difficult to devise. There is no dearth, however, of ancedotal material to suggest that such consultations are valuable.

THE CONSULTATION PERSONAE

It is, of course, meaningless to speak of consultation to a community. A community is composed of a number of discrete populations. Such populations, for example, are included on the rolls of a parish, as clients in a social agency, inmates in a jail or prison, patients of a health department, or children in a school. Members of these populations with a problem present themselves to an agency or social institution. These people are known as clients. The helping professional, i.e., minister, social worker,

127

custodial officer, school psychologist, or nurse, is the consultee. The person rendering the consultation is the consultant. The consultant works with the consultee on a client's problem. We will not discuss here the more general consultant role of "change agent"—attempting, for example, to influence legislation or public attitudes.

The mental health consultation differs from the usual psychiatric consultation in that the client (or patient) is not seen. In medicine this is not unusual. "Curbstone consultations," in the halls of hospitals, by telephone, or in the scrub rooms and lounges, are commonplace. It is a rare physician who has not presented some facet of a patient problem to a colleague and then weighed the advice or comment offered. However, the mental health consultation is more particularly concerned with the process of information exchange and not primarily with the dispensing of technical information. The reader familiar with the mental health consultation model will recognize that the consultations described here are more flexible and combine features of both consultation and patient care.

MAKING AND MAINTAINING CONSULTEE CONTACT

REFERRALS FROM AGENCIES

Some suggest that mental health consultation should be entirely on an "on call" basis, insisting that a regular contact with an agency or consultee eventually leads to relationships which must be worked through psychotherapeutically (Caplan, 1961). Our own experience has not followed this model; for several years we have maintained regular weekly contact with a number of agencies. There are real advantages to this procedure in that identification with the agency occurs, case follow-up is possible, and we are provided constant information about the value of our services. With difficult problems, maintaining a schedule of visits over a period of time permits the consultant to obtain a much clearer picture of the total structure in which the consultee works. In this arrangement, however, restraint and reaffirmation of purpose are required to avoid trying to alter the referring agency. There is an economic advantage to the regular consultation; the agency can provide and justify a specified fee for service. This is attractive to the psychiatrist in private practice since he can receive regular remuneration and schedule his consultation time.

Haylett and Rapoport (1964) outlined what they consider to be the four phases of mental health consultation. These include preparatory, beginning, problem-solving, and termination phases. Since the focus of their writings is on more comprehensive community mental health programs, their comments are not entirely relevant to our purpose. The same may be said to some extent of Caplan's (1964) approach. His formulation of the process also is essentially in the form of four phases; namely, making the contact (and contract), assessing the problem, delivering the consultation message, and termination.

MAKING CONTRACTS

The making of contracts with agencies is important. The word contract is used in the sense of making expectations clear, not in the sense of a legally binding agreement. The agency requesting service ought to have a complete understanding of what its needs are, what the consultant can offer, and in many cases, what this service will cost. A contract with an agency or consultee may require service only for a specific problem at a particular time and only for as long as that service is necessary. Haylett and Rapoport (1964) and Caplan (1961), on the other hand, have written of a service which is specifically limited yet within an ongoing relationship. For example, our local health department in Florida has four psychiatric consultants working one half day a week, each for the same agreed-upon monthly compensation. The arrangements differ, even though each psychiatrist supervises approximately 80 mental patients. Two of the psychiatrists are especially interested in direct patient care and do group psychotherapy, individual supportive work, and use chemotherapy. The other two prefer to work with the public health nurses and see patients only occasionally.

Termination has not been for us a matter of great consideration because, even though trainees may participate in consultation, various faculty psychiatrists are the continuing contacts with agencies. Termination concerns us only with regard to termination of cases presented each week. Frequently a case is presented once and then dropped for several weeks to reappear as a problem again, or a case is considered once and then never discussed again. On the other hand, clients who are severely ill may need a weekly discussion of their problems and telephone contacts during the week between agency visits. The agency is adaptable; it can accommodate these varied approaches, apportion work as seems appropriate to each psychiatrist's interests and skills, and render a high level of community service.

This is not the usual mental health consultation model. Nevertheless, we think that it fits more closely with the medical model and is particularly adapted to the psychiatrist's expertise.

Violations of the contract present problems. As with a patient in psychotherapy, alterations from the basic agreement (coming early, being late, nonpayment, and the rest) signal a difficulty which needs to be explored. Without clear expectations, demands may be made by either party which will produce discomfort and anxiety or compromise effective working relationships.

Making Contracts

DO

1. clarify and reach concensus about the needs of the consultee.
2. agree on the limit and type of service.
3. agree on fees, if any.
4. fulfill the contract.

DON'T

1. begin the consultation activity without clear expectations. (Resistance may be seen later in this area.)
2. violate the contract without prior negotiation.

IF

1. a contract cannot be agreed upon, continue negotiation in a spirit of compromise.
2. time, finances, or other commitments appear to require change, negotiate these so that bilateral agreement is reached.

PROBLEMS IN CONSULTATION

Caplan (1961) divided the kinds of problems brought by consultees into a number of categories. Three topographical areas are immediately apparent: problems within the client, within the consultee, and within an agency. Obviously a client's difficulties cannot be considered outside the field of the consultee and the agency, since they will be influenced by both.

CLIENT'S PROBLEMS

With the client, it is not always possible to make a definitive psychiatric diagnosis; indeed, this is not necessarily the aim of mental health consultation. Rather, the aim is to alter an interdependent communication system to alleviate the client's difficulty. Neither is it necessary to arrive at a specific medical diagnosis. It must generally be assumed that a medical appraisal was made, but, of course, should medical difficulties arise they should be handled by medical referral.

However, we are not opposed to seeing the client, especially in a public health setting. In some situations it is common for the psychiatrist to do a general physical examination or request particular laboratory data (chest x ray, serology, and the like). In our work at prisons, doing a physical examination is sometimes required. On one occasion a rectal examination on a patient revealed an enlarged prostate which had produced urinary obstruction with uremia and resultant behavorial difficulties. The problem, of course, presented in the reverse order as purely behavioral. Thus, any client problem in which confusion is a manifest symptom should have medical evaluation. Although such considerations are discussed elsewhere in this book, they should be held uppermost in the consultant's mind, because in working with community agencies, he often does not see the patient.

CONSULTEE PROBLEMS

The consultee's problems usually fall within two general areas: 1) lack of knowledge, skill, or information, and 2) interpersonal difficulties. When clearly identified, the first area is not difficult to manage because information can be offered or sources for help indicated, and the consultee can be directed to his supervisor for assistance.

The second problem, i.e., the consultee's interpersonal difficulties, require particular attention because in mental health consultation some of the conventional techniques of psychotherapeutic intervention must be abandoned. Even if he is so inclined, the consultee should not be encouraged to discuss his own problems. The consultant ought not risk a power struggle with the consultee or encourage a negative transference. We agree with Caplan's (1961) suggestion that a mild positive transference must be maintained. The most effective work comes out of a peer relationship with the consultee. Changing to a therapist-patient relationship compromises this association, usually with deleterious results. If ambivalence develops within the consultant-consultee relationship, it will have to be managed to the detriment of the client's interests.

Techniques from child psychiatry can be borrowed, particularly displacement of the problem. Frequently when discussing a child's problems as if they were those of another; the child can offer a solution. In working with a consultee, the problem can be displaced to the client, or reference can be made to similar cases in the past. Confrontation with, and interpretation to, the consultee must be avoided.

Interpersonal difficulties occur when the consultee is authoritarian, inflexible, or moralistic. For example, a public health nurse might, because she disapproves of the arrangement, withhold service from an unwed mother living with her children and common-law husband. Service will never be rendered if the consultant attacks or questions the nurse's values. Reality-oriented, practical goals for such a family should be doggedly pursued. A common ground of concern must be found, one devoid of conflict for the nurse, yet making use of her skills. Usually, concern for the children's physical welfare and education can be a starting point. Assisting the nurse and mother to plan together for improvements is helpful. When the client and mother are in conflict over various issues, the nurse should be helped to identify with the mother's strength and flexible attitudes; this encourages growth on the part of both client and consultee.

The techniques are similar whether the consultee's own interpersonal problems derive from neurotic or situational reactions. The consultant must not concern himself about the consultee's personal life. In the case of a particularly anxious consultee, the consultant should not mention the anxiety; it is the consultant's job to surmise where in the consultee-client relationship the anxiety arises. The concerns which the consultee presents, their form, order, and any apparent distortions or inconsistencies, are clues for the psychiatrist. Also uncritical identification with, or rejection of, the client, feelings of helplessness in meeting the client's needs, or undue optimism in the face of very difficult situations indicate problem areas.

An example of appropriate intervention for this sort of problem follows:

On routine visit to a school, the consultee learned that a ten-year-old boy was not doing well academically and also tended to fight with or withdraw from other children. The consultee advised the teacher to pay more attention to the child, spend more time with him at recess, and, in effect, be protective. Later, the consultee visited the child's mother and learned that the house was dirty and disorganized and that the boy was carrying on many of the responsibilities of running the household. In fact, the child was digging a 20-foot drainage ditch behind the house when the consultee arrived. The child was being abused in being forced to wash the dishes and do some of the cooking. The mother and father were separated, and the agency knew the mother had been hospitialized in a state mental institution because of severe personality disorganization.

The consultee referred her problem to a psychiatric consultant. The consultee told the consultant that the child had a "bad" mother, and that this should be compensated for at school.

Through peripheral sources and quite by accident, it was revealed that the consultee, herself, had a two-year-old child whom she had placed in a day care center so that she could work to support her husband through college. She had a great deal of doubt and guilt about this arrangement. Even prior to gaining this knowledge, however, the consultant felt that the consultee acted too hastily in condemning the mother and had, in effect, wanted the teacher to take over the mother's role. (The consultee even advised that the teacher walk the child home and visit him.)

The consultant took the position that this was, indeed, a difficult situation for a child. Perhaps, however, the mother needed some help in offering the child more guidance and support. He also suggested that the role required of the teacher was difficult since she had so many other children to be concerned about. He then suggested that the consultee visit the mother to assist her in household planning and to appraise her capabilities. Further, he suggested that the teacher should pay particular attention to the boy, but not single him out as an obvious favorite. Rather, he should have as much opportunity as possible to improve his peer relationships. The consultee's supervisor agreed with these suggestions and helped to carry them out.

Within a few weeks, the consultant's questions about the child were met with the reply that there were no longer any problems. The consultee carried out the suggestions and was beginning to assist the mother who had much more strength than was initially thought. The mother was doing extremely well in comparison with her past performance. The chores that the child had been doing were not so much at his mother's insistence but rather were a result of his perception of her great need for help, due to the desertion of the father, severe economic stress, and the presence of a two-year-old child needing care.

What happened with the consultee is only conjecture at this point, because, in keeping with our philosophy of not discussing consultee problems, she was not interviewed. It appeared, however, that she was able to carry out her own mothering functions vicariously and soften her self-condemnation for "deserting" her own child. From her supervisor we learned that her functioning within the agency had markedly improved.

This approach is quite different from the probing psychotherapeutic transaction. Confronting the consultee with her ambivalence toward working would probably have further increased self-questioning regarding her marriage, diminished her self-concept, and produced other problems. One might speculate that the consultee may have had considerable anxiety in her relationship with her own mother, but this is not our area of concern. Instead, our task is to use the strengths in the situation and reduce interfering factors to a minimum.

For Consultee Problems

DO

1. focus exclusively on the client's problem.
2. work out solutions within the areas of strength of the consultee and client.
3. be sensitive to areas of consultee difficulty.
4. refer the consultee to appropriate sources of information if the problem is one of lack of knowledge.
5. respect the consultee's area of skill.

DON'T

1. confront the consultee with observations or interpretations of his behavior.
2. lecture the consultee.
3. offer to do the consultee's work for him.
4. foster a relationship with the consultee which will lead to excessive dependence and ambivalence.

IF

1. the consultee makes reference to his own personal problems or client involvement, avoid these through usual interviewing techniques.
2. medical evaluation is required, as suggested by confusion or other symptoms, be sure this is carried out. In some settings make this evaluation yourself.

AGENCY FACTORS

Another problem area is the internal functioning of the agency itself. If morale is poor, financing low, staff turnover great, or if there are other personnel difficulties, these will be reflected in the consultee's work. One of the commonest symptoms of this difficulty within the agency is the consultee's feeling of helplessness in dealing with his client. Then, such statements as, "We have little to offer," may appear in his presentation to the consultant. Another symptom is the statement by the consultee that he had presented the case elsewhere but his suggestions had not been approved.

Here again, the first principle is not to attack the agency or try to explicate the problem, but rather, the consultant should use the data in helping the consultee. Judgment must not be rendered about the propriety of any administrative regulation. In any event, the consultant is rarely in a position to judge adequately the total administrative structure of an organization. Even should he be in such a position, the judgment is not properly given to the consultee but rather to the administration, and then, only if requested.

The consultant can only make matters worse and impair the consultee's effectiveness if he makes recommendations which conflict with known agency policy. If an agency cannot carry out a function which appears absolutely necessary for the client, transfer of his case should be recommended. An emergency service or walk-in clinic, for example, should not compromise its administrative structure and take on "just one" long-term case. Every rule has an exception, but the exception ought to be truly extraordinary. Making one exception leads to others and ties agencies to commitments which they are not really prepared to accept. This leads to chronic frustration and weakens morale.

An example of this problem is the public health nursing follow-up of a severely ill, previously hospitalized, marginally psychotic patient. This kind of case work is often not rewarding, and the nurse may wish to drop it over the supervisor's protest. Ordinarily, such cases should be carefully assessed with the consultee and a decrease in the frequency of the nurse's visits rather than dropping the case should be recommended. An alternative, when the patient is on medication, is to decrease or alter the dose; this provides an opportunity for increased discussion between the client and the consultant as they assess the effects of the change in dosage. Both maneuvers circumvent a direct confrontation between the consultee and his supervisor. At the same time, the client receives appropriate care. If fewer visits have no adverse effect on the patient, the supervisor is usually willing to accept additional decreases as indicated. On the other hand, if visits and changes in medication do not help the client, a curtailment of service is in order. Of course, if the nursing contacts are beneficial to the patient, then the nurse will be able to reinvest interest and time in the problem. Thus, by focusing on the client, a power struggle between the nurse and the supervisor is avoided. The opposite would be true were the consultant to enter the conflict between supervisor and consultee; power struggles and conflicts about status differences could easily arise.

Another agency difficulty occurs when the administrator is insecure and frustrates many of the consultee's plans by becoming authoritarian. Sometimes this is deliberate and overt, but often it is covert and discernible only through careful scrutiny of the problem. The temptation for the consultant to be critical of the administrator may be almost overwhelming. However, this would be a serious error. Divided loyalties and

administrative chaos would ensue. The administrator always carries ultimate responsibility, and he is aware of this. Motives, however fickle they
may seem, must be assumed to be reasonable and in good faith. As many
problems as possible should be directed to the administrator for decision.
Usually it is possible to bolster the administrator's role by making certain
that the consultee discusses any planned action with him. This is especially helpful if alternative modes of action are available and the administrator can make the final decision. Then, the administrator is both
informed of and included in an increasing number of agency activities,
and his sense of worth as well as his prestige is enhanced. The administrator becomes more certain and therefore more supportive of his staff.
His self-confidence makes him more flexible and trusting. It is an extraor-
dinarily rare person in an administrative function who does not have
considerable strength and expertise which can be exploited. If the administrator is indeed lacking in competence, he will relinquish responsibility
to capable workers, if this option is available, in order to avoid having
authority wrested from him.

For Agency Problems

DO

1. gain familiarity with the administrative structure.
2. utilize the administrative structure.
3. support the administrative framework in which the consultee functions.
4. remain aloof from the agency's policy structure.

DON'T

1. attack the agency.
2. attempt to interfere with administrative policy by overt or covert
   means.
3. suggest that consultees carry out programs contrary to administrative
   policy.

IF

1. the consultee wishes to discuss job dissatisfaction or other problems
   within the agency, avoid it. In some cases referral to the supervisor
   is appropriate.
2. there are signs of insecure administration, encourage the consultee to
   work more closely with supervisory personnel. Encourage the development of alternative plans from which supervisory personnel can
   choose.

DIFFERENCES IN CONSULTATION SETTINGS

Our work at the University of Florida developed within the following areas: the health department, child welfare department, the state prison, circuit court, probation and parole, school for the retarded, school for delinquent girls, school for the deaf, in seminars for general physicians, seminars for ministers, and the university student health service. Obviously, all these areas of consulting activity will not concern every psychiatrist. Such matters as mental retardation, juvenile delinquency, or forensic psychiatry require special knowledge or interest. Consequently we selected two areas (public health and prison) where general psychiatrists can work without special skills. The principles of consultation are much the same in all settings.

The health department, with its multiple functions, offers the broadest experience. Departments in most Florida counties have mental health divisions. Their activities are varied but usually fulfill the responsibility of following patients discharged from mental hospitals. They may also render emergency service. From the department, the mental health worker and the public health nurse work closely with other community agencies, including schools and the juvenile court. The mental health worker is often a nurse with special interests and training. The public health nurse visits the mental health patient as she does all others on her roster, patients being assigned by district rather than by type of case.

The psychiatrist's role as a consultant varies, even within a particular setting such as a health department. His role depends on whether the nurse presents a patient (at her discretion), or only a problem about a patient, school teacher, welfare worker, or family. On the one hand, there is direct patient contact, while on the other the psychiatrist assumes the mental health consultant role. When a patient is presented, the nurse usually attends the interview; families are strongly encouraged to accompany patients. Some psychiatrists will not find this model comfortable, but in our experience, it has been effective and well accepted. This model works well because the patient clearly remains the nurse's responsibility; the psychiatrist does not preempt a relationship that he cannot follow through.

The problem of confidentiality may bother the consultant. In a small community there is almost none, and this is accepted as a way of life. All agencies freely exchange information. For the consultant, at any rate, lack of confidentiality does not mean lack of discretion.

Prison work differs from other activities. The severe authoritarian system is the antithesis of the flexible health department system. Although mental health consultation principles are important, the consultant more frequently must assume the clinical role. Also, effective care is more difficult to render in a prison setting. The goals of the institution must be understood. Efforts to alter the prison system will only result in frustration for the consultant and activate severe resistance on the part of the institution. It is interesting that few psychiatrists work in prison settings for long periods. In this setting, an understanding of the administrative structure is more important than explication of a contractual arrangement.

In a prison, the custodial function is paramount. All activity must take this into consideration. Ordinarily, the psychiatrist has little voice in deciding the degree of custody (i.e., minimum, medium, or maximum), even though the degree of custody of an individual patient affects the services the consultant can render. We have seen strange paradoxes regarding the custody status of inmates. Individuals under maximum custody are often not released on parole, but must serve their sentence to expiration. At that time, however, they are released directly to the community without supervision. On the other hand, the petty offender may be released to parole supervision and guidance long before his sentence expires. We have advocated release of serious offenders to parole so that the necessary rehabilitation efforts can be carried out.

We would advise most psychiatrists to approach prison consultation with caution unless the setting is a medical facility like the one California developed at Vacaville. Nevertheless, prison consultation provides generous rewards in patient contact. More than one inmate retains lasting impressions of a "free man" who has interest, is consistent, has no axes to grind, is open and undefensive, does what he says he will do, and does not promise what he cannot deliver. An outside consultant, in contrast to the regular prison physician, has an advantage with inmates in that he is not identified with the institution and is not dependent upon it for his rewards.

Although the clinical model has been paramount, we found many situations requiring the mental health consultation model. This has occurred with other physicians, custodial officers, psychologists, and other prison workers. There is a difference, however, in that the psychiatrist has usually been called upon because of his clinical expertise. It is important to clarify early what role will be appropriate to the problem.

SUMMARY

With changes in the practice of psychiatry resulting in greater community involvement, the psychiatrist's consulting activity does not always follow the classical medical model. Likewise it does not follow entirely the mental health consultation model which has been developed with all mental health professionals in mind.

The psychotherapeutic model is also not entirely appropriate. In our community consulting activities we found ourselves blending various models with the recognition that the physician consultant still retains some skills which are peculiar to his area of activity. If his medical skills are of no value in the consultation role, then a consultant without these skills should be retained. The psychiatrist who desires to enlarge his area of activity and responsibility beyond the diadic physician-patient relationship and into the community should recognize that his usual approach to problems will not be entirely adequate or appropriate. The considerations outlined in this chapter serve as an introduction to this area of activity.

REFERENCES

CAPLAN, G. An approach to Community Mental Health. New York, Grune & Stratton, Inc., 1961, pp. 20–23.
———— Principles of Preventive Psychiatry. New York, Basic Books, Inc., Publishers, 1964, p. 41.
HAYLETT, C. H., and RAPOPORT, L. Mental health consultation. *In* Bellak, L., ed. Handbook of Community Psychiatry. New York, Grune & Stratton, Inc., 1964, pp. 319–340.

SECTION SIX   Diagnosis and Management

18   SYMPTOMS, DISEASES, AND DIAGNOSES

Remember that psychiatric disease and organic disease may not only simulate each other but may coexist.

Rossman (1963)

Daily, the consultant is beset with requests to confirm, reject, or establish diagnoses. His diagnostic job is complicated because, unlike the attending staff, 1) he must weigh a greater body of accumulated data from the medical work-up, including other physicians' opinions—which may be diverse—and a variety of laboratory findings; 2) his psychiatric diagnoses, or lack thereof, can seldom be confirmed by "objective" procedures; and 3) there is the element and burden of finality: The consultant is often the last diagnostician in the chain of patient evaluation.

Too frequently, he is asked the "either-or" question: Is this patient's illness organic or functional? However, as we have stressed in this book, the problem is more often "both-and." Such an emphasis on the concurrence of medical and psychiatric illness is relatively new. With the advent of scientific medicine, training in differential diagnosis received a high priority. The clinician was taught to exercise his skills as a logician (judging symptoms, recalling knowledge, and searching texts for advice) so he could delineate the patient's clinical picture and, hopefully, arrive at a single diagnosis.

The law of parsimony (subsuming all symptomatology under one diagnosis) prevailed. This was an outgrowth of the new scientfic medicine which emphasized diagnostic exactitude and reacted to the chaos of the previous era when syndromes, and even single symptoms, were given separate diagnostic labels. For example, "fever" was once a disease, and such a label was meaningless or at best only slightly descriptive. Now, differential diagnosis is firmly established in the medical curriculum. However, the pendulum swung so far in this direction that diagnosis by exclusion resulted. Recently the law of parsimony has been attacked. Phillip Sullivan (1963) states: "The possibility of two or more concurrent diseases is always present," and Palarea (1965) adds: "One must proceed with caution in applying the law of parsimony. . . . The presence of concurrent significant medical and psychiatric illnesses appears to be the rule rather than the exception."

Comparative studies support this thesis. Lovett Doust (1952) found there was a higher incidence of both somatic complaints and physical illness in the medical histories of psychiatric patients than in a control sample of the general population. Also, his psychotic patients reported more physical illness than the neurotics, implying that a greater degree of psychological disability is paralleled by a diminished capacity to resist physiological stress. Roessler and Greenfield (1961) confirmed Lovett Doust's work by finding there was a higher incidence of somatic disease in psychiatric outpatients (mostly neurotics) than in a control group of medical outpatients. They concluded: "Psychiatric patients do visit medical clinics more frequently than controls, but they do so because they suffer a greater frequency of 'real' illness."

Further evidence comes from other sources. Brodman et al., the authors of the Cornell Medical Index (1952), found that the same patients who reported increased psychiatric symptomatology reported more medical symptomatology. A controlled study by Matarazzo et al., from the University of Oregon (1961) showed that an increased number of medical symptoms correlated positively with an increased number of psychiatric symptoms in both medical and psychiatric inpatients and outpatients. The authors say: "*The number of medical symptoms is a good predictor of psychiatric symptomatology, and vice versa.*" (The italics are the authors.) Thus, these clinical investigations provide ample evidence that when an individual becomes ill with various presenting symptoms, the illness reflects difficulties in both his biologic and psychosocial adaptation.

In the most definitive work in this area, Hinkle and Wolff (1957) present a comprehensive evaluation of illness in relatively healthy populations. Illness was not randomly distributed among their subjects; instead, some had many more illnesses than others. Those who had the greatest number experienced a wide variety in many body systems. Also, there was a positive correlation between an increased number of major illnesses and minor illnesses, and vice versa. Hinkle and Wolff state further: "Those people who had the greater number of bodily illnesses, regardless of their nature, and regardless of their etiology, were the ones who experienced the greater number of disturbances of mood, thought, and behavior."

Illnesses were not scattered throughout their subjects' lives; instead, they usually appeared in clusters, even in the healthier persons. Clusters occurred when the person was experiencing significant difficulty in his attempts to adapt to the conflicting demands of his total environment. From their work, Hinkle and Wolff conclude that illness "is a state of the total organism and that when a human moves from a state of 'health' into a state of 'illness,' the 'illness' is likely to be manifested by a variety of syndromes appearing concurrently or consecutively, their nature being dependent upon the various factors acting on the organism at that time."

Mering and Earley (1966) report that throughout most of the Western world there are difficulties with the diagnosis of the "problem patient." In West Germany undifferentiated health aberrations account for approximately 30 percent of the total patient visits to physicians. These authors also refer to English and Dutch studies: About one half of all medical admissions could be attributed to psychosocial malfunctioning, or the patients had problems extending beyond the somatic conditions for which they were hospitalized. In the United States, Kaufman and Bernstein (1957) found that 30 percent of the patients who visited a medical clinic had nonsomatic complaints as contributing, accompanying, or dominating factors in their illnesses.

Thus the consultant's problems with diagnosis are compounded as he is forced to disregard the once simple and more comfortable dichotomous view of the patient and instead grapple with the new data about illness which evidence the complexity of the disease process.

MEDICAL ILLNESS APPEARING AS A PSYCHIATRIC DISORDER

One of the consultant's greatest concerns is that he will misdiagnose. In particular, he fears that he will diagnose as psychiatric a medical illness which needs treatment, and that his psychiatric diagnosis will be accepted with such finality that the patient's medical problem will be overlooked. Some work substantiates the reality of this concern. Rossman (1963) studied 115 patients given psychiatric diagnoses and referred for consultations who were later found to have had medical illnesses. There was no correlation between the type of medical illness and the nature of the psychoneurotic manifestations: Thyrotoxicosis appeared as an anxiety reaction, a psychoneurotic reaction, a depressive reaction, or as a personality disturbance; Addison's disease resembled vague nervous system reactions or depression. Rossman lists a number of factors responsible for misdiagnosis: the lack of abnormalities in the physical examination or the laboratory findings; the vagueness of neurotic symptoms (nervousness, headache, tension, irritability, fatigue); the overemphasis of environmental stresses; the presence of very rare illnesses; the fact that some medical illnesses were in an early stage; and an inadequate medical work-up or an inaccurate history. Very importantly, he notes that some neurotic patients and some with simple schizophrenia really cannot give an accurate medical history. Of course, overlapping symptoms are also responsible for misdiagnosis. Finally, some patients are so annoying that they keep the physician "off balance." Palerea (1965) emphasizes that a breakdown in communication is also responsible for misdiagnosis; the consultee-oriented consultation should remove some communication difficulties.

Burton (1966) says, "With the increased currency of psychiatric principles among the laity and the members of the profession, we have all become hyperaware of the psychically induced physical symptom. As our sophistication in this area has increased, our index of suspicion for the psychiatric symptom physically engendered has often been disastrously low." In one of her cases, a man with aortic insufficiency presented with anxiety and shortness of breath; in another, a woman showing episodes of dissociation and apathy was found, after receiving five years of psychotherapy, to have a left temporoparietal meningioma.

The three types of medical illnesses which most frequently present with psychiatric symptomatology that obscure diagnosis are the endocrine disorders, epilepsy, and brain tumors.

ENDOCRINE DISORDERS

Because hormones exert their effects on many organs and systems, the manifestations of endocrine disease are usually numerous, frequently vague, and often bizarre. Endocrine dysfunctions make their appearance gradually; consequently they are difficult to diagnose in their early stages, and the patient with ill-defined, general symptomatology may easily be labeled "neurotic." These disorders occur often in midlife, usually around the time of the climacteric when the patient's perspective on his life (past, present, future) is changing and when interpersonal difficulties and life's disappointments are readily apparent. At this time of life, too, the patient is aware that his body is no longer functioning as in the past; he may be altogether too willing to accept declining prowess and symptomatology as only natural by attributing it to age.

For these reasons, many patients with endocrine disorders are mis-diagnosed; they are perceived as psychiatric and their endocrine disease is neither fully investigated nor adequately treated. For example, Palerea (1965) reports a series of 196 patients with psychiatric diagnoses who were later found to have medical illness; hypothyroidism was the most frequent (12 patients). The appearance of depression causes the greatest confusion; depression, more than any other psychiatric diagnosis, is applied to patients with endocrine disorders.

PITUITARY. Patients with pituitary disease frequently complain of changed libido (usually, but not always, decreased), apathy, and distress about changes in the body image which occur with diseases such as acromegaly, Simmond's disease, or Cushing's syndrome.

THYROID. Although hyperthyroidism is usually associated with the symptomatic manifestations of anxiety (trembling, the appearance of fright, weight loss, palpitations, fear, and severe nervousness), in a few of these patients depression is predominant, particularly in the later stages. In hypothyroidism, generalized nervousness is a common complaint early in the course of the illness; the clinical appearance of depression, however, is found in almost all cases of hypothyroidism at some time later in the course of the disease. The hypothyroid patient complains of lassitude, apathy, and inability to concentrate; when this is combined with both the myxedematous appearance and the sagging musculature of the face and body the patient is stamped "depressed."

PARATHYROID. Diseases of the parathyroid glands also appear as psychiatric syndromes. Depression may mask hyperparathyroidism. More commonly, the electrolyte disturbance which results (especially if there are renal complications) may produce an acute brain syndrome with the typical features of delirium. The hypoparathyroid patient may also appear depressed; or muscle spasms and bizarre sensations due to tetany convince the physician that the patient is having a conversion reaction or that he is just plain "neurotic."

ISLETS. The disorder of the pancreas which most frequently leads to psychiatric symptomatology is hyperinsulinism due to an adenoma or to hyperfunction of the Islets of Längerhans. Hypoglycemic attacks present the well-known symptoms of episodic irritability, confusion, difficulty with concentration, transient disorientation, muscle spasms, and even convulsions in severe cases. These patients are sometimes diagnosed "neurotic," schizophrenic, or as addicts.

ADRENALS.   Diseases of the adrenal glands must not be overlooked. Typically, a pheochromocytoma is first manifested by intermittent attacks of severe anxiety, with headache, trembling, and a drastically elevated blood pressure. Patients with hypercorticism develop the Cushing-syndrome appearance with distortions of the body-image and personality changes. In the early stages, personality changes may be paradoxical (the previously shy individual becomes extroverted); in the later stages, depression, irritability, and apathy are common. In Addison's disease the early symptoms, typically, are weakness, lassitude, and asthenia. Mild anxiety, which arises because the patient does not know what is happening to him, and general weakness pervade the clinical picture so that unless the clinician is alert to the possibility of this endocrine disorder a psychiatric diagnosis is made.

EPILEPSY

In dealing with these patients, the consultant will find that diagnostic errors are made in different directions. The manifestations of epilepsy may be regarded as totally psychiatric. Because epilepsy usually makes its appearance in adolescence or in young adulthood (when the person is undergoing rapid physical and psychological changes, or when he is venturing into new tasks in life such as college, marriage, or career), the symptomatology may be attributed to the stresses of his changing life. Or conversely, too great a premium may be placed on the report of a slight abnormality in the electroencephalogram so that a patient's neurosis may be falsely attributed to an epileptic disturbance, and he receives anti-epileptic medications rather than needed psychotherapy.

This kind of either-or thinking is lamentable. The personality and its manifestations in disease states are the functions of the brain, the central integrating organ. It is highly unlikely that the cerebral disturbance which we call epilepsy will not produce mental symptomatology and personality disturbances. In turn, these symptoms aggravate the individual's problems with living; obviously, the clinical picture will be complex and there is danger that a diagnostic vicious cycle is set in motion. However, there is little need for undue emphasis on differential diagnosis; the patient's epileptic disturbances can be treated by medications, and his problems in living can be approached psychotherapeutically.

Burton (1966) notes: "Three manifestations of epilepsy . . . are the episodic psychoses, depression, and vague malaise . . . and likewise an episodic psychosis may resemble acute schizophrenia." It is well known that acute anxiety or syncope may precipitate seizures.

Psychomotor and atonic seizures are apt to be misdiagnosed unless the clinician keeps them in mind when he sees a patient who has had an abrupt onset of aberrant behavior and some disturbance in consciousness. In temporal lobe epilepsy, or what is often called psychomotor epilepsy, the patient is confused and negativistic. Automatisms are frequent and may last for even a few minutes. Varied disturbances of consciousness occur; visual, auditory, and uncinate hallucinations are common. Psychopathic behavior with poor impulse control is also frequent. Other variations in the clinical picture are seen; in discussing the psychic aspects of cerebral attacks, Richardson (1952) describes a patient whose severe trembling and agitation resembled neurotic anxiety. The consultant should also bear in mind that other forms of epilepsy, such as the focal seizures of Jacksonian epilepsy, may be difficult to diagnose. The atonic seizure must be differentiated from a convulsive disorder due to hypoglycemia, carotid sinus sensitivity, the Stokes-Adams syndrome, barbiturate withdrawal, or cranial trauma.

BRAIN TUMORS

Although not presenting the greatest difficulty in differential diagnosis, the possibility that the patient has a brain tumor is the most worrisome problem for the consultant. There is no psychiatric syndrome that is characteristic of brain tumor. Brock and Krieger (1963) emphasize that personality changes (brooding, irritability, and suspicion) may herald the onset of a brain tumor, and that when these changes are hidden by the mask of depression, the underlying organic process may not be visible until late in the course of the illness. There are some guidelines for diagnosis: 1) Localization of the tumor influences the symptomatology. Tumors in the frontal or temporoparietal lobes are likely to evidence personality changes as the presenting symptoms. The frontal lobe syndrome consists of personality change, often with euphoria, childishness, inattention, and loss of judgment. Tumors involving the temporal lobe may produce a more insidious personality change; but severe anxiety, marked irritability, and even visual or auditory hallucinations occur. Damage to the parietal lobe may be manifested by disturbances of sensation and focal seizures, as well as by anxiety, low tolerance to frustration, and depression. Tumors in the occipital area usually produce severe headaches and disturb the patient's vision. Tumors of the pituitary affect libidinal drives and body-image. 2) The personality change is seldom abrupt and is generally first seen as an exaggeration of the premorbid personality traits. The shy patient with a schizoid personality who previously had a tendency to withdraw from social situations will reveal an accentuation of these patterns; while a highly suspicious person may become paranoid. On occasion, however, the personality change is paradoxical; the patient will display a reversal of previous personality characteristics, e.g., the hypomanic person becomes withdrawn. 3) Depressive symptomatology is frequently encountered. But in general the most prominent feature of the "depression" is retardation rather than a lowering of the mood or somatic symptomatology, except for headache.

THE RECOGNITION OF SYMPTOMS BASED ON EMOTIONAL AND MENTAL DISTURBANCES

The major part of this discussion has been devoted to a recognition of the concurrence of organic illness and emotional distress, with an emphasis on the consultant's problems in diagnosing organic disease obscured by mental symptomatology. However, one should briefly consider the symptoms presented by medical patients in whom there is no evidence of organic disease. The magnitude of this problem is unquestioned. Einhorn (1957) reports that approximately 30 percent of all patients going to practicing physicians are suffering from illnesses that are purely psychogenic. He reminds us that psychoneurosis is essentially an illness of the total organism; therefore it is rare to find any patient without some somatic symptomatology.

In his article, "Is this Symptom Functional?" Phillip Sullivan (1963) studies the question most frequently asked, implicitly or explicitly, of the consultant. He lists criteria for evaluating the patient's symptomatology: "1) Is the patient's symptom consistent with a known organic disease and with the total clinical picture? 2) What were the circumstances of onset, including emotional and interpersonal factors? 3) What meaning does the patient attach to his symptom? 4) What advantage does he gain from his symptom? 5) Can his psychiatric illness be diagnosed on the basis of positive findings, and is the patient's symptom consistent with such a diagnosis?"

HOW TO HANDLE THE "EITHER-OR" QUESTION

1. The consultant should bear in mind the data which indicate that many of his consultation patients have "both-and" problems.

2. After evaluating the medical work-up, he can suggest tactfully, when necessary, that further medical evaluation is in order (see BASIC MEDICAL WORK-UP).

3. He should not strain to subsume a whole barrage of symptomatology under a psychiatric or any single diagnosis.

4. A psychiatric diagnosis should always be based on positive findings, not on exclusion.

5. The consultant should never hesitate to admit that he is in a quandary; he can discuss the need for follow-up visits and further evaluation over a period of time with both the referring physician and the patient.

6. A thumb-nail guide to the psychiatric symptoms accompanying physical illness is in APPENDIX B.

REFERENCES

BROCK, S., and KRIEGER, H. The Basis of Clinical Neurology, 4th ed. Baltimore, The Williams & Wilkins Co., 1963.

BRODMAN, K., ERDMANN, A., LORGE, GERSHENSON, and WOLFF. The Cornell medical index health questionnaire, III. The evaluation of emotional disturbances. J. Clin. Psychol., 8:119, 1952.

BURTON, R. C. Symptomatology—organic or psychogenic. New York J. Med., 66:1304, 1966.

EINHORN, E. H. Recognition of symptomatology based on emotional and mental disturbances. New York J. Med., 57(15):2509, 1957.

HINKLE, L. E., and WOLFF, H. G. Health and the social environment: Experimental investigations. Leighton, A., Clausen, J., and Wilson, R., eds. Explorations in Social Psychiatry. New York, Basic Books, Inc., Publishers, 1957, pp. 105–137.

KAUFMAN, M. R., and BERNSTEIN, S. A psychiatric evaluation of the problem patient. J.A.M.A., 163:108, 1957.

LOVETT DOUST, J. W. Psychiatric aspects of somatic immunity: Differential evidence of physical disease in histories of psychiatric patients. Brit. J. Soc. Med., 6(49), 1952.

MATARAZZO, R. G., MATARAZZO, J. D., and SASLOW, G. The relationship between medical and psychiatric symptoms. J. Abnorm. Soc. Psychol., 62(1):55, 1961.

MERING, O., and EARLEY, L. The diagnosis of problem patients. Human Organization, 25 (1):21, 1966.

PALAREA, E. P. Medical evaluation of the psychiatric patient. J. Amer. Geriat. Soc., 13:14, 1965.

RICHARDSON, C. Psychic aspects of cerebral attacks. Med. Clin. N. Amer., March:557, 1952.

ROESSLER, R., and GREENFIELD, N. S. Incidence of somatic disease in psychiatric patients. Psychosom. Med., 23:413, 1961.

ROSSMAN, P. L. Organic diseases simulating functional disorders. GP, 28:78, 1963.

SULLIVAN, P. Is this symptom functional? J.A.M.A., 185(10):747, 1963.

19 THE PERSONALITY DISORDERS

Although diagnosing personality disorders is difficult for all physicians, when the consultant identifies these disorders and evaluates their influence on illness and management, he makes a fruitful contribution to patient care. Kahana and Bibring (1964) emphasize that the psychological management of physically ill patients requires a knowledge of personality structure with its manifold symptomatology. Failure to diagnose personality disorders quickly is responsible for many of the difficulties which staff members experience with their patients. Patients with personality disorders are referred for psychiatric consultation late in the period of hospitalization, often after severe interpersonal struggles have already developed (Schwab et al., 1965).

Problems with the diagnosis of patients' personality disorders arise from a variety of factors: 1) Intrinsically, the symptoms are exclusively behavioral and interpersonal, defying precise measurement. It is difficult to determine, during the stress of the illness, whether the patient's behavior is pathological. 2) Current concepts of personality disorders are nebulous and embryonic; thus, they are incompletely understood, even by psychiatrists. 3) The physician is trained to direct his attention to physical findings or overt symptoms of mental illness; as a consequence, he is not sensitive to these patients' less tangible symptomatology. 4) The physician is unwilling to utilize or even acknowledge his own feelings about the patient. His feelings of hostility or irritability are important clues for diagnosis; but when he disregards his feelings because of guilt or because they seem "unscientific," he dulls his diagnostic sensitivity.

CLASSIFICATION

In discussing personality disorders, formally and informally, several languages are used. Most familiar is the common descriptive language

150

which conveys distinctions in types with such labels as "the complaining patient," "the angry patient," "the argumentative patient," etc. Kahana and Bibring (1964) offer a language which parallels psychoanalytic models. They outline seven categories with suggestions for appropriate management:

THE DEPENDENT, OVERDEMANDING (ORAL) PERSONALITY

Because of this patient's insatiate needs, expressed by demands and tears, the physician must set limits. But to do so, he must offer minor concessions to satisfy some of the demands for special attention.

THE ORDERLY, CONTROLLED (COMPULSIVE) PERSONALITY

The characteristic ritualism and self-discipline this personality exhibits, particularly under the stress of illness, may be utilized for therapy. A logical approach, inviting the patient to participate in therapy (e.g., counting his calories) helps him maintain a sense of equilibrium.

THE DRAMATIZING, EMOTIONALLY INVOLVED, CAPTIVATING (HYSTERICAL) PERSONALITY

Reassurance, and some occasional gestures of appreciation for the patient's attempts to be attractive, are helpful. Discussions of the patient's anxieties are useful and need not be highly structured.

THE LONG-SUFFERING, SELF-SACRIFICING (MASOCHISTIC) PATIENT

For this patient, suffering and love-gaining are associated. Recovery is facilitated when it is linked with helping others.

THE GUARDED, QUERULOUS (PARANOID) PATIENT

A friendly attitude, relatively detached and tolerant, which recognizes the difficulties underlying the patient's complaints, is most effective.

THE PATIENT WITH THE FEELING OF SUPERIORITY (NARCISSISTIC)

This patient's sense of superiority is threatened by illness. He wants to feel that he is being cared for by a physician of eminence. Reassurance about his own value comes from hearing the doctor assert that he is an experienced and recognized physician.

THE PATIENT WHO SEEMS UNINVOLVED
AND ALOOF (SCHIZOID)

This patient attempts to deny threatening illness. The medical staff should make few demands for socialization, at the same time preventing complete withdrawal.

Nosologic classifications according to the *Diagnostic and Statistical Manual of Mental Disorders* are required for completing the face sheet on the chart when the patient is discharged from the hospital or clinic. There are major subdivisions.

PERSONALITY PATTERN DISTURBANCES

These patients' personalities are characterized by pervasive, lifelong, and seemingly inherent patterns of disturbance which give the examiner the impression that there is a constitutional basis for the disorder.

THE INADEQUATE PERSONALITY

Patients with inadequate personalities are usually easy to diagnose, but sometimes the label is applied indiscriminately. Differential diagnosis includes simple schizophrenia and even chronic depression.

To identify the inadequate personality, the physician must find evidence of limited physical and psychological adaptability to stress. These patients lack vitality and stamina; they appear to have intellectual, affective, and physical deficiencies.

Many of these patients haunt public hospitals, clinics, or physicians' offices. Their inadequacy is somatized. They have realistic problems in living (poor nutrition), and continued medical care provides an acceptable excuse for their inadequacy.

When they are hospitalized for medical and surgical illnesses, they may not respond to treatment as quickly as expected. Anxiety is then aroused in the staff, and consultation may be sought. The request often reads, "What is wrong with this patient? He just doesn't seem to get well." The consultant can help the referring staff with these patients by advising them to set limited goals for recovery. They must accommodate to the slowed rate of recovery.

When the medical staff makes the diagnosis, consultations may be sought for confirmation and for assistance with disposition, such as referral to social agencies. The social worker can help with arrangements for convalescent care.

THE SCHIZOID PERSONALITY

Anxiety, emotional detachment, and social withdrawal typify these patients. Many suffer from autistic thinking, and they do not express their feelings directly. The withdrawal and apathy disturb the medical or surgical staff who do not understand why their attempts to interact with these patients are met with dull, flat responses. These patients are considered "spooky"; their medical and surgical care may suffer. Under the stress of illness, pathological responses genereally increase; but in some cases, the care provided by the staff leads to a temporary lessening of psychopathology. Sometimes syndrome shift occurs and the stress of physical illness temporarily mobilizes the patient's resources (Kissen, 1963; Schwab et al., 1965).

The consultant helps by explaining the nature of this personality disorder to the staff and by emphasizing the necessity for a concrete approach to these patients. This entails specific explanations of all procedures and the setting of limited goals. Sometimes, consultations are not requested for schizoid patients because their tendency toward quietness and seclusiveness conceals the psychopathology.

THE CYCLOTHYMIC PERSONALITY

These individuals have a marked tendency to extreme fluctuations in mood: withdrawal, moodiness, and pessimism during the depressive phase; overresponsiveness, extroversion, and outward gaiety during the hypomanic phase. Rapid swings in mood, particularly toward depression, disturb the medical and surgical staff who fear that procedures or their interactions with the patient precipitate these oscillations. Consultations are then requested to treat the depression and to evaluate the risk of suicide. Conversely, mild and early expressions of hypomania are often not perceived as pathological; consultations are requested only when these patients become overactive, neglect medical advice, and disregard admonitions.

Diagnosis is not difficult, but the consultant must promptly call the staff's attention to the nature of the disorder; instituting treatment forestalls severe depression or mania. Frequently, clarifying the diagnosis, specifying procedures, and discussing the prognosis are enough; the staff's uncertainties regarding illness were stimulating the patient's mood fluctuations.

For the depressed patient, treatment usually means antidepressant medications and sometimes E.C.T. In the manic phase, phenothiazines usually suffice, but occasionally E.C.T. is necessary. However, drugs and somatic therapies are not always needed. Psychotherapeutic confrontation which accepts mood variations and focuses mainly on diminishing their intensity is sufficient. The psychotherapy involves certain tactical maneuvers: 1) reviewing previous episodes to assess their extent (When the consultant can report that previous mood swings were self-limited, the staff and the patient are reassured. For the few cases in which the mood swings reach psychiatric proportions, psychotherapy alone is not adequate.); 2) exploring underlying feelings; and, 3) setting firm limits for the hypomanic patient.

THE PARANOID PERSONALITY

Patients with paranoid personality patterns are detected early by the medical and nursing staff because their misinterpretations, suspiciousness, and recalcitrant attitudes produce interpersonal difficulties. The staff generally develop a guarded, wait-and-see attitude toward these patients who may become flagrantly paranoid when their rigid behavioral patterns are stressed by illness and disrupted by hospitalization.

Providing management for these patients, particularly while they are moderately or severely ill, taxes the ingenuity of the consultant. He has to use flexible and varied therapeutic approaches. When suspicion and distrust have accumulated to the point that the patient is isolated by the entire staff, the consultant may have to become the patient's "only friend." Also, enlisting the cooperation of a family member whom the patient trusts dispels fear. Recommendations to the attending staff should underscore the importance of the team approach so that a single staff member is not overwhelmed by the cloud of suspicion which pervades the situation. Reality must be emphasized; opportunities for misinterpretation reduced; and all procedures clarified. A sensible, even businesslike approach is helpful. Many of these patients are intensely afraid of being labeled "crazy," and they will reveal their fears to the empathic consultant, whereupon paranoid attitudes diminish. Short, daily follow-up visits are mandatory.

PERSONALITY TRAIT DISTURBANCES

This classification pertains to disturbances which are not as severe as the personality pattern disorders. Although trait disturbances produce the great majority of management problems, they are frequently undiagnosed.

THE EMOTIONALLY UNSTABLE

This group exhibits intense and usually unpredictable emotional reactions to slight stimuli. Between outbursts and when stress is minimal, emotional instability does not appear. Illness exaggerates the disturbance. In the hospital the patient makes excessive demands for care, concerns himself with status, and responds inappropriately. He is alert to any inconsistency in the routine and uses it to justify his behavior. Because his reactions are so overt and because his outbursts of uncontrolled anger or excessive weeping upset the staff, psychiatric consultation is commonly requested. The patient is erratic, keeping the staff "off balance." Opinions about the patient vary. The nurse who has seen him only during stable periods may not understand her colleagues' impressions that he is difficult to care for, flighty, and irritable.

The consultant's basic approach should be directed toward the hostility, guilt, or anxiety underlying the emotional outbreaks. Direct questions such as, "What are you really afraid of?" or, "What do you think about your illness?" yield favorable results. The immediate behavioral problem is of secondary import, although the consultant must eventually convince the patient that his uncontrolled emotions are detrimental and handicap the staff's efforts to care for him. Brief follow-up visits continue the consultant's personal relationship with the patient and ensure cooperation.

With the more severely disturbed, seriously ill patient, whose disruptive behavior is destroying necessary treatment programs, the consultant may have to create a dependent relationship. This relationship, tailored to gratify basic needs and encourage limited regression while he is in the hospital, enables the patient to moderate his actions. As his medical condition improves, the consultant will have to diminish this dependency prior to discharge from the hospital.

Working with the staff is frequently more difficult than working with the patient. The staff cannot understand the patient's unpredictability; they are fearful of the overt emotional reactions; distrust and alienation prevail. The consultant's explanation of the source of the patient's fear, guilt, and hostility helps the staff assume a more sympathetic attitude. Follow-up visits assure them that the burden is shared. As a result, they are able to approach the patient with less anxiety.

THE PASSIVE-AGGRESSIVE

This category contains three subtypes which are variations on a single theme, the dependence-independence conflict. According to the balance struck between utter dependency and outright aggressiveness, these subtypes are: 1) the passive-dependent, 2) the passive-aggressive, and 3) the aggressive.

Consultants are now more frequently requested to see patients with passive-aggressive disorders. Difficulties with exact diagnosis persist because the normal is not sharply delineated from the pathological.

THE PASSIVE-DEPENDENT.   These patients are helpless, clinging, and dependent. When their accustomed attachments are severed by illness they appear childlike and resourceless. Or, passivity and dependency may be their main responses to life-threatening illness, for example, those with myocardial infarctions become excessively fearful of any renewed activity during convalescence. Also, dependency is a prominent feature of hospital-oriented patients who view the hospital as a sanctuary. Hospitalization may be their only solution for deteriorated personal relationships.

Although the staff is aware of increased dependency, they usually do not request consultations unless the patient fails to make progress. Then they ask the consultant to "get the patient moving"; the consultant must be supportive. Usually, the dependency is transferred to him as he works with specific fears and provides increased support during critical periods. To avoid drastic overdependency on him alone, the consultant must obtain cooperation from the family, minister, and friends. He should visit the patient regularly. With the staff, he should emphasize the necessity for a consistent approach. Occupational therapy or physical therapy consultations are valuable; they furnish independent activity which gives the patient evidence that he is not helpless.

Psychotherapeutically, the consultant has to do more than merely confront the dependency problem. Underlying fears—of loss of esteem, invalidism, or death—must be discussed.

THE PASSIVE-AGGRESSIVE.   This type of personality disorder is expressed through petulance, procrastination, and lack of cooperation. When these patients are severely ill, their passivity becomes dominant. This passivity is accepted by the staff as normal. However, during convalescence, when they are expected to engage more actively in treatment programs, their aggressive characteristics come to the fore. Their aggressiveness is camouflaged by verbal compliance, and the medical staff does not detect the underlying psychopathology.

Further, these patients' complaints appear in myriad forms so that the medical work-ups involve diagnosis by exclusion. Severe interpersonal difficulties arise as the staff responds with frustration and hostility to the passive-aggressiveness, or when face-saving diagnoses are not found. These patients seldom produce disunity among the staff; they are almost uniformly disliked.

Passive-aggressive patients are not referred until their maneuvers have produced extreme frustration in the staff or until obvious discrepancies between symptomatology and diagnosis appear. Therefore they are generally referred for psychiatric consultations late in the period of hospitalization.

After clarifying the immediate management problems and determining the basic causes for concern, the consultant must alter the treatment program so that the patient, and not the staff, assumes the fundamental responsibility. The consultant must confront the patient with the antitherapeutic effects of his passive-aggressiveness. Demands or restrictions imposed by the staff only serve to increase his passive-aggressive retaliation. Labeling these patients is helpful to the staff because it relieves their uncertainty.

THE INDEPENDENT TYPE. This is a subclassification of the passive-aggressive reaction; however, it appears in such a well-defined form among many patients that it requires special attention. These patients deny their dependency, asserting that they know more about the care they should receive than the attending staff. They derogate the importance of instructions about their care and disregard admonitions to cooperate. Instead, they insist on following their own inclinations, at first in good-natured fashion; but when they are threatened by severe illness or the demands of the staff, they may sign out of the hospital against medical advice. Consultations are requested for these patients only when a management problem flares.

The consultant has no problem identifying these patients. Their denial is apparent; they deny the illness itself. Therefore, confronting them directly with the consequences of their behavior (e.g., its adverse effect on the outcome of the illness) is useless.

The consultant must keep in mind the seriousness of the basic disorder which generates such a drastic defense. When denial is shattered, there may ensue a loss of self-esteem, overwhelming dependency, flagrant hostility, or even personality disorganization.

The consultant must first solve the immediate management problem (e.g., the patient's refusing to remain in bed or insisting on signing out). He must effect a compromise between the patient and the staff so that the patient does not lose face while complying. Asking the patient to cooperate for the sake of the staff, and not for himself alone, is a tactic the consultant can sometimes employ with success. Expressions of personal concern by the staff help. At the same time, the consultant's efforts must be directed beyond the immediate crisis; often, the patient is friendless or worried about his status in the family. Consequently, calling in the family for an interview enables the consultant to mobilize their interests in the patient. Success with these patients depends on helping them maintain their self-esteem which has been jeopardized by the illness.

THE AGGRESSIVE.   Chronic irritability, outbursts of severe aggressiveness, and even destructive behavior identify these patients. The diagnosis may be erroneous when it is not based on careful observations, including serial views of the patient's relationships with situations and individuals over a prolonged period of time.

The patients may openly belittle advice about self-care. When management problems erupt, they are acute; consultations are requested promptly, often on an emergency basis.

The consultant, aware that this reaction has concealed aspects (dependency, yearnings for care and sympathy, and extreme concern about isolation), should respond to the underlying needs for a dependent relationship. He can help the patient feel that he is accepted; then, the emergency subsides. In some situations, the consultant may have to be the patient's "only friend." Their relationship can be used to carry him through the period of hospitalization. This is necessary because usually the interactions with the referring staff are so badly traumatized that it is difficult for them to do more than provide basic care.

THE COMPULSIVE

These patients are rigid, overly concerned with detail, and filled with self-doubt. When they become ill, their compulsive mechanisms for maintaining homeostasis are strained. In the hospital, they are excessively worried by even minor lapses in the hospital routine. Their anxiety mounts; frictions with the staff develop. Consultations are requested when the compulsive defenses fail or, conversely, when compulsive mechanisms are exaggerated to the extent that the staff can no longer meet the patients' demands.

The consultant should not attempt to modify the fundamental personality structure during hospitalization. He should help the overtly anxious patients, whose compulsive defenses are failing, to rebuild them. Encouraging these patients to participate in, and even develop, their own management programs and to set goals for convalescence are useful techniques. When the patient remains helpless, he cannot use his compulsive mechanisms to advantage; therefore activities, e.g., occupational therapy, should be recommended. The consultant must inform the staff about this approach and emphasize their contribution to the treatment program through punctuality, precision, and specific explanations of the reasons for and mechanics of all procedures.

For those patients whose compulsiveness is exaggerated, the consultant must deal with their underlying fears and rely heavily on an empathic relationship to diminish the symptoms. He should explain the compulsive symptomatology to the staff and assure them that it is evanescent.

THE HYSTERICAL PERSONALITY

This is a common personality disorder for which no specific diagnosis is listed in *The Diagnostic and Statistical Manual*, but the consultant may use the code # 000-X5Y Personality Trait Disturbance (Hysterical).

Although this label has been officially discarded, it should still be used in practice; it is descriptive and applicable. The hysterical personality is an overly reactive one, characterized by a thoroughly histrionic quality. Compliance alternates with hostility. The patient communicates with gestures and body language which may contradict verbalizations. The staff has difficulty evaluating complaints or deciding which message is valid. For the referring physician, the problem is complex. For the seductive female who enmeshes the staff in sympathetic involvement psychiatric consultation may not be requested. Generally, however, the pathology is striking; notwithstanding the staff's attempts to cater to demands, a slight lapse of care or faulty response will evoke an irritable or vindictive reaction from the patient. The manipulations, opposing one staff member to another, and the enigmatic communications create irritation, confusion, and hostility in the staff.

Frequently, even the consultant becomes discouraged. Quantitatively, the disturbance is pervasive, and qualitatively, its variability resists formulation. Because the consultation provides another chance for the patient to "go on stage," it is hard to identify the patient's true concerns.

The consultant functions most effectively by: 1) making specific plans to start the patient in long-term psychotherapy. When such plans are established, the intensity of the hysterical response diminishes; the patient realizes something definitive will be done for him, and simultaneously, the staff approach the patient more consistently. 2) visiting the patient. These visits sustain continuity and offer an opportunity for ventilation, an important escape valve for hysterics. 3) defining the personality disturbance for the staff. This relieves anxiety and guilt about their feelings toward the patient.

THE SOCIOPATH

The sociopathic personality disturbances are lifelong behavioral disorders characterized by: 1) the patient's need for immediate gratification of desires, 2) his failure to learn from experience, and 3) his belief that he is not ill—he regards his symptoms as egosyntonic, not ego-alien. The behavioral difficulties appear in childhood or adolescence and continue as fixed patterns in later life. Because this disorder is not distressing to the patient, unless his antisocial activities lead to arrest or other sanctions, he does not seek psychiatric help. Although family and friends at first urge him to obtain counseling, later they "wash their hands of him," and no longer press for rehabilitation.

Physicians in general hospitals only rarely refer sociopaths for consultations. However, referrals from community agencies, particularly custodial and law enforcement agencies, are frequent. When hospitalized, sociopaths are usually cooperative because their needs for attention and care are met. Physicians refer them for psychiatric consultations for only one of three reasons: 1) When the past history reveals a long record of sociopathic behavior, the conscientious physician asks the consultant to determine whether psychotherapy will be beneficial. (These requests are infrequent because the patient conceals his past in a fabric of lies and distortions.) 2) When the patient's demands for unusual types of care (narcotics or special food) precipitate arguments with the staff, immediate management problems arise. Or, 3) when the patient's wish for a face-saving diagnosis or a gratifying treatment plan is unfulfilled, he may lose his calm facade and flare up aggressively.

The consultant's chief task is to establish an accurate diagnosis. The absence of anxiety, the manipulations, and the narcissistic and infantile aspects of the personality (minus a superego) permit rapid diagnosis in the great majority of cases. Pseudo-psychopathic schizophrenia must be ruled out. Sometimes, the older sociopath is psychotic, particularly when brain damage due to trauma or alcoholism is superimposed.

Management entails firmness, setting absolute limits, and rapid clarification of the incident which precipitated the request for consultation. Long-term psychotherapy is seldom helpful.

SEXUAL DEVIATION

In a general hospital, sexually deviant patients are seldom referred to consultants for either diagnosis or treatment. They conceal their sexual histories from their physicians, and the deviancy is masked by the fact of medical illness. The sexual deviation is a way of life, egosyntonic, without the painful and distressing symptoms of neurosis. Freud (1905) said: "Neuroses are, so to say, the negative to perversion." Many of these patients wish to retain their deviant identity, even taking pride in it because it allows membership in what they consider to be an elite group.

Consequently, those few deviants who seek psychotherapy go directly to a psychiatrist and do not take their problems to other physicians.

On those few occasions when consultations in the hospital or clinic are requested, it is because of the following: 1) A physician may wish the psychiatrist to evaluate the advisability of psychotherapy. By determining the patient's capacity for change through psychotherapy, the consultant can furnish the referring physician some guidelines about prognosis. 2) Occasionally, a consultee overreacts when he finds that his patient is a sexual deviant; the patient is referred for "psychiatric attention." The consultant must scrupulously avoid touching on the consultee's turmoil. As simply as possible, he should supply the consultee with specific recommendations for the patient. 3) Very rarely, a patient engages in sexually deviant behavior while hospitalized. When this occurs, the patient is either psychotic or his psychopathic impulses are unusually strong. If he is psychotic, the consultant must first establish the diagnosis, usually an acute brain syndrome or schizophrenia, see PSYCHIATRIC EMERGENCIES, and institute appropriate treatment, see ORGANIC BRAIN SYNDROMES. For the sociopathic patient with poor impulse control, the consultant, in conjunction with the staff and the administration, must define absolute limits restricting further deviant behavior while in the hospital.

REFERENCES

FREUD, S. Three essays on the theory of sexuality. *In* The Complete Psychological Works of Sigmund Freud. London, The Hogarth Press, 1905, Vol. VII, pp. 123–245.

KAHANA, R. J. and BIBRING, G. Personality types in medical management. *In* Zinberg, N. E., ed. Psychiatry and Medical Practice in a General Hospital. New York, International Universities Press, Inc., 1964, pp. 108–122.

KISSEN, D. M. The significance of syndrome shift and late syndrome association in psychosomatic medicine. J. Nerv. Ment. Dis., 136:34, 1963.

SCHWAB, J. J., CLEMMONS, R. S., FREEMON, B. S., and SCOTT, M. L. Problems in psychosomatic diagnosis: II. Severity of medical illness and psychiatric consultations. Psychosomatics, 6:69, 1965.

20 PSYCHIATRIC EMERGENCIES

With the assistance of Leon Marder, M.D.

BACKGROUND

Psychiatric emergencies are defined as urgent conditions which demand immediate action. Recognizing the emergency as such, however, is not always a simple matter. Labeling the patient an emergency depends on the physician's frame of reference, his comprehension of the events which precipitate the need for action, and the patient's physical and psychological condition. Emergency requests for consultation may come from the patient, his relatives, or social agencies, as well as from conventional medical sources such as the emergency room, inpatient unit, or outpatient clinic.

Emergency situations may be classified broadly as 1) those in which death or violence is a potential hazard, 2) those in which there is an acute maladjustment which, when treated properly and quickly, prevents more serious or chronic illness, and 3) those in which the patient's discomfort stimulates him to seek immediate help.

COMMON EMERGENCIES

Ungerleider (1961) analyzed 378 psychiatric emergencies seen by the staff at the University Hospitals in Cleveland. He classified the presenting problems: 1) a psychotic break—20 percent, 2) thoughts of and attempts at suicide—19 percent, 3) severe depressive symptoms—18 percent, 4) anxiety symptoms and somatic symptoms—7 percent each, 5) disorientation or confusion—6 percent, 6) disturbances of consciousness—4 percent, and 7) a miscellaneous group—19 percent (covering a wide range of problems including homicidal thoughts, hyperactivity, alcoholic intoxication, drug requests, bizarre behavior, marital difficulties, and so on). He analyzed the time factor; over one third of the emergencies presented acute problems which arose on the same day the patients were seen; one fifth presented semi-acute problems which had existed for one to seven days; and one tenth presented problems of one week's to one month's duration.

The concept of crisis intervention is particularly applicable to the management of psychiatric emergencies. As used by Lindemann (1956), Klein and Lindemann (1961), and Frankel et al. (1966), the word "crisis" implies a challenge to the patient, family, or community, created by an altered set of circumstances. When the crisis is mastered successfully, the patient has an opportunity for enriching his personality and developing adaptive responses. But Frankel continues: "Failure to meet the challenge results not infrequently in a maladaptive response which . . . [may burden] the personality with a handicap." He also points out two corollaries of crisis intervention: This is an opportune time to interest the patient in seeking help for more fundamental problems, and to strengthen the patient's motivation to enter therapy.

Caring for the psychiatric emergency is one of the major tasks of the consulting psychiatrist, but the number of emergencies varies with the situation in which he works and the service which has been established. When the psychiatrist is on call to the emergency room, especially one which provides care for a large population and encourages patients to seek psychiatric help, many requests will be handled.

We have found, however, that both inpatient and outpatient emergencies are drastically reduced in number when an effective consultation program is in operation. There are fewer inpatient emergencies when the consultant, who has a close relationship with the medical and surgical staff, makes rounds on their services and works regularly in the outpatient clinics in a general hospital. The close liaison resulting from these endeavors forestalls the development of critical situations. Also the medical staff learns how to cope with potential emergencies.

TYPES OF EMERGENCIES

DELIRIUM

This acute brain syndrome is a common psychiatric disorder. The patient suffering from delirium needs prompt and effective treatment; accurate diagnosis and proper management preclude the development of an emergency (see ORGANIC BRAIN SYNDROMES).

SUICIDE

Expressed thoughts of suicide or attempts at suicide are always emergencies; even the "hysterical" patient may succeed in killing himself. Because most suicidal attempts are made by depressed persons, the diagnosis of depression is usually the first important step in preventing suicide. The popular concept that "people who talk about it won't do it" is fallacious. Most suicidal patients ask for help beforehand. Studies (Stoller and Estess, 1960; Pitts and Winokur, 1964) show that the great majority of the people who committed suicide had communicated their intentions to do so to significant people near them and had asked for help, usually in the 24 hours before the suicide.

Many physicians either become excessively anxious about, or too casually dismiss (probably as a defensive maneuver), patients' talk about suicide or unsuccessful attempts. In fact, there is some contempt for the "bungling" of the unsuccessful suicidal patient. But he is the only one the physician sees; the successful one does not require further medical care.

RECOGNIZING THE RISK. Not all suicides can be prevented, even under ideal conditions, but the risk can be lessened by early recognition, close supervision when it is obvious that suicide is possible, and a decisive therapeutic program. Assessing the risk in any depressed patient is mandatory. The danger is greatest with the most seriously depressed, providing the patient is not stuporous. When the patient is in the depth of the depression, he is usually too apathetic to perform the act; the risk is greater when he is going into the trough of the depression or just emerging from it. The sad, smiling individual and the reasoning person who makes calm statements about suicide are the chief suspects.

The depressed patient close to suicide shows many of the typical features of depression: low spirits, apathy, and somatic complaints. It is particularly important to ascertain if this patient views suicide as "the only way out" of the dilemma for which he is seeking a resolution. Also, his problems are frequently realistic and critical; some solution is absolutely necessary. When a patient makes plans for suicide and states that "this is the only solution," the risk is very great.

Suicidal attempts are also made by people with personality disorders characterized by impulsiveness, exhibitionistic trends, and immaturity. The attempt may follow a lover's quarrel, interpersonal or vocational disappointments, or it may be part of a rage state. A mixture of hostility and passivity, anger, and despair is present. Alcohol or drugs are influential because they release impulsiveness and lessen control. Many of these attempts at suicide may be understood by the expression: "You'll be sorry when I'm gone." While some of these attempts at suicide are not life-threatening and are only manipulations, accidental death does occur.

Unfortunately, there are no infallible criteria for estimating the risk of suicide, but the following factors signal increased risk:

1. Definite plans for suicide (making a will or changing the insurance plan).
2. Earlier attempts at suicide.
3. Family history of suicide.
4. A feeling of rejection—when the patient feels he is no longer of any use, or when he lacks an occupation.
5. A markedly anxious tone to the depressive picture with sudden attacks of anxiety and acute worsening of the depression.
6. Too rapid, superficial improvement following drugs or E.C.T.
7. Isolation, loneliness, and uprooting—the prospect of having to live with few human contacts.
8. Increased hostility.
9. No religious ties or loss of faith in higher values.
10. Financial worries—the threat of bankruptcy, loss of earning power and savings.
11. Alcoholism and drug addiction.
12. Severe, painful, physical illness with prolonged sleep disturbance.

MANAGEMENT OF SUICIDAL PATIENTS. There is one principle basic to the management of suicidal patients: *Something of an active, constructive nature must be done for the patient at once.* Usually, this means hospitalization with supervision. When it is not possible to hospitalize the patient, other resources must be mobilized immediately. At these times, the family, a friend, or the minister should be called in to assist the patient with the problem and provide supervision, care, and comfort so that he is under direct observation until a more definitive approach to his illness can be developed. It is necessary for the psychiatrist to inform these other people that the risk of suicide is great and that they are undertaking a serious obligation in agreeing to stay with the patient and supervise his activities. Nevertheless, when the patient sees this demonstrable evidence that others are interested in him and will care for him, the likelihood of suicide diminishes.

Hospitalization usually suspends the risk, but not always, particularly if the suicidal impulse is very great, if there is serious medical illness, or if there is some clouding of the sensorium. Accordingly, hospitalization must include a thorough medical evaluation as well as psychiatric intervention. Many of these patients need continued observation while they are in the hospital; suicide precautions should be instituted. These precautions are:

1. The patient's room should be located near the nursing station and away from stairwells and elevators. The windows should be of safety glass or covered with protective screening. The furniture in the bedroom and the bathroom should be fixed and simplified so the patient cannot use any piece for self-destruction.

2. Constant observation by a member of the nursing staff or the family is essential. When this is not possible, placing the patient in a room with others helps.

3. The patient's personal belongings should be removed completely. Items like belts and coat hangers are particularly dangerous.

4. Everything brought into the room (gifts, the food tray, toilet articles) should be thoroughly inspected.

5. Adequate sedation should be administered.

Continued psychiatric care is necessary for these patients. They need a supportive environment which helps them replenish their resources for struggling with the problems of life. However, one of the most crucial aspects of their care, in the hospital or outside, is the continued support and encouragement they receive from others. When the patient realizes that he does not stand alone and that others do not view his problems as insurmountable, his desire to live rather than to die is strengthened.

Obviously, if the patient is seriously depressed, specific treatment is required. E.C.T., antidepressant medications, and individual psychotherapy are part of both the immediate and long-range program.

ACUTE EXCITEMENTS

The acutely excited, disruptive, and possibly violent patient is obviously difficult to manage. The differential diagnosis includes: 1) acute alcoholic intoxication, 2) intoxication produced by medications, singly or in combinations, 3) acute psychogenic disorders (the manic phase of the manic-depressive illness, a rage state, or acute catatonic excitement), and 4) various organic syndromes. The frequency of head trauma in alcoholics complicates diagnosis. Every patient must be examined for evidence of cranial trauma, and particularly for extradural or subdural hemorrhage.

THE ALCOHOLIC. *Diagnosis.* In addition to the history, important diagnostic signs are: odor of alcohol, flushing, the alcoholic tongue, and abdominal tenderness over the liver.

When these signs are not obvious, the frequently overlooked syndrome, acute pathologic intoxication, should always be suspected. This syndrome is a basic disorder of the C.N.S., probably a form of psychomotor epilepsy. A limited amount of alcohol, even one or two drinks, precipitates acute excitement, impulsiveness, aggressiveness, and amnesia for the episode. Treatment for acute pathologic intoxication must be directed toward the underlying neurologic problem and entails complete abstinence.

Management. Hospitalization, bed rest, and simple, calming contact with these patients helps to quiet them. Sometimes a soothing tub should be used. As an alternative, chlordiazepoxide-HCl (Librium), 50 to 100 mg intramuscularly is effective. The most commonly used medication is paraldehyde, 10 to 15 ml orally or 8 to 10 ml intramuscularly. Barbiturates are contraindicated because of their adverse effects in combination with alcohol. Treatment also includes intravenous fluids, vitamins, and specific medications as indicated.

Drug Intoxication. Excitement is produced by drugs, especially combinations of stimulants (amphetamines) and sedatives (barbiturates). Unless the consultant can obtain a history of drug usage from the patient or relatives, he may easily confuse the excitement with that due to other causes. Searching the patient and his effects helps to clarify the diagnosis. The possibility of concurrent medical illness must always be kept in mind.

Management. Hospitalization is necessary in order to separate the patient from his family or friends whose responses (derived from underlying conflicts) are contributing to the excitement. Gastric lavage is indicated, although frequently the drugs have already left the stomach. The patient should be observed for several hours to determine whether a stuporous or comatose condition is developing. The consultant must be cautious about prescribing any further medications. But after the direction of the reaction is ascertained, and after the patient's medical condition is evaluated, medications such as paraldehyde or a phenothiazine can be used for sedation (see APPENDIX D—MEDICATIONS).

The Acute Psychogenic Reactions. The excitatory phase or the frenzy accompanying an acute psychotic break may appear in the earlier stages of any of the following illnesses: acute undifferentiated schizophrenic reaction, manic excitement, acute paranoid reaction (when the patient is turning on his imagined persecutors), or catatonic excitement.

A rage state may be seen in a sociopath as a result of frustration (see DIFFERENTIAL DIAGNOSIS).

Management. Immediate hospitalization reduces stimuli and protects these patients from themselves and others. Hospital management does not necessitate the use of restraints or even isolation. Instead, a quiet room with a structured environment suffices, particularly when care is administered by a nurse who is accustomed to working with excited patients (see prescription for THE STRUCTURED ENVIRONMENT below).

When there is active resistance, the consultant should summon the aid of trained personnel to help move the patient to quiet quarters in the hospital; he should not attempt to do this alone.

Medications, in large doses, are required. After a test dose of 25 mg of chlorpromazine (Thorazine) is given, the dosage should be increased to 100 mg intramuscularly every two to four hours until the excitement subsides (see MEDICATIONS).

The Structured Environment.

1. A protected single room (safety glass or screen) with no decorations (remove pictures from walls); furniture should be simple and functional (unsuitable for violence to self or others).

2. Locate room near nursing station, but away from stairwells, elevators, and noise.

3. Reduce stimuli: no television or radio. Keep procedures to a minimum.

4. Soft, diffuse 24-hour lighting which eliminates shadows.

5. Keep one person (nurse, attendant, or close relative) with patient at all times. Change personnel as infrequently as possible.

6. Specific, concrete explanations to the patient.

7. No visitors.

ORGANIC SYNDROMES. Moderate to severe excitement occurs with some organic illnesses, particularly in certain phases of both acute and chronic brain syndromes. Immediate medical evaluation is essential. Head injuries, metabolic disorders (e.g., hyperthyroid crisis), toxic or febrile conditions, and epileptic states may produce agitation and severe excitement. Management hinges on skillful medical treatment and the principles which are outlined in THE ORGANIC BRAIN SYNDROMES.

THE ACUTE PSYCHOTIC REACTIONS

THE MANIC-DEPRESSIVE PSYCHOSIS. The manic-depressive psychosis is a primary mood disorder with resulting disturbances of thought and behavior. Fluctuations of mood with overenthusiasm and easy disappointment characterize the prepsychotic period. Because the patient uses personal relationships for his own gains, with little understanding of the needs of others, he meets rejection. A vicious cycle is set in motion; his demands on others increase leading to further rejection and disappointment, which in turn makes him more demanding. Such conflicts interfere with his functioning. Then the patient will swing like a pendulum either to the manic phase (in which he exults in an orgy of grandiose self-assertiveness, using mechanisms of denial to overcome guilt), or to the depressive phase (in which his rage and guilt make him feel unworthy, unloved, and fit only for self-destruction).

Management. For the manic patient, emergency hospitalization is mandatory. His irrational and impulsive behavior endangers others as well as himself. Firmness, coupled with sympathy and tolerance, is the correct psychotherapeutic approach. Medications have supplanted E.C.T. as the treatment of choice. The consultant should recommend a phenothiazine, in large dosage, e.g., chlorpromazine (Thorazine) 600 to 1,000 mg per day. Lithium is now considered by many to be the medication of choice. Dosage is 3 to 6 lithium carbonate tabs (each corresponding to 8 mEq of lithium) per day. Check blood at least weekly to attain and maintain plasma level of 1.5 to 2.5 mEq per liter. Higher levels cause toxicity. Renal insufficiency or cardiac disease are contraindications. (See Malitz, S., and Wharton, R.: "Lithium in Manic-Depressive Psychosis," in *American Handbook of Psychiatry, Vol. III*, ed. by Arieti, S., pp. 509–511, 1966). But, somatic therapies such as E.C.T. or sleep therapy should be employed if the patient does not respond to medication within two to three days. Intensive psychotherapy should be continued concomitantly with any somatic therapy. Occasionally the patient swings suddenly from mania to severe depression; here the risk of suicide is great.

ACUTE SCHIZOPHRENIC REACTIONS. The acute schizophrenic episode is a crisis situation. Repressed conflicts of many years erupt. Hallucinations may command the patient to suicide or homicide. Or, there may be panic and confusion as the patient attempts to distinguish between external reality and his inner impulses. Patterns of behavior and mood vary widely as he responds to instinctual forces and utilizes psychotic defenses. At one moment he may appear reasonable; at the next he is antagonistic and suspicious of all attempts to control or help him.

Management. The management of the acutely disturbed schizophrenic patient requires hospitalization for safety, as well as to reduce the likelihood or intensity of chronicity. A therapeutic milieu with a structured environment is obligatory. Phenothiazines, such as chlorpromazine (Thorazine), in large dosage, 600 to 1,200 mg per day, furnish emergency control (see MEDICATIONS).

PARANOIA AND THE PARANOID STATES. The term "paranoid" is commonly used to describe suspiciousness as a character trait. But the truly paranoid patient reveals systematized delusions of persecution. The delusions are seldom bizarre; instead, they are related to everyday matters: marital infidelity, social injustices, or plots against life and fortune. The possibility of violence is always present; it is difficult to evaluate and can only be estimated in terms of the history of previous reactions to frustrations. A more passive person, unused to violence, is less likely to be homicidal than one whose reaction pattern has been overtly aggressive.

Emergency management is identical to that described above for the acute schizophrenic patient. Because of the danger of homicide, special care must be taken to restrict visiting privileges.

POSTPARTUM PSYCHOSIS. The diagnosis "postpartum psychosis" is applied descriptively to a group of acute psychotic reactions. These take several forms, appearing as a delirium, a schizophrenic reaction, or more commonly, as a psychotic depression. They occur in some women as early as five to six days after childbirth and in others as much as three to four months later. Even in the milder cases, there is depression and some degree of personality disorganization as evidenced by a change in habits (a previously neat and tidy woman becomes careless and sloppy). In the more severe cases, elements of the psychotic reaction are closely related to parturition. Common manifestations are rank indifference toward the baby, excessive ruminations, delusions, hallucinations, and verbalized fears of harming the child.

Management. Immediate psychiatric hospitalization is a must. Because of the severity of the reaction and because its dynamics involve guilt about childbirth, there is always danger that the distraught mother will harm the child and herself. Definitive treatment depends on the consultant's specific diagnosis, usually depression or schizophrenia.

THE HOMICIDAL PATIENT

There were 8,122 homicides in the United States in 1958. Although many of the murderers were seen by psychiatrists after they were jailed, it is believed that very few ever discussed their plans with psychiatrists beforehand, or were in psychotherapy immediately prior to the act. In fact, there is very little in the psychiatric literature about the potential murderer.

Some statistics on this subject (MacDonald, 1961) indicate that most murders happen at a particular time of the day, day of the week, and season of the year. Most are committed at night, especially between 8 p.m. Saturday night and 2 a.m. Sunday morning. More than 50 percent occur on Saturdays and Sundays, and many are committed on holidays. More murders occur in the summer than in the winter, and most take place in the home, rather than on the streets or in public places.

Sociocultural factors are important. Males murder five times as frequently as females; most murderers are between the ages of 30 and 35 (younger than their victims); Negroes murder more often than do Caucasians; and most murderers come from the lower socioeconomic strata of society.

The developmental history of the murderer is usually characterized by emotional deprivation, family pathology, and cruelty. A pathognomonic triad has been described: bed wetting, fire setting, and cruelty to animals. Most murderers have abnormal electroencephalograms.

The victim has a statistically greater chance of being killed by a member of his family than by a stranger. Some people are "victim prone" just as others are "accident prone"; they may set up their own murders by tormenting or challenging the aggressors. Depressed persons may be seeking punishment, and thus become victims; or masochists may invite the aggression which leads to murder.

The risk of homicide is great if there is evidence of: 1) psychosis with a thought disorder characterized by a persecutory delusional system, 2) a previous record of violence, 3) sexual conflict, rivalry, and jealousy, 4) a hatred of authority, 5) recent brooding, moodiness, and withdrawal, 6) obvious sociopathy, 7) alcoholism or drug effect.

Regardless of this patient's appearance—usually a rage state, but occasionally a deceptively quiet paranoid expression—any evidence of homicidal intent is always an emergency. Most murderers are either paranoid schizophrenics, or conscienceless sociopaths.

Management. The consultant must arrange for immediate hospitalization or emergency custodial care. Ascertaining who the intended victim is and safeguarding that person are not sufficient; the psychotic may change quickly and his delusional system may vary so that even a casual bystander becomes the victim.

1. Set firm limits.
2. Mobilize community resources.

3. Separate the patient from family members.

4. Always keep in mind that the homicidal patient is also suicidal.

THE ACUTELY DISTURBED PSYCHONEUROTIC REACTIONS

As an emergency, the acutely disturbed psychoneurotic patient exhibits one of the following: 1) acute, overwhelming anxiety, with phobias and panic, or somatic manifestations, or both (e.g., hyperventilation syndrome); 2) a conversion reaction; or 3) a dissociative reaction. Differential diagnosis is not difficult, but the consultant should search for associated organic illness.

ANXIETY REACTIONS.   The patient suffering from severe anxiety tells the consultant readily of his extreme fears which are usually focused on his body. The psychophysiologic concomitants of anxiety are manifold. In addition to nervousness and extreme tremulousness, these patients complain of bizarre sensations, dry mouth, difficulties with respiration, pain in the chest, abdominal distress and so on (see ANXIETY).

Management.   Management requires an immediate medical work-up and rapport with the patient. Most of these patients respond to reassurance concerning their medical condition, particularly when informed that they will be taken care of. Their anxiety diminishes even before diagnostic procedures, such as obtaining an electrocardiogram, are completed.

Rapport enables the patient to reveal his fears and the consultant to discuss definite plans for psychotherapy. This is crucial because the emergency increases the patient's motivation for getting help, and also psychotherapy is more effective if instituted before these reactions become patterned and chronic. The consultant should provide antianxiety medications for the severely anxious patient (see MEDICATIONS).

CONVERSION REACTIONS.   *Diagnosis.*   Diagnosing the acute conversion reaction may be extremely difficult. Even the so-called classical reaction may mask a neurologic lesion, and elements of the conversion reaction may be complicated by organic illness. Exact diagnosis can be made only after the patient has a definitive neurological evaluation and after sufficient time elapses for the consultant to understand the course of the illness. Diagnosis of conversion reaction should *never* be made by exclusion.

The symptoms are divided into three groups: 1) hyperactivity or excessive function as tics, seizures, uncontrollable movements of various parts of the body and so on; 2) loss of function by paralysis, anesthesia, or sensory loss such as hysterical blindness; and 3) pain. The symptoms usually defy accepted anatomic and physiologic limits. The choice of the symptom symbolizes the conflict and also provides a temporary solution for it. Additionally, there is secondary gain, and the patient displays "la belle indifference."

Classically, these reactions occur in patients with hysterical personalities, but it is important to note that conversion reactions are seen in other personality types and in the depressed (Chodoff, 1954). Also, the conversion reaction may be the schizophrenic patient's last-ditch defense against a complete breakdown.

Every consultant should read "Contemporary Conversion Reactions: a clinical study (Ziegler et al., 1960, 1962).

Management. Management involves a go-slow approach. These patients should be hospitalized for diagnostic evaluation. The consultant should not focus his efforts on removing the symptoms; too often, when a symptom is removed by active measures (confrontation or hypnosis), it is supplanted by another symptom(s) of greater severity, or an underlying schizophrenic process emerges.

The consultant should support the patient and assure him that the symptoms will gradually disappear. Employing face-saving measures (e.g., physical therapy for the "paralyzed" limb) enables the patient to relinquish the symptom after a week or two. During the course of the medical work-up, the consultant has an unusual opportunity to explore the patient's personal history and current life situation in order to define areas of conflict which can be approached psychotherapeutically. Medications are usually unnecessary and, indeed, may be contraindicated because they reinforce the belief that the symptom is medically, not situationally, determined. The "magic" attributed to medications blends with the patient's psychopathology while more reality-bound measures such as physical therapy do not.

DISSOCIATIVE REACTIONS. The dissociative reaction is a severe personality disturbance. It may appear as amnesia, a fugue state, a twilight state, or it may simulate delirium. Extreme cases show panic; for all practical purposes, the patient is acutely psychotic. Depersonalization and dissociation occur. The severity of the symptomatology is an index of the seriousness of the basic illness, for example, somnambulism has a better prognosis than depersonalization. The possibility of neurologic disease such as trauma, brain tumor, or encephalitis must always be kept in mind.

The immediate management program is similar to that outlined for the conversion reaction. But medications, such as phenothiazines or a sedative, are usually needed (see MEDICATIONS). Obviously, plans for long-term psychiatric treatment should be made while the patient is in the hospital or the emergency room.

THE "SUITCASE SYNDROME"—SIGNING OUT AGAINST MEDICAL ADVICE

These patients complain either that the physician is not giving them adequate medical care or, conversely, that he overestimates the seriousness of their illnesses. The former group derogate the care they are receiving and provoke active hostility from the staff. Then they can state that their grievances are real and that they are justified in signing out of the hospital. With uncanny accuracy, they find flaws in the hospital procedures (e.g., having to wait for x-rays, and so on). The latter group is more psychiatrically ill. To preserve their defenses, they use denial to minimize the seriousness of their medical illnesses and prognoses. Or, sometimes, they cannot tolerate the passivity and dependency required for convalescence.

When the psychiatric consultant receives this emergency call, the staff wants him to 1) dissuade the patient from leaving the hospital, or 2) make sure that the patient has willingly consented to sign the appropriate papers releasing them from responsibility. When the consultant gets to the patient's room, he finds the suitcase packed and the patient ready to leave. In all of these cases there has been a failure between the staff and the patient to arrive at consensus about the severity of the illness and about the necessary treatment.

Management. The consultant must work directly with the patient to achieve a compromise by employing face-saving measures which allow the patient to stay in the hospital and maintain his dignity. Then, the consultant has to determine to what extent he should confront the patient's excessive denial. Premature confrontation may either shatter his defenses (resulting in psychosis) or strengthen his denial.

The consultant's work with the staff may be equally difficult. When the situation has deteriorated so that the patient is leaving the hospital, the staff is usually ambivalent; on one hand, they are concerned about his condition, on the other, they are glad to be rid of a troublesome patient. The consultant must interpret the patient's behavior to the staff so that they can deal with it as an illness.

REFERENCES

CHODOFF, P. Re-examination of some aspects of conversion hysteria. Psychiatry, 17:75, 1954.
FRANKEL, F. H., CHAFETZ, M. E., and HOWARD, T. B. The treatment of psychosocial crises in the emergency service of a general hospital. J.A.M.A., 195(8):626, 1966.

KLEIN, D. C., and LINDEMANN, E., Preventive intervention in individual and family cirsis situations. *In* Caplan, G., ed. Prevention of Mental Disorders in Children. New York, Basic Books, Inc., Publishers, 1961, pp. 283–306.

LINDEMANN, E. The meaning of crisis in individual and family living. Teachers College Rec., 57:310, 1956.

MacDONALD, J. M. The Murderer and His Victim. Springfield, Ill., Charles C Thomas, Publisher, 1961.

MALITZ, S., and WHARTON, R. Lithium in manic-depressive psychosis. *In* Arieti, S., ed. American Handbook of Psychiatry, III. 1966, pp. 509–511.

PITTS, F. N. and WINOKUR, G. Affective disorder, III.: Diagnostic correlates and incidence of suicide. J. Nerv. Ment. Dis., 139:176, 1964.

STOLLER, R. S., and ESTESS, F. M. Suicide in medical and surgical wards of general hospitals. J. Chronic Dis., 15:592, 1960.

UNGERLEIDER, J. T. The psychiatric emergency, analysis of six month's experience of a university hospital's consultation service. Arch. Gen. Psychiat. (Chicago), 3:593, 1961.

ZIEGLER, FREDERICK, IMBODEN, JOHN, and MEYER, EUGENE, "Contemporary conversion reactions: A clinical study." Amer. J. Psychiat., 116:901–910, 1960.

ZIEGLER, FREDERICK and IMBODEN, JOHN, "Contemporary conversion reactions." Arch. Gen. Psychiat., 6:279–287, 1962.

21　ORGANIC BRAIN SYNDROMES

Where have I been? Where am I?—Fair daylight?—
I am mightily abused—I should e'en die with pity,
To see another thus.—I know not what to say.—
I will not swear these are my hands: let's see;
I feel this pin prick. Would I were assured
Of my condition.

. . . .

I fear I am not in my perfect mind.
Methinks I should know you, and know this man;
Yet I am doubtful: for I am mainly ignorant
What place this is; and all the skill I have
Remembers not these garments; nor I know not
Where I did lodge last night.

King Lear IV, vii

BACKGROUND

During the last 25 years, psychiatrists turned their attention toward psychodynamics and psychotherapy, away from the organic brain syndromes. But now this shift is causing concern. First, more and more patients are suffering from the organic brain syndromes. And second, consultants are noting physicians' errors in diagnosis. In a review of 600 consecutive psychiatric consultations, Reding and Daniels (1964) found that 10 percent of the patients suffered from organic brain syndromes and that in 50 percent of this group the correct diagnosis had not been made by the referring physician. They listed common reasons for difficulties with diagnosis: 1) an incomplete mental status examination, 2) inattention to nurses' notes, 3) failure to question relatives about recent changes in the patient's behavior, 4) a tendency to overemphasize psychodynamic factors, 5) the absence of a sharp borderline between the manifestations of aging and a pathological syndrome, 6) the physician's anxiety, and 7) failure to give proper emphasis to EEG changes, particularly decreased alpha frequency.

Reding and Daniels state that early diagnosis has distinct advantages: 1) It institutes prompt treatment for the reversible cases, 2) it alerts the staff to the possibility of a patient's unexpected behavior, and 3) it provides an indicator of the course and the risk of procedures.

Patients with organic brain syndromes have poorer prognoses than other general medical patients. Considering only first admissions to Barnes Hospital, St. Louis, Guze and Cantwell (1964) reported the mortality rate for patients with organic brain syndromes was 17 percent compared with the general rate of 3.7 percent. Age was not the major factor accounting for this increased mortality; 13 percent of the patients under the age of 50 with organic brain syndromes died. Other studies (Corsellis, 1962 and Stewart et al., 1962) indicate that when the organic brain syndrome is encountered, it is of serious import.

Most of our current understanding of organic brain disease is based on the work of Hughlings Jackson (1958) and Kurt Goldstein (1959). Jackson conceptualized the central nervous system as hierarchically arranged so that when there is loss of function at one level, function of the next lower level then emerges, unrestrained by the integrating and inhibiting influences of the higher centers. Jackson (1958) stated that organic brain disorders produce both negative and positive symptoms: negative ones due to a loss of function, and positive ones that develop as other structures or functions compensate for the loss. For example, symptoms such as hallucinations and delusions "represent the survival of the patient's then fittest state." Goldstein (1959) advanced Jackson's concepts, stressing that the loss of the abstract attitude is the basic lesion in organic brain disease. These conceptualizations are fundamental for an understanding of both the acute and the chronic syndromes.

ACUTE BRAIN SYNDROMES (DELIRIUM)

Delirium, the acute brain syndrome, is one of the most common psychiatric illnesses. It occurs as a frequent reaction to a wide variety of primary disease processes. Throughout history, it has been known as a complication of infectious diseases, metabolic disorders, and cardiovascular illnesses, as well as a reaction to drug withdrawal, intoxication, trauma and surgery. The presence of delirium always indicates diffuse biochemical or structural impairment of brain-tissue function.

The clinical picture is the result of two sets of factors, the causative and the personality. It is always dangerous to specify a single etiologic factor. Berblinger (1962) states that there is no other psychiatric syndrome in which multiple etiologic factors are so important.

Lack of sleep and sensory deprivation are contributory causes. The variety of tranquilizers and sedatives available to the public today is a further complication which interferes with precise diagnosis. Also, drug combinations (of tranquilizers, sedatives, antispasmodics, or steroids) obscure etiologic exactness. In one study, Guze and Cantwell (1964) found that drugs were responsible for 20 percent of the cases of delirium in medical patients. The superimposed effect of drugs on other contributing factors may be critical. Thus, a combination of etiologic agents upsets an already precarious balance. In many cases, dehydration and electrolyte imbalance are also fundamental causes. Diuretics, now commonly used by many people for various reasons, have recently been added to the list of causes of delirium (Wohlrabe et al., 1965).

Because the onset of delirium is gradual, the predelirium stage frequently passes unrecognized. The course is progressive, and unless treatment is vigorous and adequate, death may result. Delirium is seen most often in elderly medical patients, particularly those with circulatory disturbances affecting the C.N.S., and those who have been taking moderate or large amounts of alcohol, sedatives, or drugs prior to hospitalization. In surgical patients, delirium usually develops as a withdrawal reaction three to five days post-operatively, or in the early stages of recovery from trauma.

Variations in development and susceptibility are due to the patient's individual capacity to withstand stress. Some people develop delirium easily; others are quite resistant. The very young and the very old are more susceptible because their homeostatic mechanisms are more fragile.

In the 19th century, a characteristic clinical picture was outlined for each causative agent producing delirium; minute variations of the delirium syndrome were described in endless detail. For example, dark-colored hallucinations were attributed to morphine intoxication, bright-colored ones to bromides, and micronopsia to alcoholism. However, Bonhoeffer's classic study (1908) demonstrated the essential uniformity of the delirious reaction, regardless of etiology. Hoch (1912) substantiated Bonhoeffer's findings and confirmed that no specific noxious agent produced a singular, defined reaction. Wolff and Curran (1935) studied 106 delirious patients and found no evidence of a specific relationship between a particular etiologic agent and either the form or the content of the resultant disturbance. Engel and Romano (1959) draw attention to the basic similarity of all delirium by terming it "a syndrome of cerebral insufficiency." As a result of these studies, scientific interest in the fine discrimination of delirious symptomatology has diminished.

Some variability in the clinical picture, of course, is determined by the patient's emotional state, previous personality adjustment, and repressed feelings. For example, a delirious alcoholic's repressed homosexuality may emerge in an exaggerated manner. Thus, the content of the delirium, to some extent, reflects the patient's conflicts and his personality structure.

DIAGNOSIS

The early diagnosis of delirium hinges on finding a changed state of consciousness. An altered state of consciousness is a sign as objective as the color of the skin in jaundice or the chest contour in emphysema. Depression of consciousness to stupor or coma is readily apparent, but the diagnosis of lesser changes requires a careful mental status examination.

Intellectually, capacities for attention, concentration, and endurance are diminished, and abstract thinking is impaired. Simple calculations are done poorly. However, Engel and Romano (1959) state that the number of errors up to three in the serial seven's is less important than the manner in which the patient does the test; the observer should note irritability, obvious strain, delay, and the like.

Emotionally, instinctual drives are expressed overtly because of decreased control. The affect is usually sad or labile.

Neorologically, the purposeless movements are similar to those seen with cerebral lesions which involve release from higher cortical inhibitions. Reflexes are brisk or unchanged.

Serial EEGs are helpful in establishing the diagnosis. In delirium, the changes are diffuse, thus differentiating it from the focal changes produced by a brain tumor or a cerebral thrombosis. Diffuse slowing to six to eight per second frequency is an early sign; as the delirium deepens the frequency will decrease progressively, even within 24 hours. As the patient improves, the frequency returns to normal.

Differential diagnosis includes depression, the aging process, and the acute undifferentiated schizophrenic reaction. Precise diagnosis thus depends on a history which gathers information about the patient's behavior during the preceding days and weeks. The influence of multiple etiologic factors must always be kept in mind.

SYMPTOMATOLOGY

The symptomatology is divided into distinct stages:

STAGE I—PREDELIRIUM. This stage is difficult to diagnose; only the subtle and discriminate functions are impaired. Predelirium is characterized by apprehenison and restlessness, not outright fear and agitation; but, to a sensitive observer, the patient looks anxious. Examination of the sleep pattern has particular value for early diagnosis; the sleep is both intermittent and poor in quality; continued sleep deprivation leads to full-blown delirium. Very slight disorientation is present intermittently, but may not be obvious because it is only in the temporal dimension. The patient knows where he is and who he is, but he is unsure about the exact time of day, or he does not perceive the passage of time accurately (Pollack et al., 1965). For example, although the nurse was in the patient's room only ten minutes before, he may say that several hours have elapsed since he saw her last. The patient has difficulty grasping the exact meaning and the importance of the doctors' and nurses' communications. He betrays his apprehension by interrupting their conversations with him to ask fearfully how he is getting along. Temperature, pulse. and respiration may be elevated.

STAGE II—EARLY DELIRIUM. This stage is characterized by outright fear, increased motor restlessness, and obvious signs of anxiety: tachycardia, dilated pupils, and manifest excitement. The sleep pattern is grossly disturbed, and fluid and food intake are insufficient. There is disorientation in time, but not usually in place. (Disorientation is found in over 80 percent of all cases of delirium; it occurs first in the sense of time and next in place, while disorientation for person is the last to appear, and then only in the advanced stages.) The patient may have intermittent periods of lucidity which obscure precise diagnosis. His general physical condition is deteriorating. Temperature, pulse, and respiration are abnormal.

STAGE III—FRANK DELIRIUM. The patient is obviously confused; there is disorientation as to time and place. Fear is manifest, agitation is rampant, and the patient is uncooperative. Hallucinations and delusions are common. Misinterpretations involve the immediate surroundings: mistaking the window for a door, or the bedcovers for everyday clothing. Although hallucinations of all types occur, visual hallucinations are most common. Auditory hallucinations are about 50 percent as common as visual, while tactile and olfactory hallucinations are the rarest. Confabulation is found in 15 percent of the cases; it usually consists of simple elaborations about leaving the hospital. The delusions and misinterpretations are poorly organized and readily forgotten. Fear of torture or of being killed is the most frequent of these misinterpretations; panic may lead to suicide as the patient attempts to escape. His physical condition is worsening.

STAGE IV—IMPENDING EXHAUSTION.   The patient's condition is deteriorated. He displays occasional bouts of frenzy but generally is quieter, only because of exhaustion. Establishing contact with the patient is extremely difficult. The pulse is weak and thready and there are neurologic signs: ataxia, slurred speech, tremors, and abrupt convulsions. This stage may be irreversible.

STAGE V—STUPOR.   The deterioration is marked. Coma may be interrupted by convulsions. Usually, the patient dies.

The consulting psychiatrist, working with other physicians, has the opportunity to help with diagnosis in two ways: First, by calling attention to the predelirium stage when prompt treatment obviates severe management problems; and second, by detecting a particular type of patient, seen more frequently in the last few years, whose clinical picture is perplexing to all physicians. A typical case history follows:

A young or middle-aged person presents a number of complaints of recent onset which simulate a neurologic disorder: ataxia, weakness, slightly slurred speech, visual complaints, and headache. Examination reveals signs which are difficult to evaluate: a little fever, slight pupillary inequality, unequal reflexes, and transient episodes of mild confusion. The clinical picture changes every few hours; at one time the patient appears cooperative and is not confused, at another time he is less cooperative and looks more ill. The differential diagnosis includes encephalitis, brain tumor, systemic disease, or a degenerative neurologic disorder. The patient appears to be in the very early stage of delirium.

Repeatedly, in these cases, careful history-taking from a family member or a search of the patient's personal effects will reveal overdosage or misuse of various drugs, singly or in combinations. In fact, drug misuse is the first thing we think of when patients show this bizarre clinical picture which continues to defy any exact diagnosis.

Close cooperation between consultants and other physicians increases the effectiveness of treatment programs.

GUIDELINES FOR MANAGEMENT

1. Evaluate the patient's general condition by a physical examination and a mental status examination (orientation as to time, place, and person; simple arithmetic; and so on) to determine the precise stage. This should be noted to gauge change.

2. Review all orders and discontinue every medication and procedure not absolutely essential.

3. Search for causes. The most common possibilities include: infections (pneumonia, g. u. tract, wound); cardiovascular diseases with diminished cardiac reserve (impending congestive failure, thrombosis, pulmonary embolism); metabolic disorders (nitrogen retention, electrolyte imbalance, dehydration); diseases of, or trauma to, the CNS (convulsive disorder, intracranial neoplasm, subdural hematoma); intoxications (sensitivity to medications, alcohol). Electrolyte imbalance, dehydration, and vitamin deficiency may underlie any or all of the above causes. Always suspect that drugs or alcohol may have been taken prior to hospitalization, and search the patient's personal belongings.

TREATMENT

1. Explain all procedures to the patient in simple terms. Keep one person (nurse, attendant, or relative) with the patient at all times. Change personnel as infrequently as possible. Repeated reassurance, stated concretely and specifically, is essential.

2. Protect the patient from suicide: remove sharp instruments, peg the windows, observe the exit from the room. Avoid restraints if at all possible.

3. Keep light on at all times. Delirium is worse at twilight or at night. Place lights so that unusual shadows do not appear.

4. Simplify the environment. Remove pictures or unfamiliar apparatus from the room; they lead to illusions. Bring in familiar objects from the home if necessary (see STRUCTURED ENVIRONMENT IN PSYCHIATRIC EMERGENCIES).

5. Medications: a) Phenothiazines are the medications of choice, orally if possible. Immediately give chlorpromazine (Thorazine) 25 mg at once orally or intramuscularly and observe closely for signs of hypotension. Keep patient in bed. Check vital signs every 10 to 15 minutes for one to two hours. If there are no adverse reactions within 45 minutes, give an additional 50 mg orally or intramuscularly. Repeat dose in two more hours, and thereafter give 50 to 75 mg orally every three hours, or 25 to 50 mg intramuscularly every three to four hours. The patient should show improvement in 8 to 12 hours; then, 50 to 75 mg of chlorpromazine

should be given every four to six hours. Maintenance dose is 200 to 500 mg daily for five to seven days; then gradually reduce. Avoid sedatives, particularly barbiturates; they increase the patient's problem with perception and understanding, and their action is potentiated by phenothiazines. Do not use epinephrine. If a vasoconstrictor is needed, use levarterenol (Levophed), remembering that it counteracts phenothiazine action.

(b) If chlorpromazine is contraindicated or not tolerated because of its epileptogenic qualities or because of liver damage, use perphenazine (Trilafon); it may be preferred anyway. Dosage is 5 mg intramuscularly repeated in three to four hours, and then 4 to 8 mg orally or intramuscularly every six hours for three more doses. Maintenance dose for four to five more days is 12 to 20 mg per day, then taper off for three to four days. Thioridazine (Mellaril), in the same dose as chlorpromazine, is another alternative. Precautions for all phenothiazines are the same.

(c) Chlordiazepoxide-HCl (Librium) 50 to 100 mg parenterally every four to six hours for three doses may be a satisfactory substitute if phenothiazines are contraindicated. Do not give more than 300 mg in a 24 hour period. Maintenance dose is 25 to 50 mg every six hours for three to four days; then reduce gradually. If there is not a favorable response in 12 hours, switch to phenothiazine.

6. Maintain adequate nourishment. Intravenous fluids are usually necessary to correct the electrolyte imbalance and dehydration, but all procedures and instrumentation should be kept to an absolute minimum. Encourage nourishing liquids every hour when the patient is awake.

7. Give vitamins, orally if possible. Otherwise, give Bejectal w/Vitamin C, 2 ml intramuscularly or in the intravenous fluids. Repeat for several days. Maintain on vitamins for at least one or two months.

8. Restore adequate perception by a hearing aid, glasses, and so on. Diminished perceptual acuity contributes to delirium.

9. Treat constipation with cathartics; avoid enemas.

10. Analgesics, such as meperidine (Demerol) 25 to 50 mg parenterally every four hours may be needed to alleviate pain which prevents sleep and contributes to the delirium. Phenothiazines potentiate narcotic action; but if the patient is in pain, Demerol should be used cautiously in small doses.

11. Anticonvulsants may be indicated, particularly if there is a seizure history or a problem with alcohol or drug withdrawal. Give diphenylhydantoin (Dilantin) 100 mg every six to eight hours for 12 days. Phenothiazines may be epileptogenic.

12. As the patient recovers, maintain all medications for a few days, and then reduce gradually. Explain in detail what occurred. Many patients suffer unnecessary guilt and shame following an episode of delirium

because they are unsure of what they did or said. Review all happenings with the patient.

PREVENTION

Delirium frequently follows medical and surgical procedures. It is prevented by maintaining fluid and electrolyte balance, giving adequate amounts of analgesics, and providing sedation which ensures sleep. Sedation during the daytime, however, is usually contraindicated. If the patient is in pain, he should receive analgesics during the day and analgesics with sedation at night.

THE CHRONIC BRAIN SYNDROMES

Although the chronic brain syndromes are irreversible, both the symptomatology and the severity of the condition are variable not only from patient to patient, but also for each individual from time to time. Etiologic agents are innumerable; in fact, they are classified in broad groups such as constitutional (congenital), infectious, traumatic, circulatory, and so on. As is true of the acute brain syndromes, there are usually multiple etiologic factors in each case, and chronic intoxications are important causes. The personality structure and etiologic agent(s) determine the form and the content of both the acute and the chronic syndromes; however, the chronic develops more slowly. Certain features are characteristic of all patients with chronic brain syndromes.

CHARACTERISTIC FEATURES

First, the abstract attitude is impaired (Goldstein, 1959). This loss is characterized by stimulus-bound and field-oriented responses. Thought is concrete; this is revealed by the patients' speech and their inability to understand subtleties of language. Also, they have difficulty with shades of meaning and with symbolization. Under careful observation, these patients are stereotyped, lack initiative and spontaneity, and react to stress in patterned ways regardless of the particular stressful factors involved.

Second, emotional expression is defective; either emotional lability or a general flattening of the affect results.

Third, personality changes occur. These may be dramatic, as exemplified by a change from compulsive neatness to careless disarray. But the change may be in an opposite direction; the patient may become more compulsive as he strives to maintain an arranged, understandable world about him. Cardinal features of the early stage are: a blunting of the ethical sense, a loss of judgment (which may appear in business affairs), and difficulties with interpersonal relationships resulting from an insensitivity to others.

Fourth, there is a progressive loss of memory. It appears in diverse forms: trouble with immediate recall, poor retention, or inability to remember the distant past. The memory loss is spotty; the patient remembers certain facts very well while others, which would seem to be more significant, are forgotten.

Fifth, data perception and integration fail as the illness progresses. In the early stages, this is reflected by a change in established reading habits, or a withdrawal of interest from complex activities which tax perception and memory (e.g., card playing). In advanced stages, of course, there is disorientation, first in the temporal dimension. Distorientation in terms of place and person occurs only late in the course of the chronic brain syndrome when the patient is also manifesting confusion.

Sixth, affective and thinking disorders are superimposed on the brain syndrome. Anxiety, depressive, or paranoid reactions add to the disability produced by the brain damage.

TYPES

The arteriosclerotic and the senile brain disease are the two most common types; there are differences between them. The arteriosclerotic has an erratic, stormy course. As the lesions produce damage, the patient's condition worsens abruptly but then may level off or even show some improvement. The arteriosclerotic patient retains his concerns for his health, family, finances, and so on; he is painfully aware of his disability and displays anxiety. In contrast, the course of senile brain disease is characterized by a slow, gradual decay over a number of years. The patient shows less overt anxiety because awareness diminishes slowly and evenly. Differential diagnosis for the arteriosclerotic depends on finding signs of focal neurologic impairment and other evidence of cardiovascular disease.

Chronic brain syndromes caused by alcoholism are common. In the florid stages, the patient may show Korsakoff's psychosis with disorientation, memory loss, confabulation, and polyneuritis.

Presenile dementia, either Pick's disease or Alzheimer's disease, is rare. Diagnosis may be difficult because of the early age of onset, the late 40's or early 50's. There are few characteristic features; in fact, these diseases may be variants of arteriosclerotic brain disease appearing at an early age. In evaluating patients with chronic brain syndromes at this age, the consultant must keep these disorders in mind, and he must rely upon extensive neurologic evaluation for the exact diagnosis. Brain tumor, trauma, and degenerative disease of the CNS must be ruled out.

DIAGNOSIS

The basic clinical features of the chronic brain syndrome are: memory loss, emotional lability, disorientation, and personality changes. Finding the exact etiologic agent(s) requires complete medical and psychiatric evaluations. Psychologic testing is helpful. The consultant can use the Bender-Gestalt Test to advantage. The differential diagnosis includes chronic undifferentiated schizophrenia, depression, and neurologic disorders ranging from brain tumor to familial or degenerative diseases of the CNS.

TREATMENT

Flach and Regan (1960) state: "The crucial factor in the treatment of patients with organic reactions is the recognition that the organic lesion exists in a total personality setting . . . The organic lesion is an added factor which is superimposed on the basic personality of the patient and upon any other psychiatric illness that the patient has." Although the chronic brain syndromes are by definition irreversible, the consultant can provide assistance to the consultee for the care of these patients. Skillful management enables many of them to live comfortably for a number of years; it does not always entail institutionalization.

The principles of treatment are:

1. Use all available therapy after adequate medical evaluation. Special attention should be given to the patient's bodily complaints (constipation, insomnia, arthritic aches and pains). Measures which improve his perceptual acuity (hearing aid, new spectacles, removing cataracts) enable him to maintain better orientation and to adapt more responsively to his environment.

2. Establish a doctor-patient relationship characterized by flexibility and rapport. For example, sometimes the patient requires weekly visits, while at other times, infrequent visits suffice. Treatment programs cannot be rigid.

3. Make a realistic appraisal of the medical status. The patient should be urged not to exceed his capabilities or overextend his already strained reserves. Instead, he must place a greater reliance on familiar activities which are not too demanding.

4. Simplify the environment at home and in the hospital. The patient should not be overwhelmed by a barrage of stimuli. Also, to help the lagging memory, he should carry a notebook and keep calendars in convenient places.

5. Treat superimposed affective disorders. Definitive treatment for anxiety or depression improves the general condition.

6. Use appropriate medications. They include vitamins and sedatives, as well as specific medications for established illnesses.

Lastly, the doctor-patient relationship should be imbued with hope; hope for attaining comfort, ease, and continued usefulness.

CATATONIC STATES IN ORGANIC BRAIN DISEASE

Classical catatonic states are sometimes encountered in patients with organic brain disease produced by: frontal lobe lesions, tumors, vascular lesions, encephalitis, degenerative states, and poisons (Kraepelin, 1909–1913; Rochlin, 1935; Bleuler, 1948; Mayer-Gross et al., 1960; Schwab and Barrow, 1964).

These catatonic states must be differentiated from catatonic schizophrenia and also from akinetic mutism (Cairns, 1929; Brain, 1964). Akinetic mutism appears in patients with lesions near the third or fourth ventricle and in patients with damage to the reticular activating system (Haymaker, 1956).

When produced by organic factors, the onset of the catatonic symptoms is abrupt. The clinical picture shows either catatonic stupor or excitement, or rapid shifts from one to the other.

Management requires: treatment of the causative factor, a structured environment, and the cautious use of phenothiazines.

REFERENCES

BERBLINGER, K. W. Psychiatric perspectives in medicine, part II. Psychosomatics, 3(2):42, 1962.

BLEULER, M. Investigations from the borderline of psychopathology and endocrinology. Arch. Psychiat. Nervenkr., 118:271, 1948.

BONHOEFFER, K. Zur Frage der Klassification der Symptomatischen Psychosen. Berlin Klinik Wschr., 14:2257, 1908.

BRAIN, W. R. Clinical Neurology, 2nd ed. London and New York, Oxford University Press, Inc., 1964, p. 463.

CAIRNS, H. W. B. Observations on the localization of intracranial tumors. Arch. Surg., 18:1936, 1929.

CORSELLIS, J. A. N. Mental Illness and the Aging Brain. London, Oxford University Press, Inc., 1962.

ENGEL, G. L., and ROMANO, J. Delirium, a syndrome of cerebral insufficiency. J. Chronic Dis., 9:260, 1959.

FLACH, F. F., and REGAN, P. Chemo-Therapy in Emotional Disorders. New York, McGraw-Hill Book Company, 1960, p. 225.

GOLDSTEIN, K. Functional disturbances in brain damage. In Arieti, S., ed. American Handbook of Psychiatry. New York, Basic Books, Inc., Publishers, 1959, Vol. 1, pp. 770–796.

GUZE, S. B., and CANTWELL, D. P. The prognosis in organic brain syndromes. Amer. J. Psychiat., 120:878, 1964.

HAYMAKER, W. Bing's Local Diagnosis in Neurological Diseases. The C. V. Mosby Co., 1956, p. 293.

HOCH, A. Psychogenesis in dementia praecox. Med. Rec., 73:452, 1908.

——— Review of Bleuler's schizophrenia. Rev. Neurol. Psychiat., 10:259, 1912.

JACKSON, H. Selected Writings of John Hughlings Jackson. New York, Basic Books, Inc., Publishers, 1958.

KRAEPELIN, E. Psychiatry, 8th ed. Leipzig, 1909–1913.

MAYER-GROSS, W., SLATER, E., and ROTH, M. Clinical Psychiatry, 2nd. ed. Baltimore, The Williams & Wilkins Co., 1960.

POLLACK, I. W., OCHBERG, F. M., and MEYER, E. Effect of deprivation of sight of subjective time sense. Psychosom. Med., 27:71, 1965.

RACHLIN, H. A follow-up study of Hoch's benign stupor cases. Amer. J. Psychiat., 92:531, 1935.

REDING, G. R., and DANIELS, R. S. Organic brain syndromes in a general hospital. Amer. J. Psychiat., 120:800, 1964.

ROMANO, J., and ENGEL, G. L. Med. Clin. N. Amer., p. 629, 1944.

SCHWAB, J. J., and BARROW, M. V. A reaction to organic flourides simulating classical catatonia. Amer. J. Psychiat., 120(12): 1196, 1964.

SCHWAB, J. J. The treatment of delirium. In Conn, H. F., ed. Current Therapy. Philadelphia, W. B. Saunders Co., 1966.

STEWART, M. A., TUCSON, V. B., GUZE, S. B., and SATHERFIELD, J. H. A study of psychiatric consultations in a general hospital. J. Chron. Dis. 15:331, 1962.

WOHLRABE, J. C., et al. Delirium and complex electrolyte disturbance. Dis. Nerv. Syst., 26:44, 1965.

WOLFF, H. G., and Curran, D. Nature of delirium and allied states, dysergastic reaction. Arch. Neurol. Psychiat., 33:1175, 1935.

22 SOMATOPSYCHIC RELATIONSHIPS: REACTIONS TO ILLNESS

Emotional reactions to illness may be described as the silent areas in medical practice.

Bartemeier (1961)

A psychosomatic disorder is usually described as an illness preceded by psychic conflict of major etiologic importance. A somatopsychic reaction is similarly described as the psychic consequence of somatic illness. Delineating such exact cause and effect relationships, however, is generally unrealistic; it implies mechanistic concepts of health and illness.

Psychoanalytic interest in somatopsychic processes springs from Ferenczi's 1916 case study entitled "Disease—or Patho-neurosis" (1952). Reporting on personality disorganization following orchiectomy for the treatment of tuberculosis, he postulated that some neuroses result from somatic illness. Basing this theory on Freud's discussions of narcissism, Ferenczi stated that in such cases the libido is withdrawn from the outer world and is directed to the diseased or injured organ as well as to the ego. Further, he pointed to postpartum psychosis as a pathopsychosis of this type.

Groddeck's work (1961), which received little publicity until recently, differs somewhat in that he insists, absolutely, on the unity of the organism and on the contribution of the vital life force—the "it"—to the production of all disease.

The psychoanalytic concept of ego development is fundamental to our understanding of somatopsychic relationships. Schilder (1951), Engel (1953), and Menninger (1954) reaffirmed Freud's thesis that "The ego is first and foremost a bodily ego" (1961). This primacy of the somatic elements of the ego explains its involvement in physical illness; involvement even to the point that other ego functions are affected. Neurosis may follow. These theories are supported by neurophysiologists. For example, Herrick *Brains of Rats and Men* (1963), thinks that through evolution, the development of manual skills stimulated the further development of the human cerebral cortex (and ego).

Ehrentheil (1959) proposes a simple classification of somatopsychic relationships: 1) intracranial processes including diseases located within the confines of the skull, such as injuries or tumors, which lead directly to psychic symptomatology; 2) extracranial processes influencing brain function, in which the brain is affected by toxic, metabolic, or other influences, following liver diseases, cardiovascular illnesses, the use of ACTH, and so on; and 3) psychologic reactions to somatic diseases, including the psychoneuroses superimposed on illnesses such as heart disease and cancer.

These somatopsychic concepts can be broadened to include all reactions to illness. They cover the entire range of psychiatric disturbances (brain syndromes, personality disorders, neuroses, and psychoses). In addition, an individual's reactions to illness or physical disability create problems related to his productivity at work, status in the family or society, and convalescent management. Medicine's relative inattention to patients' reactions to illness has been remarked by Bartemeier (1961): "the fantasies commonly associated with physical symptoms, the occurrence of illness are rarely brought to the attention of the physician. . . . and the beliefs, even the convictions that some patients hold about the cause of their illness or its significance, may interfere with recovery or complicate management."

Nancy Swift (1962) notes that the psychologic reactions to illness are determined by four main factors: 1) the nature of the illness, 2) the age of the patient, 3) the personality of the patient, and 4) the environmental circumstances in which the illness occurs. In discussing the emotional problems of the chronically ill, Anshin (1962) describes time perspectives. He says: "When the longitudinal consideration of the patient's life history is given emphasis, the physician will learn *what* reaction to expect in the patient, he will realize *why* the patient reacts in a particular fashion, and finally *where* to look in the current situation so as to make changes bettering the patient's adjustment to life and illness."

Anshin thinks patients generally respond to illness in one of three ways: 1) with a continuation of a previous personality disorder, such as excessive dependency; 2) with an acute reaction manifested as depression, anxiety, anger, or fear; or 3) with a transition into a psychotic state which may be abetted by drug intake.

The most common reactions to illness are anxiety and depression (see Chapters 24 and 25), regression, and denial. However, these reactions seldom exist in pure culture; they overlap. The patient has at his command a variety of mental mechanisms which he uses singly, or in combinations, depending upon his ego strengths, patterns of adaptation to stress, personality dynamics, ability to change, his perception of the illness, and the degree to which others force behavioral modes upon him. The consultant must determine how these reactions are individualized, to what degree they are adaptive, and when psychotherapeutic intervention is necessary.

REGRESSION

The continuum, ranging from regression to denial, encompasses most of the reactions to illness. Regression is probably the more natural and salutary response. In an essay on this subject Meerloo (1964) describes the concept of retrogenesis, taking a step backward in order to leap forward. Some degree of regression, at least a limitation of activity and a preoccupation with self, takes place with most illnesses. However, regressive states are usually feared by the physician and the family because of the danger that the patient will obtain so much secondary gain that he will persist in a stage of helpless dependency. Further, behavioral changes accompanying regressed states produce interpersonal difficulties; regressed patients may appear infantile or dependent, characteristics generally disdained by our society. Psychiatric assistance is necessary when both the degree and the quality of the regression are such that they: 1) antagonize therapeutic programs, 2) retard convalescence, and 3) produce interpersonal difficulties.

Knowing that the staff's fears of prolonged regression are exposed in their dealings with these patients, and that these fears complicate management, the consultant can provide guidelines for managing patients who respond to illness with marked regression. When the consultant explains the necessity for limited regression and its health-promoting benefits and assures the staff of his continued availability, he reduces their fears. For example, it is mandatory that the patient with an acute myocardial infarction remain partially regressed for three to six weeks following the attack. If regression persists, the consultant must work to alleviate the patient's anxieties and to minimize the secondary gains. He must explore mechanisms and avenues by which the patient may obtain gains more healthfully. Interviews with the family, sometimes including the patient, can be effective for: 1) understanding family conflicts and expectations of the patient (for all concerned), 2) resolving problems

pertaining to secondary gain, 3) educating the family and patient together so that there is consensus about the nature of the illness and the
prognosis, and 4) rearranging domestic conditions and habits.

Interviews with the patient, the consultant, and the staff together may
also be necessary, and can be designed to serve these same purposes.

DENIAL

Denial, the negative illness as it is termed by Meerloo (1964), is
probably the most serious reaction to illness; it is fraught with difficulties
for the consultant. Denial indicates a fragile character structure, so fragile
that negation of the illness-imposed threat to the integrity of the organism
is necessary in order to maintain homeostasis. Excessive denial is deleterious to medical care. Titchener and Levine (1960) found that it was responsible for unnecessarily delayed surgery in many patients who ignored
obvious lesions until they were inoperable or until cure was not possible.

Denial also has implications for the doctor-patient relationship. It
precludes agreement between the patient and the physician about the
severity of the illness; and, when such accord is lacking, cooperation is
replaced by dissension. Denial is responsible for many patients' signing
out of the hospital against medical advice. When a patient's denial is
shattered, psychosis or open hostility may appear.

Providing therapeutic management for the hospital or clinic patient
who uses excessive denial is a difficult task. The consultant must obtain an
understanding of processes which defy generalization. Irrational fears
and unconscious mechanisms underlie extreme denial. These range from
fears about the diagnosis and prognosis, through anxiety concerning loss
of status, to masked hostility toward oneself and others. Based on his
evaluation of the strength of the denial and the patient's need for maintaining it, the consultant must make a decision. He has two choices: 1)
to challenge the denial system directly, or 2) to permit the patient to
maintain the denial in slightly modified form, in order to gain short-term
cooperation.

If the consultant takes the first course, he can minimize the risk of
personality disorganization or of flagrant hostility toward the staff by
establishing a continuing relationship through daily visits. When the patient is severely ill, or when personality disorganization is likely to follow
surrender of the denial, the consultant should choose the latter course.
When in doubt, or when there is an emergency situation, he should use a
cautious, day-by-day approach.

The consultant should explain to the staff the nature and extent
of the patient's denial processes and express his opinion of the patient's

capabilities for altering his behavior. Then, the consultant and the staff can work out a modified, usually less restrictive, treatment program which can be offered to the patient as a face-saving compromise.

Other maneuvers involve: 1) supplying secondary gains for the patient as he begins to acknowledge his illness, and 2) dropping any challenge of the denial while enlisting the patient's cooperation "for the sake of the family or staff."

OTHER REACTIONS

Besides regression and denial, Anshin (1962) lists other common reactions to illness: 1) The enforced inactivity of illness increases the need to be watched over and cared for. Dependency is accentuated, particularly in patients who have always felt isolated and rejected. He says, "Some patients have a life-long history of seeking overprotection; they tend to prolong their illnesses while exaggerating their dependent needs." 2) Others who seem aggressive and independent deny dependency; they become frightened by their needs and, when treated kindly, they react violently. Such patients should not be made to feel helpless. Anshin says, "By understanding how patients either overemphasize or resist dependency, physicians may give them comfort and understanding, and at the same time, encourage some feelings of independence and self-sustainment." 3) Lonely and mistrustful patients become argumentative and angry; their hostility may be projected in a delusional manner on the institution, the family, or their doctors. 4) Chronically anxious persons react to illness with increased anxiety. Pain is a special aspect of this reaction; it may be exaggerated to obtain dependency needs, or denied to achieve a "martyr" status. 5) Reactions to illness also include hypochondriasis, somatization, and psychologic invalidism. 6) Compulsive persons protect against anxiety by repetitive rituals of thought and deed; they may become depressed when they are robbed of these defenses or when their self-esteem is shattered. 7) Emotionally unstable, immature, impulsive persons react poorly to stress, becoming garrulous, dramatic, or grandiose. 8) All patients, to a degree, use their illnesses to manipulate physicians and other involved persons.

Starrett (1961) studied paraplegic patients; pure anxiety was found at the beginning of the illness when the body-image was disrupted. Later, the patients displayed defenses against this anxiety—predominantly, denial, hostility, and depression.

Brown (1950) found that indifference and apathy were the two symptoms most commonly seen as personality responses to chronic disabling illnesses. He recommends increased symptomatic therapy to combat the apathy: heat, massage, the use of unessential drugs, recreation, occupational therapy, physical activity, and social events.

In describing the psychologic problems of terminal cancer management, Rothenberg (1961) emphasizes that an elemental factor for the cancer patient is the loss of control. In fact he says that the word "cancer" or "crab" captures the popular conception of the disease—an uncontrollable process which is slowly devouring one. He says: "The single most frightening aspect of the terminal cancer experience, to both the patient and the staff, therefore, is the inability to control the process." Loss of control is accompanied by blame and guilt for all concerned. Rothenberg also discusses the grief and the sense of failure which pervade terminal cancer care. The profound sense of bodily failure accentuates the symptoms. Lastly, Rothenberg discusses isolation; communication is disrupted with cancer patients to a greater extent than is true in almost any other illness. He concludes: "Attention to this interpersonal factor is crucially important as the patient's feelings of isolation from loved ones and life, and his concern with the isolation of death, are probably the most painful psychological experiences in terminal cancer."

ATTITUDES AND VALUES

To understand patients' reactions to illness, we must also consider their attitudes and values; indeed, they may influence the reactions. One of our studies of personality variables and attitudes revealed that when a general medical inpatient population was divided into four diagnostic groupings, unique sets of attitudes characterized each of the groups (Goldman and Schwab, 1965).

The attitudes of the seriously. often terminally ill, patients were highly rigid and unrealistic. These patients denied that their illnesses had any basic effects on them and their families. Although very ill, they perceived their "core stability" as unchanged. Under the stress of major illness, they maintained a psychological status quo—probably to avoid thinking about the consequences of the illness.

The moderately ill patients assessed their illness as nuisances, serious but not catastrophic, and not involving the "core" of their lives. They acknowledged the effects of their illnesses and considered the consequences realistically. They perceived themselves as only temporarily handicapped. They were in contact with their personality resources and appeared to be using them to meet the imposed stress of illness.

The attitudes of those with vague and poorly defined illnesses were more complex. They complained about their illnesses, yet denied being anxious about them. They were ambivalent, contradictory, and less specific about their illnesses than patients in the other groups. Attitudes held by these patients raise the question: Do they need help in refocusing their attention from aggravation to anxiety?

The patients with psychiatric diagnoses were highly anxious, perceiving their illnesses as severe and all-pervasive. They seemed to be sacrificially motivated to recover, stating that they were willing to change home, business, length of life, and personal convictions, in order to get well. A sense of basic inadequacy was revealed; they regarded the remnants of their adequacy as being even more diminished by the superimposed illnesses.

General conclusions concerning broad diagnostic groupings of medical inpatients and their attitudes furnish only tentative guidelines for optimal management. Clinical experience vouches for the many individual exceptions undoubtedly present in any group of human beings. Whether such expressed attitudes were reactions to illness, concomitants of illness, or persistent personality attributes can be ascertained only by prospective studies.

Most of the medical patients in the last group, those with psychiatric diagnoses, were referred for psychiatric consultations; very few in the other three groups were. Thus, in general, only patients who exuded anxiety received consultations, while those who denied anxiety and the need for help were not referred. Obviously, patients with vague and poorly defined illnesses present major clinical problems; many should have psychiatric evaluations. Also some of the patients who held unrealistic attitudes and others who used excessive denial should have been seen by consultants. Because these patients conceal their anxiety, physicians must be aware of the more obscure manifestations of their distress.

Traditionally, changes in patients' attitudes and behavior as an accompaniment of, or reaction to, medical illnesses have been described in humanistic terms. But with the development of contemporary psychiatry and the focus on somatopsychic relationships, there is now an emphasis on patients' responses to illness in psychodynamic terms: depression, anxiety, denial, changed self-concept, and disturbed interpersonal relations. However, reactions to illness must be understood from a perspective which encompasses both humanistic and psychiatric views.

REFERENCES

ANSHIN, R. N. Emotional problems of the chronically ill. J. Amer. Geriat. Soc., 10:447, 1962.

BARTEMEIER, L. H. Psychiatric aspects of medical practice. Emotional reactions to illness. Maryland Med. J., 10:240, May, 1961.

BROWN, J. R. The holistic treatment of neurologic disease. Med. Clin. N. Amer., July:1019, 1950.

EHRENTHEIL, O. F. Some remarks about somato-psychic compared to psychosomatic relationships. Psychosom. Med., 21:1, 1959.

ENGEL, G. Homeostasis, behavioral adjustment and the concept of health and disease. In Grinker, R., ed. Mid-Century Psychiatry. Springfield, Ill., Charles C Thomas, Publisher, 1953.

FERENCZI, S. Disease or pathoneurosis. In Theory and the Technique of Psycho-analysis. New York, Basic Books, Inc., Publishers, 1952, pp. 78–89.

FREUD, S. The Ego and the Id (Vol. XIX of the Complete Psychological Works). Strachey, J., and Freud, A., (translators and editors). London, The Hogarth Press, 1961.

GOLDMAN, J., and SCHWAB, J. J. Medical illness and patients' attitudes: Somatopsychic relationships. J. Nerv. Ment. Dis., 141(6):678, 1965.

GRODDECK, G. Book of the It. New York, The New American Library of World Literature, Inc., 1961.

HERRICK, C. J. Brains of Rats and Men. New York, Hafner Publishing Co., Inc., 1963.

MEERLOO, J. A. M. Illness and Cure. New York, Grune & Stratton, Inc., 1964, p. 44.

MENNINGER, K. A. Psychological aspects of the organism under stress: Part I: The homeostatic regulatory function of the ego. J. Amer. Psychoanal. Ass., 2:67, 1954.

ROTHENBERG, A. Psychological problems in terminal cancer management. Cancer, 14:1063, 1961.

SCHILDER, P. The Image and Appearance of the Body. New York, International Universities Press, Inc., 1951.

STARRETT, D. Psychiatric mechanisms in severe disability. Rocky Mountain Med. J., 58:42, 1961.

SWIFT, N. I. Psychological reactions to illness. Physiotherapy, 48:172, 1962.

TITCHENER, J. L., and LEVINE, M. Surgery as a Human Experience: The Psychodynamics of Surgical Practice. New York, Oxford University Press, Inc., 1960.

23 THE DYING PATIENT

In the past, the care of the dying patient fell upon the family, the physician, and the clergy. Each one had a defined role; the family's responsibility was to provide care, the physician's to alleviate suffering, and the clergyman's to look after the patient's soul. The current demands on physicians to assume roles which were formerly sociocultural or theological, and the greater accessibility to hospitals, have combined to enlarge the physician's responsibilities. As a result, the psychiatric consultant is more and more being called upon to assist in the hospital management of the dying patient.

Eissler (1955), Feifel (1961), Aldrich (1963), and others have written at length about the dying patient. Eissler (1955) elaborates on the intricate mechanisms which can be used to help dying patients preserve whatever meaning and dignity they have developed through life. Aronson ("Treatment of the Dying Person," 1959) lists four rules: 1) Do not tell the patient something that might induce psychopathology; 2) Never allow hope to die too far ahead of the patient; 3) Do not minimize the gravity of the situation; 4) Structure the period before death in such a way that there will be no time for the patient to sit idly awaiting death. In criticism, Dovenmuehle (1965) replies that carrying out these rules is antitherapeutic because the patient may be encouraged to preserve illusions.

It is obvious that most dying patients do not need psychiatric consultations. Brosin (1965) is impressed with how well-mannered many dying people are. In the same report, Weinberg (1965) states: "In the vast majority of the people in our culture it (death) certainly has not struck a paralyzing and immobilizing terror." However, our changing cultural attitudes toward death have been recently attacked. Wedge (1965) offers the proposition "that death in our society and in our time may have replaced sex as the subject for repression—social repression." Such books as Jessica Mitford's *The American Way of Death* (1963) not only expose the multibillion dollar death industry, but focus our attention on some of the fictions which are almost uniformly accepted.

For the medical profession, there are three major problems: 1) detecting the patient who will have the greatest difficulty with dying, 2) deciding what to tell the patient with a critical illness, i.e., the physician's approach to the patient, and 3) developing guidelines for psychotherapy with the dying patient.

EVALUATING THE DYING PATIENT'S NEED FOR CONSULTATION

There is little systematized research to provide criteria for evaluating how patients face their terminal illnesses and react to dying. In general, it is believed that he who lives well dies well; but it has also been noted that seriously depressed patients and even psychotic patients have died peacefully. Thus, it is necessary to question today's standards for defining the patient who requires psychiatric consultation during his final days. Those who are management problems, those with flagrant anxiety, those who are unwilling to cooperate in continued-care programs and those who are lonely due to disruption of family and other personal relationships, need psychiatric help or increased assistance. These are obviously pragmatic indices of the need for special care, but until there is greater investigation of this entire subject, we do not have more substantial guidelines.

WHAT TO TELL THE DYING PATIENT ABOUT HIS PROGNOSIS

The physician may find that his own reactions to death interfere with his work with the patient. Choosing to become a physician may be a characterophobic defense against fears of death—a reaction formation. In a sense, this represents our identification with the aggressor. Feifel (1965) developed this hypothesis, quoting Kasper's (1959) belief that the physician takes his own fears about death, poses them as intellectual questions, and tries to answer them for other people.

What the physician should tell the patient with a hopeless prognosis is a subject which the medical profession and its colleagues debate endlessly. Most physicians resolve this problem by developing a personal schema for informing patients about impending death. Some physicians rather brusquely tell all their patients of the expected outlook, while others never inform any, saying little or nothing, falsifying the prognosis, or employing euphemisms. However, most physicians try to be selective and use differential approaches, depending upon their estimate of what the patient wishes to know, how he will receive it, and the practical necessity for offering such information. Feifel (1965) reports that in a sample of 52 persons whom he studied, 82 percent wished to be informed precisely of their prognoses in order to settle their affairs or at least maintain their essential dignity as human beings, saying, "I have the right to know." Feifel (1965) also reports that 69 percent to 90 percent of the physicians were not in favor of telling their patients if they are dying; in contrast, 77 percent to 89 percent of these patients wanted to know.

In most instances, the physician's task boils down to the problem of the patient's denial. Should the denial system be uncovered so that underlying concerns can be worked with? In his report on the attitudes of patients with advanced malignancies, Feder (1965) describes the extreme denial manifested. But he feels strongly that the important point is, "Once you have said to the patient—however you say it—that you recognize that his is a serious and potentially fatal illness, you have established a relationship upon which you can base future communications at various levels."

Most physicians believe that imparting some quality of hope, or, at least, not leaving the patient with an absolute sense of hopelessness, is imperative. Of course, the question arises: What is hope? Is it hope for recovery from illness, hope for prolongation of life, hope for one's self, or hope for others? The physician's expressions of uncertainty sustain hope while arousing anxiety; defined statements may allay anxiety by providing certainty, but hope may be the casualty. Nevertheless, many of the writers in this field do not give sufficient consideration to the patient's capacity for understanding and responding to what the doctor tells him. A patient who clings to denial can continue to use this mechanism effectively, regardless of the information relayed to him by physicians.

Aldrich (1963 and 1965) says that the physician's need for self-protection causes him to avoid close personal relationships with dying patients. He thinks that in working with the dying patient, physicians frequently act as if the diagnosis of a serious condition inevitably means a hopeless prognosis. Aldrich recommends that physicians structure their statements about serious illness so that the patient can make his own choice between denial and acceptance.

GUIDELINES FOR PSYCHIATRIC CONSULTANTS

1. Individualize each patient. The psychiatrist must obtain an understanding of what each patient thinks about death. Depending on age, religious background, and other human factors, such as the desire to live,

or the willingness to give up, dying and death have different meanings for different individuals. The psychiatrist should discuss the patient's religion with him and find out whether he would like to see a clergyman. A last-minute confession or even a death-bed conversion to a religious faith is common and may result in an enhanced sense of well-being. When the patient expresses views on death which touch on its religious significance or on reunion fantasies, basic death-anxiety can certainly be explored without depriving the patient of all hope.

2. Evaluate the anxiety-denial complex. The referring physician may be mistaken about the need for concealing the prognosis or for strengthening the patient's denial system. The consultant should assess the importance of denial to the patient. The need for denial may vary from day to day or week to week. Even though the patient insists on maintaining a moderate degree of denial, thus reducing anxiety, he should be encouraged to articulate what dying means to him. He then begins to modify some of his illusions about the fatal prognosis.

Dying is looked upon as an "ultimate crisis," a critical situation; with help, the individual can develop resources for facing it with dignity. Weisman and Hackett (1961) state: "The fear of dying is a matter distinct from anticipation of death. The fear of death, of which so many patients speak, is in fact a specific attitude toward the process of dying and is not related to the fact of death." Thus, the psychiatrist's major task is to understand the patient's view, evaluate his coping mechanisms, and see him often to prevent the isolation which may ensue.

3. Avoid isolation; preserve communication. This is perhaps the only single generalization that is applicable to the management of the dying patient in Western culture. "Sitting up" with the dying patient is traditional; it indicates concern, maintains relationships, and diminishes the progressive sense of aloneness.

4. Provide support; allow the patient to verbalize his hopelessness and fear. Most people wish to die with propriety and are fearful that their behavior will be destructive to others. With the consultant's support, the patient can gain confidence about the appropriateness of his behavior. Also, he can become engaged in resolving problems, requite guilt-producing actions of the past, and view life in perspective.

5. Maintain body-comfort and "live" body image. Pain should be alleviated, but the patient should not be narcotized into oblivion. For, to feel nothing is to be dead. Most importantly, the patient should be physically touched, because touch implies tenderness and acceptance; it is a way of communicating love and concern for comfort. For example, frequent back rubs and massages provide physical care and aid psychological well-being. Cosmetic care of the patient should not be neglected; this

is particularly important for a woman. Minor ailments such as rashes should be treated promptly. In evaluating depression in medical inpatients, we (Schwab et al., 1965) found that the seriously ill reveal intense somatic preoccupation; the findings underscore the necessity for responding to these patients' bodily needs and disturbed physiologic functioning, as well as providing relief for their suffering.

The therapist who works with patients in a catastrophic situation may find to his surprise that there are real rewards in the work that he did not expect. Further, one discovers something that is rarely mentioned in the textbooks of psychology and psychiatry. One sees clearly the strength and dignity of human beings, the deep altruism, the positive qualities that exist at all levels of personality. Working with people who are under the hammer of fate greatly increases one's respect for them and makes one proud of being a human being.

LeShan (1964)

REFERENCES

ALDRICH, C. K. The dying patient's grief. J.A.M.A., 184:329, 1963.
—— Discussion. Death and Dying, GAP Report, 5(9):645, 1965.
ARONSON, G. T. Treatment of the dying person. *In* Feifel, H., ed. The Meaning of Death. New York, McGraw Hill Book Company, 1959, pp. 251–8.
BROSIN, H. W. Discussion. Death and Dying, GAP Report, 5(9):642, 1965.
DONENMUEHLE, R. H. Affective response to life-threatening cardiovascular disease. Death and Dying, GAP Report, 5(9):607, 1965.
EISSLER, K. R. The Psychiatrist and the Dying Patient. New York, International Universities Press, Inc., 1955, pp. 1–86.
FEDER, S. L. Attitudes of patients with advanced malignancy. Death and Dying, GAP Report, 5(9):614, 1965.
FEIFEL, H. Death-relevant variable in psychology. *In* May, R., ed. Existential Psychology. 1961, pp. 61–74.
—— The function of attitudes toward death. Death and Dying, GAP Report, 5(9):632, 1965.
KASPER, A. M. The doctor and death. *In* The Meaning of Death. New York, McGraw-Hill Book Company, Inc., 1959.
LeSHAN, L. L. Psychosomatic Aspects of Neoplastic Disease. Kissen, D. M. and LeShan, L. L., eds. Philadelphia, J. B. Lippincott Co., 1964.
MITFORD, J. The American Way of Death. New York, Simon and Schuster, Inc., 1963.
SCHWAB, J. J., CLEMMONS, R. S., BIALOW, M. R., DUGGAN, V., and DAVIS, B. A study of the somatic symptomatology of depression in medical inpatients. Psychosomatics, 6:273, 1965.
WEDGE, B. M. Discussion. Death and Dying, GAP Report, 5(9):648, 1965.
WEINBERG, J. Discussion. Death and Dying, GAP Report, 5(9):643, 1965.
WEISMAN, A. D., and HACKETT, T. R. Predilection to death: Death and dying as a psychiatric problem. Psychosom. Med., 23:232, 1961.

24 ANXIETY

What is new is the degree to which our era is concerned with anxiety. . . . our worry about anxiety, and our hope of doing something about it. This is not only an age of anxiety; it is also an age of anxiety about anxiety.

(Scheier, 1962)

Awareness of anxiety is increasing in the Western world; Rennie (1948) found some form of anxiety in 75 percent of his New York City sample; Andresen (1963) says that anxiety is epidemic; and, Hope (1962) observes: "As a clinical syndrome, the anxiety state outranks all other problems in general medicine." In Finn and Husten's (1966) survey of 29,412 patients in Iowa, 291 physicians reported that more than 18 percent suffered from emotional distress, and that the anxiety-tension syndrome was the commonest manifestation. Adams and Hope (1962) found that 22 percent of 4,660 patients admitted to the New England Center Hospital had psychiatric syndromes; the anxiety state was present in 21 percent of this group. Our studies (1966a, 1966b) are corroborative; 20 percent to 25 percent of the general medical inpatients had severe anxiety, and over 50 percent had moderate or severe anxiety about their illnesses and medical care. In fact, the anxiety scores of 20 percent were higher than the mean scores obtained from psychiatric inpatients. These data are in accord with Cattell and Scheier's (1961) statement: "Epidemiological estimates vary . . . [but] a conservative consensus estimate would probably place 20 percent of the American population as needing treatment for disorders in which anxiety plays a prominent role."

NATURE OF ANXIETY

Although there is unanimity about the seriousness of anxiety, there is little agreement about its nature. Because anxiety is studied from various theoretical and methodologic points of view, there is even difficulty with definition. Definitions are so numerous that they must be classified in categories: those that focus on avoidance behavior; those that emphasize measures of psychophysiologic arousal; and those that consider anxiety as a mental state, a signal to the ego, or apprehension resulting from a threat to the integrity of the organism (Sarbin, 1964).

Throughout his career Freud grappled with the concept of anxiety. Near the end, he called anxiety "the central problem in neurosis" (1936). In 1921 he had this to say: "We call it an affective state, although we are also ignorant of what an affect is." He discussed three components of anxiety, listing 1) the specific feeling of unpleasure, 2) acts of discharge (motor and autonomic functions), and 3) the perceptions of these acts.

Engel (1962a, 1962b) proposes that anxiety is the earlier of two basic biologic patterns; depression-withdrawal is the other. He says that anxiety "includes a variety of active modes of coping with stress which are designated the *flight-fight patterns* to indicate corresponding behavioral aspects (Cannon, 1939). These involve not only the biochemical and physiologic preparations for flight but also internal changes anticipating bodily injury" (Engel, 1962b). The psychophysiology is neuroendocrine, including activity of the limbic system and the hypothalamus, which leads to activation of the pituitary-adrenal cortical system and facilitates a wide range of metabolic processes involved in the long-term responses to injury (Ingle, 1952; F. Engel, 1953; Selye, 1960).

Grinker (1956) emphasizes the quantitative aspects: "Lesser quantities of anxiety are synonomous with alertness or vigilance . . . constant and automatic . . . accompanied by little psychological cognizance or awareness of somatic participation. Greater quantities of anxiety occur episodically as apprehension under conditions appropriate to the preparation for intensified activity under strain. Then there is cognizance of anxiety . . . tachycardia, increased respiratory rate . . . etc. . . . Free anxiety of greater degree, either continuously or in attacks, is neurotic anxiety. It is one of the most unendurable states to which man is subject. Temporarily it may lead to facilitation of psychological and behavioral processes, but in greater amounts it is accompanied by disorganization of functioning and to increasing disturbance leading to regression."

These are fundamental concepts. For the sake of completeness we should add that Berger (1962) propounds an organic point of view when he says that "anxiety is a disease of the brain." In contrast, others see anxiety as a patterned response which is the result of faulty learning; to them, neurotic symptoms are learned patterns of behavior (Mowrer, 1950; Eysenck, 1952). Many theorists believe that not only is anxiety a signal of danger which is protective to the organism, but also that it is a constructive force which accounts for motivation and monitors behavior.

Psychiatrists contend that anxiety is the basis of all psychopathology; as a painful affect it is a signal of danger to the ego which sets in motion a chain of defensive processes which are manifested as overt symptoms. Psychosomaticists hold that excessive or sustained anxiety produces disturbance of bodily functions or structures which result in organic illness. Conversely, anxiety should be viewed from the somatopsychic frame of reference. For example, in writing about patients with structural heart disease, Reiser (1967) says, ". . . unresolved anxiety, somatopsychic in origin, may act to aggravate the condition or to counteract the effects of medical treatment. Cyclic self-reinforcing situations commonly develop."

Physicians acknowledge that anxiety can be a contributing factor, a correlate, or a result of many disease states. They are primarily concerned with the problem of how to treat patients with acute distressing "anxiety" attacks and those with high levels of chronic anxiety who are difficult to work with because of their general nervousness, irritability, fright, and erratic behavior. Many psychologists study anxiety in terms of its psychophysiologic concomitants such as the GSR responses to stressful stimuli; others such as Cattell et al. (1961) are using extensive factor analyses of symptoms and overt behavioral manifestations.

Conventionally, anxiety is differentiated from fear. Anxiety is considered to be more subjective, a diffuse sense of apprehension which arises from internal sources; fear is more objective, a more specific reaction to defined external dangers. However, West (1963) links anxiety to fear: "Fears resulting from an unknown threat bypass the ego and are properly termed anxiety." Anxiety may also be thought of as the fear of fear. In the medical situation, the differentiation between anxiety and fear has only limited value; it is seldom apparent and may not be real. In a recent study, we (O'Leary et al., 1967) found that cardiac patients did not have higher measurable anxiety levels than other medical inpatients, but in interviews they expressed more fear, worry, and concern about illness and its effects on their lives.

We think of anxiety as both a signal of a threat to the organism and as an apprehensive, fear-like state which is expressed psychically and somatically. In his book, *The Meaning of Anxiety*, Rollo May (1950) presents a comprehensive and critical review of various theories of anxiety. In 1967 he elaborated the existential concepts. May's works should be read by everyone interested in obtaining a greater understanding of the problem of anxiety.

ANXIETY AND MEDICAL ILLNESS

Medical illness, with its threat to the organism, can provoke anxiety. Of the medical patients we (1966c) studied, we found that anxiety increased with illness for 79 percent, for 11 percent there was no change, and for 10 percent anxiety levels diminished with illness.

Other relationships between anxiety levels and medical illness came to light when these patients' illnesses were classified by types. Greater anxiety was found in patients with psychiatric, musculoskeletal, and gastrointestinal disorders, while anxiety was surprisingly low in patients with other categories of illness, particularly the cardiovascular and neurological. However, some patients in all disease categories had high levels of anxiety.

That anxiety increased with the onset of illness is consistent with our expectations. Anxiety may be one of the first reactions when illness is perceived as a threat to life and values. But, the problem of anxiety in medical patients has other ramifications. *Displacement* of anxiety may occur with medical illness and hospitalization. A typical example is the cardiac patient who expresses concern about the accuracy of his diagnosis, or the medical expense, rather than about stressful situations at home or at work which preceded the onset of the illness and will complicate convalescence. For some of the 10 percent who reported diminished anxiety, admission to the hospital and expectations of help were meliorative. For others in that group, illness probably bound their anxiety so that it was temporarily controlled; with his concept of the economic distribution of libido, Freud (1936) explains that "organic disease often relieves neurosis by binding the unmanageable quantities of libido."

In another study (1966d) we found that high anxiety, low self-concept, and poor body image appear as a *syndrome* in some medical patients, particularly women. This syndrome occurred most frequently in the medical patients with psychiatric and musculoskeletal disorders, and least often in patients with neourological and cardiovascular diseases.

There are interpersonal aspects to these medical patients' anxious conditions (Schwab, 1966b). Our patients with higher anxiety felt that their illnesses exerted deleterious effects on both their work and their self-esteem. They believed that their illnesses undermined their ability to accomplish what they desired in life. They also disclosed significantly less dependence on their physicians than did medical patients with less anxiety, but they were significantly *more* dependent on others, particularly family, friends, and clergy. The increased dependency on others and the syndrome—high anxiety, negative attitudes toward the body, and low concept of the self—were indicative of clinical psychopathology (as corroborated by abnormalities in their mental status examinations and by psychiatric evaluations).

Although physicians recognize anxiety, tension, and fear in their patients, they have difficulty gauging the seriousness of these conditions. Consequently, referral patterns are inconsistent. Physicians delay referring many of these patients because they believe that completing the medical work-up may provide sufficient clarification of the illness to reduce the anxiety and fear (Schwab, 1967a).

CONCEPTUALIZATION OF ANXIETY IN MEDICAL PATIENTS

In our work with medical patients, we conceptualize anxiety as a disturbing, even painful affect which is expressed in the following forms: 1) by psychophysiologic manifestations; 2) by increased worry and concern; and, 3) by characterologic disturbances typified by negative attitudes toward and complaints about medical care. These modes of expression appear in combinations more often than singly.

Anxiety in medical patients is accompanied by some diminished awareness, particularly of interpersonal transactions. While the patients' attention and sensitivity to anxiety-provoking cues intensify, general awareness of the environment and the persons in it decreases. Those who are highly anxious do not know how they are affecting other people, and they do not interpret others' responses adequately. Communication difficulties and impaired relationships result. For example, the patient who complains bitterly that his doctor does not "tell him enough" may not really be *able to listen* to the physician. When the anxiety-provoking stimulus is introspective bodily concern, increased attention is focused on physical processes; then, the patient's excessive complaining further obstructs the physician-patient relationship. And, because the patient is keenly aware of minor aches and pains that usually go unnoticed, or at least unremarked by the less anxious individual, he not only complains more but has more to complain about.

THE TREATMENT OF CLINICAL STATES

THE ACUTE STRESS REACTION

Because there is a precipitating event, or a discrete situational stress, psychotherapy should be directed toward helping the patient work through his reactions to the event, or toward resolving the environmental stress. Medications may be necessary, but should be given for only a short time, a few weeks. Chronic reliance on medications may produce just enough relief so that instead of seeking decisive solutions, the patient remains symptomatic, and helplessly entangled in a stressful situation for which drugs are no remedy. Often, adequate nighttime sedation is sufficient; a barbiturate (e.g., secobarbital or pentobarbital 100 to 200 mg), meprobamate 800 mg, or chloral hydrate 0.5 to 1.0 g for a few nights is effective. During the daytime, meprobamate or chlordiazepoxide may be given in moderate dosage for a short time.

ACUTE ANXIETY

Acute anxiety attacks often appear as discrete clinical syndromes; the patient displays overt apprehension and the symptoms of autonomic nervous system imbalance. He complains of severe dread and a fear that he is dying, or that he is afflicted by an unknown, terrifying condition. Panic may ensue. The physical symptoms include headache, an inability to concentrate, rapid heartbeat, shortness of breath, gastrointestinal distress, bizarre sensations of tension or pain, and generalized motor hyperactivity. The patient may be hyperventilating, complaining of numbness and tingling of the extremities and sharp twitches of pain in the chest, and showing signs such as pallor, profuse sweating, and uncontrollable muscle spasms.

Clarifying the patient's physical status and reassuring him about it usually terminates such acute attacks, but these measures do not prevent recurrence. Therefore, when such patients are first seen, the physician should explore the possible causes incisively. If the condition becomes chronic, the patient focuses his attention so exclusively on the distressing symptomatology that insightful information is difficult to obtain. Because these patients are frightened and suffering, they respond to direct questioning about the quality of their interpersonal relationships, stresses at home and at work, sexual activities, basic fears regarding adequacy, and so forth. An open discussion of causes and fears is mandatory. Intravenous sodium amytal 200 to 500 mg relieves the acute attack quickly. Meprobamate 400 to 800 mg three or four times a day, or chlordiazepoxide 10 to 20 mg three times a day alleviates the anxious condition, but provides only limited protection against recurrence. The side effects of these anti-anxiety agents include withdrawal symptoms, paradoxical reactions, drug dependency, and allergic conditions.

CHRONIC ANXIETY STATES

Chronic anxiety states manifest a wide range of symptomatology. For some patients, the repeated acute attacks lead to the chronic condition; a high level of anxiety is apparent between the acute attacks which then occur more frequently. Engel (1962a) says, "The somatic symptomatology and the physiologic changes associated with anxiety set in motion a vicious cycle—the patient begins to fear the onset of the next acute attack and his perception of somatic symptoms reinforces this signal of danger." Chronic anxiety is evidenced by the patient's tense appearance which is accentuated as the day goes on and the strains of activity, exercise, and worry take their toll. Although the anxious patient has difficulty going to sleep, he appears more relaxed in the morning; in contrast, the depressed patient is generally more apathetic in the morning and brighter in the evening. Most morbidly anxious patients will speak frankly about their worries, fears, and sustained tension; they say that they are "on edge" all the time; their agitation is betrayed by trembling and the inability to be at ease; they are preoccupied with worry over both their mental and physical conditions.

These patients are often referred for psychiatric consultation. Because the condition is both severe and chronic, medications are usually needed to alleviate the extreme discomfort which obstructs psychotherapy. If the patient displays moderate muscle tension and agitation, and if his ego strength is reasonably good, meprobamate is preferred. For the patient who seems to be more psychiatrically ill, obsessive, and has diffuse complaints, chlordiazepoxide is usually more effective. For the even more chronically ill patient who will require medication for months, phenothiazine compounds should be used; we start with 25 mg of chlorpromazine or thioridazine four times a day, check for hypotensive reactions, and then raise the total daily dosage by 50 to 100 mg every few days until the patient notices relief of symptoms, or side effects appear. The most common side effects are the dyskinesias, particularly Parkinsonism and akathisia; dystonia is now seen only occasionally, and in recent years reports of jaundice and agranulocytosis have diminished; hyperpigmentation, photosensitivity, and pigmentation of the cornea and the lens do occur. Hollister (1966) noted that some patients taking chlorpromazine for many years showed coronary artery changes on postmortem examination, but this has not been validated.

ANXIETY EXPRESSED CHARACTEROLOGICALLY

Anxiety is expressed through "neurotic" behavior and attitudes, and a host of characterologic defenses which affect interpersonal relationships. These characteristics may appear so intangible to the physician that he is reluctant to refer the patient for consultation until more obvious difficulties appear. Such "neurotic" behavior includes emotional lability, erratic and inconsistent attitudes, and impaired communication, especially between patient and physician. This difficulty with communication may be so great that the physician and his patient are unable to reach consensus about the severity of the illness or the necessity for particular types of treatment.

In an evaluation of medical inpatients' attitudes, we (1966a) found that those with increased anxiety focused their concern toward hospitalization and physicians as well as toward the illness. They had negative attitudes about hospitalization, expressing downright dislike for it. They felt insecure in the hospital, regarding it as threatening, unsafe, and confining in contrast to the feelings of security and safety expressed by those with less anxiety. Patients with greater anxiety also expressed a lack of confidence in their physicians and had less personal liking for them than did those with less anxiety. They complained that they could not really talk with their doctors; that the doctors were not listening to them, not giving them enough time, or not telling them everything. Characterologic defenses were manifold: chronic irritability, suspicion, lack of cooperation, and passive-aggressive activities, such as delaying, aloofness, and variably expressed hostility. Grinker (1959) stated: "because anxiety is so disagreeable, often unendurable, psychologic defensive manoeuvres are aroused to avoid the unpleasure. *Much of the character and personality deformation*, various symptoms comprising psychiatric syndromes, and regressions associated with chronic somatic disturbances are the consequences of prior anxiety" [the italics are the authors].

Medication is of little value for treating these patients because their defenses bind the anxiety. They consider their personality traits "normal," although these traits are distressful to others. Psychotherapy also has limited effectiveness until the interpersonal difficulties produce defined troubles. When a crisis arises, the indicated psychiatric referral is usually accepted by the patient.

ANXIETY AND SCHIZOPHRENIA

Many ambulant and borderline schizophrenic patients present with anxiety and vagueness rather than obvious psychotic symptomatology. Most respond well to psychotherapy which emphasizes specificity, concreteness, and current realities. Phenothiazines are the only medications which are beneficial. These patients require 200 to 500 mg per day of chlorpromazine (or equivalent doses of other phenothiazines), for many months. When the medication is to be discontinued, it should be reduced gradually over a number of months.

ADMIXTURES OF ANXIETY AND DEPRESSION

Patients with these conditions constitute a large and heterogeneous group who first go to general physicians seeking treatment for their emotional distress. After the patient has been referred to him, and after psychiatric evaluation, the psychiatrist will often recommend that the physician continue the care of the patient by beginning office psychotherapy. To do this effectively, the patient and the physician must agree on goals and work together to explore the causes of the distress. The physician should enlist the patient's aid in actively seeking ways to eliminate contributing circumstances; he should use the patient's suggestions as well as his own ideas. Ordinarily, the tensions at work or at home, distorted relationships, and turbulent emotions are both causes and complaints. When the patient feels better and has increased confidence in his ability to function, he can find healthful solutions. But the causative factors are not always easily discernible; frequently, they are subjective, colored by troublesome fantasies and irrational fears. It is the physician's task to elicit the patient's irrational fears openly and without humiliating him, so that they are exposed to light instead of festering in obscurity.

The choice of medication for these patients is generally directed toward the dominant affect. If the patient appears more anxious than depressed, antianxiety medications are used; when lowered mood is paramount, antidepressant medications are prescribed. But using the antidepressants rather than the antianxiety agents may be preferred; amitriptyline is often effective: 75 to 100 mg daily to begin, then gradually raise to 100 to 150 mg per day. Because amitriptyline exerts a sedating effect, it has value as an antianxiety agent during the daytime and it helps the patient sleep, particularly if the bedtime dose is doubled.

Combinations of antianxiety and antidepressant drugs are becoming more popular. Deprol, containing meprobamate and benactyzine, is the oldest of these; it seems to be beneficial for milder cases. The new combinations of amitriptyline, 10 to 25 mg, and perphenazine, 2 to 4 mg (Triavil or Etrafon), three to four times a day, are gaining favor. Reports concerning optimum effectiveness of different combinations vary. The appropriate combination must be selected for each patient on an individual basis; for example, when the patient's anxiety is great and his ego strength is poor, the combinations with larger amounts of perphenazine should be used.

GUIDELINES FOR MANAGEMENT

1. From the medical history, the consultant must ascertain whether the patient has a chronic anxiety neurosis or increased anxiety as a discrete reaction to the threat of illness and hospitalization. Evaluating the quality of the patient's responses to previous stressful situations (medical and nonmedical) enables the consultant to make this important differ-

entiation. The mental status examination is also an effective tool for diagnosing anxiety.

2. Management, while the patient is hospitalized, requires clarification of the stress which provokes increased anxiety. When the stress arises from diagnostic procedures or the prognostic implications of the illness, the consultant must work closely with the staff to provide clear answers about the patient's medical condition. Persistent uncertainty only aggravates anxiety. Even though the patient may have a serious illness, exact knowledge about it and concrete plans for treatment diminish his vague concerns and enable him to focus attention on the treatment program.

3. For those patients with increased anxiety related to medical care and hospitalization, limited regression is usually health-promoting. It permits the patient to pull together his already strained defenses and battered resources. However, time limits should be established and the staff should be informed that the consultant will continue to supervise management and that the regressed condition will not mean total dependency. Permitting regression entails limiting demands on the patient, increasing sedation, and simple catering without causing humiliation or struggle. Restricting the patient's visitors is sometimes advisable; the anxiety may be aggravated by family and friends whose solicitude only veils hostility derived from previous conflicts.

4. The consultant can help the consultee provide needed reassurance to these patients. Too often, the physician considers reassurance to be soothing statements indicating that "everything is going to be all right." However, the essence of reassurance is his relationship with the patient, and this depends on conveying to the patient the certainty that his care will continue.

5. Medications are usually indicated: antianxiety agents or sedation or both. Because sleep deprivation increases anxiety, sedation is usually required to restore healthful sleeping patterns. (See Medications).

6. For the patient with an anxiety neurosis, the consultant has to provide a temporary treatment program and at the same time ensure that the patient obtains more definitive long-term psychiatric treatment, usually intensive psychotherapy. During hospitalization, the patient is more amenable to making plans for psychotherapy.

Even in his limited contacts with the patient, the consultant must explore the problem of anxiety, find its sources, and uncover the fears and concerns which are rampant. When the consultant does this with compassion, objectivity, and interest, his efforts are usually rewarded, particularly if the patient's self-esteem improves. This need for increased self-esteem in the anxious patient is supported by research, which shows how frequently a lowered self-esteem accompanies increased anxiety. Anything which would diminish the patient's self-esteem or impair his already flawed self-concept will increase anxiety and have deleterious consequences.

The therapeutic task is to convert apprehension to comprehension, and in the literal sense of the word, when we can "grasp" fear we can usually "handle" it. . . . How then can the physician with limited time at his disposal help the patient with these kinds of complaints. First, listen to the patient. Secondly, explain to the patient. Thirdly, explore with the patient his life and feelings. Fourthly, comfort and reassure. Fifthly, . . . use drugs sparingly and do not overstudy the patient.

Wahl (1962)

REFERENCES

ADAMS, R. D., and HOPE, J. M. The anxiety state and psychasthenia. *In* Harrison, T. R., et al., eds. Principles of Internal Medicine. New York, McGraw-Hill Book Company, 1962, pp. 390–397.

ANDRESON, A. F. R. A practical approach to anxiety reactions. New York, J. Med., 63:1144, 1963.

BERGER, F. M. The treatment of anxiety: a critical review. J. Neuropsychiat., 98:103, 1962.

CANNON, W. B. Bodily Changes in Pain, Hunger, Fear, and Rage. New York, Appleton-Century-Crofts, 1939.

CATTELL, R. B., and Scheier, I. H. The Meaning and Measurement of Neuroticism and Anxiety. New York, The Ronald Press Company, 1961.

ENGEL, F. General concepts of adrenocortical function in relation to response to stress. Psychosom. Med., 15:565, 1953.

ENGEL, G. L. Anxiety and depression-withdrawal: the primary affects of unpleasure. Int. J. Psychoanal., 43:89, 1962a.

—— Psychological Development in Health and Disease. Philadelphia, W. B. Saunders Co., 1962b.

EYSENCK H. J. The Scientific Study of Personality. London, Routledge and Kegan Paul, 1952.

FINN, R., and HUSTEN, P. E. Emotional and mental symptoms in private medical practice. J. Iowa Med. Soc., 56(2):138, 1966.

FREUD, S. *In* Strachey, J., ed. The Complete Psychological Works of Sigmund Freud. London, Hogarth Press, 1921, Vol. XX, p. 132.

—— The Problem of Anxiety. New York, W. W. Norton & Company, Inc., 1936.

GRINKER, R. R. Psychosomatic approach to anxiety. Amer. J. Psychiat., 113:443, 1956.

—— Anxiety as a significant variable for a unified theory of human behavior. Arch. Gen. Psychiat., 1:537, 1959.

HOLLISTER, L. E. Psychopharmacologic drugs. J.A.M.A., 196(5):125, 1966.

HOPE, J. M. The anxiety state. Med. World, 96:99, 1962.

INGLE, D. The role of adrenal cortex in homeostasis. J. Endocr. 8:22, 1952.

MAY, R. The Meaning of Anxiety. New York, The Ronald Press Company, 1950.

—————— The existential approach. In Arieti, S., ed. American Handbook of Psychiatry. New York, Basic Books Inc., Publishers, 1967, pp. 1348–1361.

MOWRER, O. H. Learning Theory and Personality Dynamics. New York, The Ronald Press Company, 1950.

O'LEARY, J. P., COLUMBARO, R. L., SCHWAB, J. J., and McGINNIS, N. H. Anxiety in cardiac patients. J. Nerv. Dis., In press.

REISER, M. F. Cardiovascular disorders. In Freedman, A. M., Kaplan, H. I., and Kaplan, H., eds. Comprehensive Textbook of Psychiatry. Baltimore, The Williams & Wilkins Co., 1967.

RENNIE, T. A. C. Anxiety states: their recognition and management. Med. Clin. N. Amer., 597:608, 1948.

SARBIN, T. R. Anxiety: reification of a metaphor. Arch. Gen. Psychiat., 10:630, 1964.

SCHWAB, J. J., McGINNIS, N. H., MARDER, L., and CLEMONS, R. S. Evaluating anxiey in medical patients. J. Chronic Dis., 19:1049, 1966a.

——————, McGINNIS, N. H., and HARMELING, J. D. Anxiety in medical patients. Excerpta Medica International Congress Series No. 134. Psychosom. Med. Proceedings of the First International Congress of the Academy of Psychosomatic Medicine: 229–232, Palma de Mallorca, Spain, Sept. 1966b.

—————— MARDER, L., CLEMMONS, R. S., and McGINNIS, N. H. Anxiety, severity of illness, and other medical variables. J. Psychosom. Res., 10:291, 1966c.

—————— HARMELING, J. D., and McGINNIS, N. H. Anxiety, self concept, and body image: psychosomatic correlations, I. A preliminary report, presented at the IV World Congress of Psychiatry in Madrid, Spain, Sept. 5–11, 1966d, In press.

—————— Evaluating psychiatric consultation work. Psychosomatics, 8:309, November / December, 1967a.

—————— McGINNIS, N. H. The treatment of anxiety. Medical College of Virginia Quarterly, 3(2):101, Summer, 1967b.

—————— BROWN, J. M. The treatment of anxiety and depression. Postgrad. Med., In press.

SCHEIER, I. H. Experimental results to date from the standpoint of the clinician. Ann. N.Y. Acad. Sci. 93:840, 1962.

SELYE, H. The concept of stress in experimental physiology. In Tanner, J. M., ed. Stress and Psychiatric Disorder. Oxford, Blackwell Scientific Publications, 1960.

WAHL, C. W. The medical management of acute anxiety states. New Physician 2(12):430, 1962.

WEST, L. J. Psychophysiology. In Lief, H. I., Lief, V. F., and Lief, N. R., eds. The Psychological Basis of Medical Practice. New York, Harper & Row, publishers, 1963.

25 DEPRESSION

With the assistance of Judith Benninger Brown, M.A.

The term depression is used to describe a complex of symptoms that may occur in any human illness. . . . depression should be viewed as a reaction to somatic, psychological, or social stress which causes the patient to feel loss of self-esteem, status, or love, in the sense of being alone or abandoned. The patient reacts to this loss with aggression and anger which involves persons close to him as well as himself.

(Ewalt, 1960)

DEFINITIONS

Although depression is a recognized psychobiologic mode of human reactivity, the assessment of depression in medical and surgical patients is complicated for psychiatrists and other physicians. The term depression is used frequently, often without clarity and precise meaning, mainly because there is little concensus about its definition. Cleghorn and Curtis (1959) emphasize responsivity and somatic symptoms in their definition: "Depression is a response of the human organism usually characterized by sadness and despair, but in which a physical symptom or symptoms may be the only indication of the unexpressed depressive affect." Masserman (1965) equates the physiologic symptoms with the term "depressive reaction," which in turn is part of the larger category, depression. Depression, he says, is a "state characterized affectively by maintained dejection in mood, ideologically by gloomy ruminations or foreboding, and physiologically by the depressive syndrome: varying degrees of anorexia, insomnia, loss of weight, gastrointestinal dysfunctions, fatigability, and diminished sexual desire."

214

The consultant's difficulties with diagnosis are compounded because depression in medical patient appears to differ from the classical descriptions derived mainly from observations of psychiatric patients. Whether there are different types of depressive illness, or whether the medical patient's depression is merely an early phase of classical depression, melancholia, cannot be answered with finality. Engel (1956, 1962a, 1962b, 1967a, 1967b) and his colleagues (Adamson, 1965; Schmale, 1958, 1964a, 1964b, 1966a, 1966b) have been engaged in a series of long-term studies of the affects which compose the depressive syndrome, delineating sadness, helplessness, and hopelessness, and researching the relationships between these affective states and many kinds of illnesses. In view of this work, perhaps classical depression should be clearly labeled melancholia; it involves a predominance of affective symptomatology, a withdrawal of the libido from the external world, and a relinquishing of object relations. Hopelessness, rather than the affects of helplessness and sadness, prevails. On the other hand, medical patients with depression appear to have more somatic complaints and display a clinging quality—the libido is still involved in, rather than withdrawn from, object relations (Schwab, 1967a). The central feature of melancholia is diminished self-esteem traceable to disturbances of early psychosexual development which render the individual vulnerable in later life. An understanding of depression in medical patients requires some quantitative modification of this concept.

When the early disturbance is of sufficient magnitude, the patient's clinical picture is melancholia, typified by fear and sorrow, and manifested by the withdrawal of libido from the external world. Those in whom a constitutional element is present appear as manic-depressives, while the melancholia of the others appears on a continuum of severity from neurotic to psychotic. All such individuals are diagnosed as unambiguously psychiatric.

The person whose psychosexual development was less flawed, or who utilized compensatory mechanisms more effectively, becomes depressed for the first time usually during the climacteric, or when elderly. Depression occurs when he realizes that his aspirations will not be attained, and that like all other men, he is a creature of biologic existence subject to "time's wingèd chariot hurrying near." Although these individuals may appear on medical units for diagnosis, more often their symptomatology so closely resembles melancholia that they too are labeled psychiatrically depressed.

In our study (1967a), the depressed medical patient had either a developmental disturbance of even less magnitude or a previous affliction such as psychosomatic illness; the quality of his depression differed from melancholia. These medical patients reported a sense of helplessness, yet this was not abject despair; they had some hope in medical science. When the effects of adverse circumstance conjoin with the developmental disposition, the scales are weighted against him, and his self-esteem suffers. These circumstances are quite tangible: object loss, deprivation, or a reaction to medical illness. Significantly, we found definite object loss in 42 percent of the depressed medical patients and in only 20 percent of the nondepressed.* In contrast, object loss was not characteristic of Grinker's psychiatrically depressed patients, pointing up one of many differences between the medically and the psychiatrically depressed. That many of our depressed patients were of the lower class probably shows the additive influence of deprivation in lowering self-esteem. The stress of serious medical illness also figures as a contributory factor. For many of these patients, the diagnosis reactive depression is descriptively appropriate. When any or all of these factors are superimposed on even a slight disturbance of early development, the summation is sufficient to produce a loss of self-esteem; the individual reacts in the depressive mode with manifestations qualitatively different from classic melancholia. Our research (1967b) revealed another complication: Depressive symptomatology in medical patients was related to socioeconomic class, differing from class to class.

Because of the many complexities, other researchers are using factor analysis to delineate the types of depression more clearly. In their extensive analysis of the factors associated with depression, Grinker et al. (1961) described five: 1) a factor of hopelessness, with a feeling that the external world can provide no relief and a self-concept of "badness"; 2) a factor of concern about material loss and a belief that the external world could alleviate the concern, if only it would; 3) a guilt factor, by which the patient perceives the illness as his "just desserts" for wrongdoing; 4) a factor of "free anxiety"; and, 5) a factor of "envy, loneliness, martyred affliction, secondary gain, and gratification from the illness, and attempts, by provoking guilt, to force the world into making redress."

Beck's (1967) recent book on depression deserves special mention. He examines the symptomatology, the course and prognosis, and the evolution of our concepts. He delineates each symptom, presents the subtle differences among them, and arrives at precise definitions. Then, he reviews the biologic, psychologic, and psychodynamic studies of depression. Beck offers a thoughtful analysis of the changing and controversial concepts of depression. For example, he shows that while long out of vogue, Kraepelin's gigantic efforts to construct a unitary theory for the various types of depressions have a timely significance.

Beck's depression inventory, the BDI, is clinically derived; it consists of 21 graded symptom attitude categories scored by the patient. Our experience indicates that this is a highly effective measure of the

* P < .02, chi square.

severity of depression, one which can be used by physicians and researchers.

According to Beck's theoretical formulation, the depressive-prone individual suffers from disturbances in the development of his self-concept; as a result, his cognitive patterns force him to view himself, his work, and his future in an idiosyncratic way which produces the affective and behavioral symptoms. Although Beck postulates a circular feedback model with lowered mood reinforcing the cognitive disturbance, he believes that the disorder in cognition is primary. This model is plausible, but it lacks a scientific base which shows how and why the impaired self-concept is responsible for the thinking disorder. And, he has difficulty integrating into his model psychobiologic mechanisms and the possibility of a biologic etiology.

INCIDENCE

Notwithstanding these difficulties with defining, understanding, and diagnosing, depression is frequently seen in general hospital patients. Adams and Hope (1962) found that of 4,660 admissions at the New England Center Hospital, 1,045 patients presented psychiatric syndromes; depression was the most common, diagnosed in 520 patients (11 percent). In a study of 153 patients admitted to the Medical Unit of the University of Florida Teaching Hospital (Schwab, 1965a), the medical staff gave provisional diagnoses of depression to 22 percent; three psychiatrists from the consultation service reviewed the patients' hospital records and found evidence of depression in 30 percent. In another study (Schwab, 1965b) of 100 consecutive medical patients referred for psychiatric consultation, we found that the term "depression" was listed at least once in 32 percent of the patients' medical charts; 26 percent were diagnosed depressed by the psychiatric consultants. The latter percentages parallel Ripley's findings (1947) from the New York Hospital; 28 percent of his patients referred for consultations were depressed.

SYMPTOMS AND DIAGNOSIS

A review of the literature * shows that 36 symptoms are commonly held to be indicative of depression. A tripartite classification separating the array of symptoms into the affective, the somatic, and the behavioral manifestations enables us to order our thoughts. The affective include lowered

* Beck (1961), Chalgren (1953), Davies (1964), Dewan (1952), Ebaugh (1956), Engel (1962), Ewalt (1960), Hamilton (1960), Henderson (1956), Kielholz (1959), Kraines (1957), Noyes and Kolb (1958), Rice (1959), Schottstaedt (1960), and Stoeckle and Davidson (1962).

mood, pessimism, dissatisfaction, helplessness, and hopelessness; the somatic: insomnia, weight loss, palpitations, constipation, and anorexia; the
behavioral: crying, retardation, and social withdrawal. The symptoms may
also be classified according to systems as illustrated by the following: 1)
the psychobiologic—lowered mood, anxiety-tension symptomatology; 2)
the skin—dryness, changes in the hair; 3) the musculoskeletal—retardation,
general pain, fatigue; 4) the cardiovascular—palpitations, chest pain; 5) the
gastrointestinal—anorexia, indigestion, constipation; 6) the genitourinary—
loss of libido, dysuria; 7) the neurological—headaches, severe agitation,
motor restlessness; and, 8) the sense organs—disturbance of vision or pain
in, around, or behind the eyes.

Rice (1959) emphasizes that the symptoms of depression involve the
gastrointestinal tract most frequently. They cover the range of GI activity
from dryness of the mouth to constipation. The physician working with
GI patients can expect to diagnose depression frequently. But his task is
difficult because complaints of anorexia or constipation may be indicative
of the structural disease rather than depression. In one study (1968a), we
found that all of the GI patients reported a wide range of depressive symptoms, but of these, five distinguished the depressed GI patients from the
nondepressed at a level of statistical significance. These five symptoms portray a pervasive syndrome of distress. When the somatic symptoms of
headache and *chest pain* are coupled with symptoms of GI distress, all of
the body except the extremities is involved. And the marked *diminution in
interest in sex* indicates that function of another system, the genitourinary,
is affected by the depressive illness. The affective symptoms of *guilt* and
self-hate reflect the loss of self-esteem which is central to depression. Consequently, we recommend that physicians focus their attention on these
symptoms; and even more, to diagnose depression in gastrointestinal patients, they should be alert to syndromes in which loss of self-esteem and
extended somatic symptomatology are present.

Rice (1959) also calls attention to depression underlying alcoholism
and addiction. Individuals resort to alcohol as a defense against depression,
and the vicious cycle is mobilized.

We (1967b) found that many of the 36 conventional symptoms of depression are distributed ubiquitously throughout a general medical inpatient population: somatic preoccupation 86 percent, retardation 82 percent,
irritability 78 percent, anxiety-tension 76 percent, and insomnia 68 percent.
These symptoms cover a broad range of human reactivity. Their high frequency indicates that they are sometimes components of the reaction to
medical illness and hospitalization, rather than symptoms of depression.

Of these 36 symptoms only 17 were found more frequently ($p < .05$)
in the depressed medical patients than in the nondepressed (see Table 1).

Table 1. Frequency of Symptom in Total Population, Depressed, Nondepressed Groups.

Symptom	% of Total (n = 143)	% of Depr. (n = 29)		% of Nondepr. (n = 114)
Mood (Sadness)	51	86	***	42
Pessimism	24	38		21
Guilt	33	59	**	26
Crying (more than usual)	36	76	***	26
Irritability	78	93		75
Work Inhibition	72	86		68
Somatic Preoccupation	86	100	*	82
Suicidal Thoughts	16	24		12
Sense of Failure	15	18		15
Dissatisfaction	30	48	*	25
Punishment	10	10		10
Self-Hate	19	28		17
Self-Accusation	20	31		18
Social Life (Loss of Interest)	11	28	***	07
Decreased Social Life	14	14		14
Indecisiveness	22	28		20
Negative Body Image	12	21		10
Retardation	82	100	**	77
Anxiety-Tension	76	100	**	69
Loneliness	36	73	***	27
Hopelessness	07	14		05
Helplessness	22	42	**	17
Insomnia	68	86	*	64
Difficulty Falling Asleep	64	90	***	56
Waking Early	60	83	***	53
Fatigue	71	86	*	68
Anorexia	40	72	***	32
Weight Loss	31	45		28
Diminished Sex Drive	22	31		19
Upper GI (Indigestion, etc.)	53	69		49
Palpitations	31	48	*	26
Headache	42	70	***	35
Urinary Complaints	22	28		20
Lower GI (Constipation, etc.)	30	48		37
General Pain	21	28		19
Chest Pain	31	31		31

* $p < .05$; ** $p < .01$; *** $p < .001$. Chi Square, two-tailed.
Symptoms italicized meet our criteria for "clinical applicability."

In considering the clinical utility of these data, a variety of difficulties appear. First, some symptoms occurred so often among these patients that they are poor discriminators of the depressed. Also, some symptoms were reported infrequently; for example, few patients expressed thoughts of

suicide—perhaps the experience of hospitalization, involving care and solicitude on the part of the family and staff, precludes such thoughts. Therefore, to isolate the symptoms which should have greater clinical utility
we evaluated them by more rigorous criteria; the symptom must: 1) distinguish depression at $p < .05$ level; 2) be present in at least 50 percent of
the depressed patients; and, 3) be present in no more than 33 percent of
the nondepressed patients. Only four symptoms met these criteria, but the
value of the symptomatology for assessing depression became far more
evident when we divided the patients into socioeconomic classes. We
then found that 10 symptoms, discriminating depression, met our rigorous
criteria for clinical applicability (see Table 2).

Table 2. Statistically Significant Discriminators of Depression by Class

Lower	Middle	Upper
Affective		
* *Hopelessness*	* *Loneliness*	* Social Life (Loss of Interest)
* *Self-Accusation*	Guilt	
Crying	Crying	* Pessimism
Dissatisfaction	Anxiety-Tension	Dissatisfaction
Guilt	* Helplessness	Anxiety-Tension
Mood (Sadness)	Mood (Sadness)	
Somatic		
* *Palpitations*	* Diminished Sex Drive	* Fatigue
Headache	* Urinary Complaints	* Insomnia
Anorexia	* Difficulty Falling Asleep	
Waking Early	Headache	
	Anorexia	
	Waking Early	

* Unique to that Class
Symptoms italicized meet our criteria for "clinical applicability."

Grouping these medical patients into classes provided a more complete picture of depression for diagnostic purposes.

    We (1967b) also found that the demographic characteristics varied
from class to class. In our lower class, the depressed patients were younger,
most were men, and many were Negroes. In the middle and upper classes,
there were only slight age differences between the depressed and nondepressed, and a sizable portion of the depressed were married. It is fruitless
to apply conventional cliches ("depression is more frequent in women")
when class status is not considered.

    Further, the severity of medical illness related inversely to depression (p < .10).* Likewise, within each class the depressed had less severe medical illness than the nondepressed. Medical illness was most severe in the lower class patients. Importantly, depression in our medical patients occurred in all age groups.

Looking only at those symptoms which met our rigorous criteria, class profiles of depression emerged. The lower class was heterogeneous; its affective symptoms suggest a syndrome of the oppressive effect of lower class status itself. The pervasive sense of *futility* implied in the symptoms *dissatisfaction, self-accusation,* and *hopelessness* corresponds with the finding from the Midtown Manhattan Study (Langner, 1963) that persons in the lower social class expressed feelings of futility to a significant degree. Importantly, *hopelessness,* indicative of more serious depressive illness, was a symptom unique to the lower class. The tendency for lower class patients to have a more serious type of depression is supported by Hollingshead and Redlich (1958). They found that neurotic depression was twice as common in their two upper classes as in their lower, but that psychotic depressions were two and a half times greater in the lower. Our lower class depressed patients reported more somatic symptomatology than the patients in the other classes. When combined with somatic afflictions, the class condition (with its futility syndrome) may become pathological. To diagnose depression in the lower class, the clinician must be armed with a picture of depression which appears to differ drastically from that conventionally associated with the middle and upper classes.

In the middle class, *loneliness* and *guilt,* accompanied by *crying,* were each reported by 83 percent of the depressed. These symptoms reflect the philosophic syndrome of alienation, suggestive of the existential disease so often associated with neurotic disorders of this class. *Helplessness,* symptomatic of reactive and neurotic depressions, was unique to this class. No somatic symptoms met our rigorous criteria for distinguishing depression.

In the upper class only one symptom, *social life (loss of interest),* met our criteria for "clinical applicability," and only six symptoms distinguished the depressed (as contrasted with 12 in the middle class and 10 in the lower). Yet clinicians diagnosed depression frequently in this class. It appears that the medical staff, probably because of its lesser social distance, were more attentive to any manifestations of emotional illness in upper class patients.

Diagnosing depression in medical patients is fraught with difficulties.

---

* But depressions occurred in patients with all levels of severity of medical illness and existed in the following combinations: 1) as an isolated entity (20 percent), 2) in association with minor illnesses (25 percent), and 3) most often in concurrence with medical illness of substantial severity (55 percent). Schwab, 1967a.

The symptoms of chronic medical illness may simulate or, conversely, obscure those of depression. Zeal in pursuing interesting diagnoses or pressing emergencies during the work-up can block sensitivity to depression. Differentiating between depression and schizophrenia is a persisting problem. Further, physicians often report difficulty with communication, and by implication, difficulty with diagnosis, in their write-ups and discussions about lower social class patients and those from ethnic or subcultural groups very different from their own.

Although most physicians are alert to the possibility of depression, they have problems evaluating its severity, and referral patterns are inconsistent. Of the depressed medical patients in one of our studies (1967d), 17 percent of the lower class depressed, 33 percent of the middle class depressed, and 100 percent of the upper class depressed were referred for psychiatric consultation. In referring patients with depression, physicians frequently ask consultants to assess its extent, determine its significance, confirm their diagnostic impressions, and recommend treatment.

THE TREATMENT OF CLINICAL STATES

A general approach to the psychopharmacologic and somatic therapy of depression calls for beginning with the dibenzazepine compounds, such as imipramine, amitriptyline, or desipramine. These are mood elevators for the depressed; in healthy normals they induce fatigue. They have some cholinergic blocking properties, induce orthostatic hypotension, and presumably modify catecholamine activity. The atropine-like actions include: dry mouth, dizziness, blurred vision, and urinary retention. Both hypotension and headache have been reported, and a transition from depression to excitement has been observed. The dibenzazepine compounds should not be given concurrently with the mono-amine-oxidose (MAO) inhibitors; in fact, the patient should be free of all antidepressants for at least one week before switching from one to the other.

We use amitriptyline beginning with 75 mg per day and raise the dose gradually to 100 to 200 mg per day until we observe a therapeutic effect. Then, we lower the dose gradually to the maintenance level. If the patient is no better after two weeks, he should be hospitalized. In the hospital, if there is no response to amitriptyline, we advocate using a MAO inhibitor, preferably tranylcypromine, the most effective of this group. It has severe side effects, a number of deaths and acute toxicity with hallucinations and hyper-reflexia have been reported. A severe hypertensive crisis can be precipitated by the ingestion of foods containing pressor amines; for example, tyramine is the causative substance in cheese which potentiates this crisis. Thirty mg tranylcypromine per day is the recommended dosage. If the patient does not improve within two weeks, this medication should be discontinued and E.C.T. should be given for the treatment of his depression.

THE GRIEF REACTION

Grief is a normal response to loss. The sadness, lowered mood, sense of emptiness, and many physical complaints are natural. However, a prolonged grief reaction cannot be considered "normal"; it is evidence of underlying psychopathology, an ambivalent relationship with the lost object, or of circumstances which temporarily inhibited the immediate expression of emotion. Anxiety, depression, and physical illness on the anniversary of a loss is a variant of the grief reaction. Treatment for these conditions depends mainly on psychotherapy which encourages the expression of pent-up feelings. Medications should be limited to nighttime sedation. Antidepressant medications are usually ineffective; they may shift the patient's emphasis away from his grief to concern with pills. If too much reliance is placed on medications, disillusionment results and is likely to pervade the entire doctor-patient relationship. Every consultant should be familiar with Freud's classic, "Mourning and Melancholia," with Lindemann's (1944) excellent discussion of the clinical aspects of grief reactions.

CHRONIC SADNESS

The chronically sad person suffers from inveterate low self-esteem; his life is filled with pessimistic overtones; the future seems arid and bleak, and dejection, often punctuated by bouts of alcoholism, becomes his way of life. Many of these patients seek medical care because their low spirits are accompanied by physical symptoms and a lack of vigor. They appear hypochondriacal and display a shallow affect. Limited psychotherapy is usually of little benefit; the chronic depression is a lifelong defensive pattern. A trial with antidepressant medication is certainly warranted because some will respond. When there is a good result, the patient should be maintained on medication, possibly for years. Many of these patients have to be referred for intensive psychotherapy, but the psychiatrist's success with these patients is limited.

NEUROTIC AND REACTIVE DEPRESSIONS

These depressive conditions are the most common seen in patients coming to general physicians or undergoing diagnostic work-ups in medical units. The initial approach to treatment should always involve psychotherapy focused on the following: 1) eliciting the meaning of the loss; 2) evoking the expression of feelings, these are usually ambivalent; 3) exploring factors producing the lowered self-esteem which is central to the depression; 4) clarifying environmental forces contributing to the depression; and 5) providing environmental support. Concurrently, antidepressant medications should be used. The regimen previously outlined, beginning with amitriptyline and then proceeding with other medications, is the preferred course. Somatic therapy such as E.C.T. may be needed, but the combined psychotherapy and pharmacologic approach is so effective that E.C.T. is necessary for only a few of these patients.

THE AGITATED DEPRESSIONS

These severe depressive states are marked by anxiety, motor agitation, and painful restlessness. It is distressing to the physician and family to see a person with this condition. The extreme agitation makes psychotherapy an arduous task; consequently, many of these patients need psychiatric hospitalization. However, a trial with the combinations of phenothiazines and antidepressants is often successful with these patients. Combinations of amitriptyline 25 mg and perphenazine 2 to 4 mg (Elavil or Etrafon) should be given 3 to 4 times a day.

Sometimes, particularly for the elderly, these illnesses are produced largely by current environmental stresses; thus, environmental manipulation is usually necessary. Convalescence in a nursing home is beneficial.

PSYCHOTIC DEPRESSIONS

Psychotic depressions are spotted as unambiguously psychiatric since they are typical of classical melancholia. After the medical work-up rules out organic illness (see APPENDIX), immediate psychiatric hospitalization is usually necessary to prevent suicide and to ensure vigorous treatment. For treatment of the manic-depressive illnesses, see PSYCHIATRIC EMERGENCIES.

GUIDELINES FOR THE CONSULTANT

1. The depressive syndrome in medical patients resembles melancholia; unless one appreciates the differences, errors in diagnosis result. The depressive syndrome may be regarded as a natural accompaniment of physical illness or pass unrecognized because its configuration is not so sharp as that of typical melancholia.

2. The symptoms, *guilt, crying, loneliness,* and *anorexia,* are particularly characteristic of depressed medical inpatients. In addition to their affective distress, medical patients exhibit generalized somatic symptomatology.

3. The physician should become more sensitive to depression in demographic groups usually considered less susceptible. In medical patients

depression is common in all age groupings (Schwab, 1968d); males are afflicted almost as often as females, and in many low SeS (Socioeconomic Status) patients it presents as a *futility syndrome*.

4. For greater precision in diagnosis, the physician should question his patient about recent object loss, ascertain whether the symptoms are attributable to chronicity or to depression, make a careful evaluation of the patient's reaction to immediate serious illness, and maintain a holistic approach even when he is zealously pursuing the medical work-up.

5. Differentiating depression from schizophrenia has therapeutic implications (e.g., the use of phenothiazines may deepen depression).

6. The depressed patient is always a suicidal risk (see PSYCHIATRIC EMERGENCIES). The consultant must inform hospital staff explicitly of the degree of this risk.

7. Depressive symptomatology obscures medical illnesses with serious prognoses. Many patients with carcinoma of the pancreas or brain tumors present symptoms characteristic of depression. When undue emphasis is placed on the depression and other diagnoses overlooked, unfortunate errors occur. Therefore, a complete medical work-up is mandatory.

8. The medical evaluation should provide a realistic assessment of the patient's capabilities. Any limitations imposed by concurrent medical illness should be clearly outlined for the patient. Although the depressed patient should be encouraged to renew activities, these should not strain his resources but should be tailored to reinforce his sense of accomplishment; failure only deepens his depression.

9. Occupational and physical therapy programs help to mobilize the patient; they should be initiated while he is in the hospital.

10. Intensive psychotherapy is necessary for many of these patients upon discharge from the hospital. However, the family physician can handle many of these patients, particularly when the consultant supplies him with a treatment program and continues to be available.

11. Antidepressant medications are often indicated. These include amitriptyline (Elavil), imipramine (Tofranil), or a monoamine oxidase inhibitor, such as tranylcypromine (use only when the patient is in a hospital). Adding an amphetamine such as Dexedrine (5 mg t.i.d.) for the first few days seems to accelerate the effectiveness of some antidepressants (see MEDICATIONS).

12. Adequate sedation is essential. Sleep patterns reflect the patient's progress. For severe insomnia, a mixture of 200 mg sodium amytal and 200 mg barbitol at bedtime provides 7 to 8 hours of sleep. Chloral hydrate, 0.5 to 1.0 g at bedtime, is effective and may be preferred because the patient does not continue to feel sedated in the morning.

13. Psychiatric hospitalization and E.C.T. or Indokolin therapy may be necessary for severely depressed patients particularly when the risk

of suicide is great. Somatic treatments can be used effectively while the patient is on a medical or surgical unit if sufficient nursing care is insured. On occasion, with full cognizance of the risk, they can be administered to seriously ill medical patients.

REFERENCES

ADAMS, R. D., and HOPE, J. M. The anxiety state and psychasthenia. *In* Harrison, T. R., ed. Principles of Internal Medicine, 4th ed. New York, McGraw-Hill Book Company, 1962, pp. 390–397.

ADAMSON, J. D., and SCHMALE, A. H. Object loss, giving up, and the onset of psychiatric disease. Psychosom. Med., 17(6):557, 1965.

BECK, A. T., WARD, C. H., MENDELSON, M., MOCK, J., and ERBAUGH, J. An inventory for measuring depression. Arch. Gen. Psychiat., 4:561, 1961.

BECK, A. T. Depression: Clinical, Experimental, and Theoretical Aspects. New York, Harper & Row, 1967.

CHALGREN, W. Physical symptoms of depression. Minn. Med., 36:148, 1953.

CLEGHORN, R. A., and CURTIS, G. C. Depression: mood, symptom, syndrome. Acta Psychosomatica Documenta Geigy, No. 2, North American Series, 1959.

DAVIES, E. B., ed. Depression. Cambridge, Cambridge University Press, 1964.

DEWAN, J. G. Mild depressions. Med. Clin. N. Amer., March: 527, 1952.

EBAUGH, F. The depressed patient. *In* Liebman, S., ed. Management of Emotional Problems in Medical Practice. Philadelphia, J. B. Lippincott Co., 1956.

ENGEL, G. L., and REICHSMAN, F. Spontaneous and experimentally induced depressions in an infant with gastric fistula: A contribution to the problem of depression. J. Amer. Psychoanal, 4:428, 1956.

——— Anxiety and depression-withdrawal: The primary affects of unpleasure. Int. J. Psychoanal., 43:89, 1962a.

——— Psychological Development in Health and Disease. Philadelphia, W. B. Saunders Co., 1962b.

——— SCHMALE, A. H. Psychoanalytic theory of somatic disorder: Conversion, specificity, and the disease onset situation. J. Amer. Psychoanal. Ass. 15(2):344, 1967a.

ENGEL, G. L. Psychological processes and gastrointestinal disorder. *In* Paulson, M., ed. Gastroenterologic Medicine. Philadelphia, Lea & Febiger, 1967b.

EWALT, J. Somatic equivalents of depression. J. Mich. Med. Soc., 59(9), 1960.

GRINKER, R. R., MILLER, J., SABSHIN, M., NUNN, R., and NUNNALLY, J. C. The Phenomena of Depressions. New York, Paul B. Hoeber, 1961.

HAMILTON, M. A rating scale for depression. J. Neurol. Neurosurg. Psychiat., 23:56, 1960.

HENDERSON, D., GILLESPIE, R., and BATCHELER, I. A Textbook of Psychiatry, 8th ed. London, Oxford University Press, Inc., 1956.

HOLLINGSHEAD, A. B., and REDLICH, F. C. Social Class and Mental Illness: A Community Study. New York, John Wiley & Sons, Inc., 1958.

KIELHOLZ, P. Diagnosis and therapy of the depressive state. Acta Psychosomatica Documenta Geigy, No. 1, North American Series, 1959.

KRAINES, S. H. Mental Depressions and Their Treatment. New York, The Macmillan Company, 1957.

LANGNER, T. S., and MICHAEL, S. T. The Midtown Manhattan Study. Life Stress and Mental Health. New York, McGraw-Hill Book Company, 1963, Vol. II, pp. 61, 407, 462.

LINDEMANN, ERIC. Symptomatology and management of acute grief. Amer J. Psychiat., 101:141–148, 1944.

MASSERMAN, J. The Practice of Dynamic Psychiatry. Philadelphia, W. B. Saunders Co., 1965.

NOYES, A., and KOLB, L. Modern Clinical Psychiatry, 5th ed. Philadelphia, W. B. Saunders, 1958.

RICE, D. Somatic syndromes causing depressive state. Practitioner, 183:49, 1959.

RIPLEY, H. Depressive reactions in a general hospital: A study of one hundred and fifty cases. J. Nerv. Ment. Dis., 105:607, 1947.

SCHMALE, A. H. Relationship of separation and depression to disease. I. A report on a hospitalized medical population. Psychosom. Med. 20(4):259, 1958.

————— Object loss, "giving up" and disease onset: An overview of research in progress. Walter Reed Army Institute of Research, 22–24 April, p. 433, 1964a.

————— A genetic view of affects with special reference to the genesis of helplessness and hopelessness. Psychoanal. Stud. Child, 19:287, 1964b.

————— IKER, H. P. The psychological setting of uterine cervical cancer. Ann. N. Y. Acad. Sci., 125:807, 1966a.

————— IKER, H. P. The affect of hopelessness and the development of cancer. I. Identification of uterine cervical cancer in women and atypical cytology. Psychosom. Med., 28(5):714, 1966b.

SCHOTTSTAEDT, W. Psychophysiologic Approach to Medical Practice. Chicago, Year Book Medical Publishers, Inc., 1960.

SCHWAB, J. J., CLEMMONS, R. S., BIALOW, M. R., DUGGAN, V., and DAVIS, B. A study of the somatic symptomatology of depression in medical inpatients. Psychsomatics, 6:273, 1965 a.

————— CLEMMONS, R. S., FREEMON, F. R., and SCOTT, M. L. Differential characteristics of medical inpatients referred for psychiatric consultation: A controlled study. Psychosom. Med., 27(2):112, 1965b.

————— BIALOW, M. R., BROWN, J. M., and HOLZER, C. E. Diagnosing depression in medical inpatients. Ann. Intern. Med., 67(4):695, October, 1967a.

————— BIALOW, M. R., BROWN, J. M., HOLZER, C. E., and STEVENSON, B. E. Sociocultural aspects of depression in medical inpatients. Arch. Gen. Psychiat., 17:539, November, 1967b.

————— BROWN, J. M., and HOLZER, C. E. Depression in medical inpatients with gastrointestinal diseases. Amer. J. Gastroent., 49(2):146, February, 1968a.

————— BROWN, J. M., HOLZER, C. E., and SOKOLOF, M. T. Current concepts of depression: the sociocultural. Int. J. Soc. Psychiat., in press, 1968b.

————— BROWN, J. M. The treatment of anxiety and depression. Postgrad. Med., in press, 1968c.

————— BROWN, J. M., and HOLZER, C. E. Depression in medical inpatients: sex and age differences. Ment. Hyg., in press, 1968d.

STOECKLE, J., and DAVIDSON, G. Bodily complaints and other symptoms of depressive reaction. J.A.M.A., 180:134, 1962.

26 PAIN

Pain, it has been said, is one of nature's earliest signs of morbidity. Few will deny that it stands preeminent among all the sensory experiences by which man judges the evidence of disease within himself. There are relatively few maladies that do not have their painful phases, and in many of them, pain is a characteristic without which diagnosis must always be in doubt.

Adams and Resnick (1966)

The great majority of medical and surgical patients referred to the psychiatric consultant either complain of pain or speak of it as the most prominent feature in the illness. One of the tasks most frequently required of the consultant is to determine, as the consultee puts it, whether the patient's pain is "real or psychogenic."

A number of studies attest to the presence of pain in many patients with diverse illnesses. Devine and Merskey (1965) found that 65 percent of their psychiatric patients and 75 percent of their medical patients complained of pain; Edmonds (1947) notes that 47 percent of 183 patients with psychoneurosis had muscular pains and 39 percent had headaches; Klee et al. (1959) report that 61 percent of patients in a Veterans Administration psychiatric clinic complained of pain on admission.

Adams and Resnick (1966) state that in clinical practice three types of problems with pain are common: 1) patients who complain of pain, but who really have a troubled emotional state; 2) patients who are "difficult pain cases" in which no amount of investigation brings to light medical illness or psychiatric disturbance; and 3) patients with intractable pain, often caused by an established or incurable disease.

THE NATURE OF PAIN

Many writers remind us of Aristotle's concept that pain is exclusively a feeling state. This concept was accepted until the end of the 19th century when the discovery of neuroanatomic pathways focused on the physiologic basis of pain. Since, there has been undue emphasis on the dichotomy: "real" pain due to stimulation of pain receptors, and "psychogenic" pain which is a function solely of the CNS. However, Sherrington described pain as being the psychic component of a protective reflex. Cooper and Braceland (1950) say that pain must be approached as a "Gestalt problem." Engel (1958) describes pain as an experience, not a sensation; one element of pain is the "peripheral signature" (pain associated with particular pathologic processes), and the other element is the "individual psychic signature" (patients' private concepts of how their bodies function, and all the psychic processes involved in the final pain experience). Hardy (1963) concurs, saying "Pain sensation is but part of the total pain experience and indeed may not even be a major feature."

Psychoanalysts have tended to regard complaints of pain, without a structural basis, as conversion symptoms (Breuer and Freud, 1955, and Fenichel, 1945). Recent work is supportive. Merskey (1965) found that persistent pain is more often associated with hysteria-anxiety than with depression or schizophrenia. In discussing contemporary conversion reactions, Ziegler et al. (1960) report that pain is found as a conversion symptom more commonly now than in the past; in fact, pain was the primary complaint in 74 of 134 consecutive patients with conversion reactions.

Both Bleuler (1960) and Jaspers (1963) described pain appearing in the nature of a hallucination or a somatic delusion. Other psychoanalysts indicated that pain is an affect (Fenichel, 1945, and Engel, 1958). Engel says, "We must acknowledge that pain, in the final analysis, is a psychic phenomenon."

Hart (1947) suggested a close relationship between ego and cortical functions. He said that reception, interpretation, or projection in response to painful stimuli are functions chiefly of the cerebral cortex. Accordingly, he postulated, it is logical to assume that as a function of the corticothalamic organization the ego displaces guilt through peripheral somatic pain.

Petrovitch (1958) studied associations with pain and found that painfulness concepts embrace a considerable range and variety of experiences: specific physical injuries and ailments (gunshot wound or broken bone) and also situations which are primarily psychologic or emotional in nature (death of a loved one, disappointment, and others).

Pain is an individual experience; it has limitless associations (e.g., trauma, deprivation, eroticism, grief-tension, or satiation); it is impossible to define and difficult to describe; it is related to man's noblest and basest emotions. Also, there are many social and cultural variations [Ross (1962)]. Zborowski (1952) found that Jews and Italians tended to display emotional responses to pain, while there was less emphasis on such complaints among "Old Americans." There are other specific variations. Even today the people in the hills of Kentucky use the idiom, "I am punishing" when they are attempting to describe pain. Interestingly, Webster lists the Latin origin of *pain* as "penalty," "punishment," and the Greek as "penalty," "payment," "to pay." Szasz (1959) emphasizes the symbolic and communicative aspects of pain. He stresses that when the patient tries to describe pain, he speaks in one language, while the physician is usually speaking in another; therefore, the physician must become a translator.

THE MEANING OF PAIN

Engel (1958) says: ". . . pain belongs to the systems concerned with protecting the body from injury. We may assume from birth on, the individual builds up a library, so to speak, with pain experiences originating from a variety of peripheral stimulations which he experiences in the course of life." He lists six special meanings of pain: 1) Pain warns of damage to the body and is part of the protection system; 2) Developmentally, pain is involved in human relationships—even in infancy, pain leads to crying and a response from the mother; 3) Early in childhood, pain and punishment become linked; 4) Pain early becomes associated with aggression and power—the child learns he can inflict pain; 5) Pain is connected with object loss, real or symbolic, especially when there is guilt; and 6) Pain is associated with sexual feelings.

Pain is used by patients as a complaint to gain access to physicians, to disguise feelings of grief or aggression, and to obtain benefits such as sympathy or attention. It is a common feature of certain psychiatric syndromes: first and foremost, conversion-hysteria, second, psychophysiologic reactions, and third, depression (general pain may be the only complaint the patient can muster in an attempt to communicate his feelings of despair). Pain is an essential complaint in the syndrome that is labeled "hypochondriasis." Pain is usually the malingerer's chief complaint; the novice malingerer will state that he has many aches and pains which are diffuse and variable; in contrast, the sophisticated malingerer steadfastly insists that he has only one pain (one that he knows is difficult to evaluate, such as headache, or the simulated kidney stone). Pain appears occasionally in schizophrenia and may be a somatic delusion. Most authorities agree that once the psychic organization for pain is established, continued stimulation from peripheral pain receptors may no longer be necessary. In hospitalized patients, pain is a common language and one which is universally accepted as being indicative of illness. Cooper and Braceland (1950) note four principal situations which provide a suitable background for the perpetuation of pain: 1) the need to cover drug addiction, 2) compensation-neurosis, 3) post-traumatic neurosis, and 4) perpetuation of psychoneurosis with elements of secondary gains.

In discussing the pain-prone individual, Engel (1958) says that he usually shows some of the following: a predisposing background to the use of pain, a history of suffering and defeat, intolerance of success, a propensity to solicit pain, a strong aggressive drive which is unfulfilled, development of pain when a relationship is threatened or lost, a location for the pain which is determined by an unconscious identification with others, and guilt.

GUIDELINES FOR THE CONSULTANT

1. "Real or psychogenic pain?" In view of the above discussion of the nature and meaning of pain, this question (which is frequently asked of the consultant) is obviously too dichotomous. It usually disguises the consultee's more fundamental question: "Inasmuch as we cannot find sufficient structural illness to account for this patient's complaints, does he have an emotional illness which is responsible; or, can you make a psychiatric diagnosis which will explain the complaints of pain?" When he encounters this patient, the consultant fears: 1) that his diagnosis of psychiatric distress will be accepted and that consequently a pathologic, pain-producing process will be overlooked; 2) that the patient has emotional problems but how can he say for sure that they are producing the symptoms; or, 3) that he just can't answer.

Generally, pain originating from emotional illness without a defined organic basis has the following characteristics: The patient's description is excessive and his affect inappropriate; pain is poorly localized, and its radiation is inconsistent and diffuse; the patient expresses vague suffering; precipitating factors are nonspecific—instead, the patient just "has it all day" or "on the weekend" (the Sunday neurosis usually indicates marital discord); factors which relieve the pain are not related to physiology, such as change of posture, but instead are related to events and interpersonal happenings, or it "just goes away" (see Gould, 1962).

These generalizations have limited value because the exceptions are so numerous. The consultant must always accept the patient's complaints; in fact, he should assure the patient that pain is always real and never imagined. This assurance gains the patient's confidence and allows him to initiate a personal description of the symptom which may clarify its meaning. Certain questions are helpful in eliciting the full import of the pain. Is the pain a sensation? If so, to what is it akin (a needle prick, a burning, a bruise)? Very often the patient will describe it as tension, a tightening, a constricting feeling, or a "pressure." Then the consultant must discover if the patient is really trying to describe anguish.

What produces the pain? When? What relieves it? When? What is it associated with?—Activities? Hours? Days? People? Who? Other associations? Ask the patient for fantasies and dreams; does he experience pain in his dreams? What do others do when the patient has pain? What does the patient do—obtain medication, rest, relief from strain? Is it an excuse for not meeting supposed or real obligations?

Finally, what is the meaning of pain to the patient? Express confidence that he can put his own ideas into words and that his ideas are important.

Always, of course, the consultant will have to rely on his clinical judgment to answer the consultee. He should not hesitate to ask for time, for studies, for follow-up, for obtaining greater understanding, or just for reflection. In his continued work with the patient, the consultant should encourage ventilation; abreaction is usually pain-relieving.

2. Do not dismiss complaints of localized, persistent, or severe pain as psychogenic. Although the consultant may have been asked specifically to make the "either-or" diagnosis about the patient's pain, when it is severe, persistent, or localized, it is injudicious to announce that it may be psychogenic even when there are positive factors in the patient's psychosocial existence which might account for neurosis. Here, the consultant should insist that he be given an opportunity for follow-up visits. When medications are needed, tranquilizers should be used during the day and sedatives only at night. Nonaddicting analgesics should be used during the day or at night, keeping in mind that phenothiazines potentiate their action and that the dependent personality is apt to develop some dependency on any medication.

3. Always beware of the problem of addiction. The patient may already be addicted, or addiction will supervene if continued symptomatic treatment for the pain involves drugs.

4. Management of the suspected addict.

(a) Medication. Study medication chart to determine how much narcotic (usually Demerol or codeine for the hospitalized patient) the patient received during the last few days. Substitute 5 mg of methadone orally for every 50 to 75 mg of Demerol or 60 mg of codeine. Usually 10 mg of methadone every 12 hours is sufficient; reduce methadone by 5 mg daily. If abstinence symptoms appear (profuse sweating, vasomotor instability, or even convulsions), maintain present dosage of methadone for two more days before reducing it further; also, give anticonvulsant medications, Dilantin 100 mg three or four times a day. Concurrent use of phenothiazines may be helpful; Thorazine or Mellaril 50 mg three or four times a day.

   (b) Brief psychotherapy while the patient is in the hospital.

   (c) Make definite plans for continued psychotherapy after the patient is discharged.

5. Management of the patient who may or may not be addicted but whose demands for medication distress the staff.

   (a) Medication. If the patient is addicted (or it is suspected that he is), explain the problem of addiction to him frankly, ask for his cooperation, and institute the methadone regimen described above. For these patients it is generally best to prescribe Thorazine or Mellaril 25 to 50 mg three or four times a day whether or not the methadone regimen is used.

   (b) Substitute care and attention for medications. The consultant should visit the patient briefly each day. Obtain assistance from nurses, students, the chaplain, or a social worker. Many of these patients are desperately lonely and afraid; having someone to "talk to" takes the place of medications. Increasing visitors, or even asking family members to stay with the patient beyond visiting hours is helpful; on occasion we have realized that these patients are really asking for a relative or friend (who may not live nearby) to visit them, and we have called in a distant "mother" or a favorite aunt.

   (c) Increase activities. Intensive occupational therapy and physical therapy programs are beneficial.

6. Intractable pain. If the patient is not suffering from diagnosed organic illness (tabes dorsalis, radiculitis, neuralgia, and so on), psychiatric hospitalization with milieu therapy is mandatory. If a medical or surgical inpatient has intractable pain and is addicted to narcotics, the consultant may wish to postpone treatment of the addiction until the patient is transferred to a psychiatric unit. On these occasions, the consultant must discuss the long-term plans with the staff as well as with the patient; otherwise, they may be so fearful and guilty about contributing to the addiction that management, while awaiting transfer, becomes very difficult. If the patient has organic illness which accounts for the pain, the consultant can recommend nonnarcotic analgesics, phenothiazines, and psychotherapy. Sometimes neurosurgery (cutting a nerve root) or psychosurgery (lobotomy) is necessary; lobotomy may be helpful but, as Freeman (1959) says: "Lobotomy relieves suffering rather than pain. . . . Furthermore, it makes the pain an experience of the moment, without the dreaded anticipation . . . and its continual reverberations through

the whole being of the patient." In all cases, the patient should have adequate trial of intensive milieu therapy before the decision for neurosurgery or psychosurgery is made.

7. For teaching others how to evaluate pain, the consultant can use Cooper and Braceland's (1950) precepts: 1) understand the patient and the emotions which initiate or exaggerate his reactions to pain; 2) consider the context in which the patient lives and works (marital status, economic difficulties, and former methods of reacting); 3) take time to explain to the patient how emotional problems influence somatic reactions and facilitate pain; 4) realize that frequent or injudicious injecting, massaging, and the like serve to fix the symptom; 5) take the necessary time to hear what the patient has to say; 6) know that hostility begets hostility; 7) realize that reassurance is a short-lived therapeutic device; and 8) value psychiatric judgment as ranking in importance with medical and surgical judgment.

REFERENCES

ADAMS, R. D., and RESNIK, W. H. Cardinal manifestations of disease: Pain. *In* Harrison, T. R., ed. Principles of Internal Medicine, 5th ed. New York, McGraw-Hill Book Company, 1966, pp. 10–17.

BLEULER, E. Textbook of Psychiatry, 10th ed. Springer-Verlag New York Inc., 1960.

BREUER, J., and FREUD, S. Studies on Hysteria, Standard Edition, Complete Psychological Works of Freud. London, Hogarth Press, 1955.

COOPER, I. S., and BRACELAND, F. J. Psychosomatic aspects of pain. Med. Clin. N. Amer., p. 981, 1950.

DEVINE, R., and MERSKEY, H. The description of pain in psychiatric and general medical patients. J. Psychosom. Res., 9:311, 1965.

EDMONDS, E. P. Psychosomatic pain—articular rheumatism. Ann. Rheum. Dis., 6:36, 1947.

ENGEL, G. L. "Psychogenic" pain. Med. Clin. N. Amer., p. 1481, 1958.

FENICHEL, O. The Psychoanalytic Theory of the Neuroses. New York, W. W. Norton & Company, Inc. 1945.

FREEMAN, W. Psychosurgery. *In* Arieti, S., ed. Handbook of Psychiatry. New York, Basic Books, Inc., Publishers, 1959, pp. 1521–1540.

GOULD, J. The assessment of pain in clinical practice. Brit. J. Clin. Pract., 16:31, 1962.

HARDY, J. D. Pharmacodynamics of human disease: 3. The pain threshold and the nature of pain sensation. Postgrad. Med., 34:579, 1963.

HART, H. Displacement of guilt and pain. Psychoanal. Rev., 34:259, 1947.

JASPERS, K. General Psychopathology, 7th ed. Hoenig, J., and Hamilton, M. W., trans. Manchester, Manchester University Press, 1963.

KLEE, G. D., OZELIS, S., GREENBERG, I., and GALLANT, L. J. Pain and other somatic complaints in a psychiatric clinic. Maryland Med. J., 8:188, 1959.

MERSKEY, H. The characteristics of persistent pain in psychological illness. J. Psychosom. Res., 9:291, 1965.

PETROVITCH, D. V. A survey of painfulness concepts. J. Clin. Psychol., 14:288, 1958.

ROSS, J. A. Social class and medical care. J. Health Hum. Behav., III:35, 1962.

SZASZ, T. S. Language and pain. *In* Arieti, S., ed. American Handbook of Psychiatry. New York, Basic Books, Inc., Publishers, 1959, pp. 982–999.

ZBOROWSKI, M. Cultural components in responses to pain. J. Social Issues, XIII:16, 1952.

ZIEGLER, J. J., Imboden, J. B., and Meyer, E. Contemporary conversion reactions. A clinical study. Amer. J. Psychiat., 116:901, 1960.

SECTION SEVEN   A Teaching
                    Program

27   CONSULTATION-LIAISON
         PROGRAM

*It is a sobering fact to remember that today we are training physicians
to become psychiatrists who will be practicing in the year 2000. We are
preparing the psychiatrist for a role which we do not yet clearly understand except that we do recognize he must be prepared for a changing
role in a changing world.*

(Mendel and Solomon, 1968)

Psychiatric consultation services are expected to meet the traditional
functions of patient care, education, and research. Too often, however,
these services respond only to the pressing needs for patient care. Demands for service can exceed the capabilities of the program so that little
attention is paid to teaching and research activities.

The consultation-liaison program developed in 1962 at the University of Florida Teaching Hospital differs from others in its greater
emphasis on the educative functions as an important segment of the psychiatric resident's training. Our teaching program was designed to fulfill
the specific objectives of education and training. We think that education must be distinguished clearly from training. In writing about this
distinction, Ewalt (1965) says that the function of a teaching program
for residents is to encourage curiosity, promote independent thought,
and stress that knowledge changes. We think the program should be
geared first to education, "the leading forth," and second to training,
with its narrower aspects: the acquisition of knowledge, skills, and practical experience.

BASES FOR OUR PROGRAM:
HISTORICAL AND THEORETICAL

It is generally accepted that the role of the psychiatrist is in transition. The recent articles by Lipowski (1966), books by Zinberg (1964), Kaufman (1965), and Mendel and Solomon (1968), and the number of symposia (1965, 1965, 1966) devoted to consultation activities, indicate that psychiatry is abandoning the classical isolation of the past. The psychiatrist's close association with all medical and paramedical specialties and his entrance into community activities also point to this change.

In the American Psychiatric Association's 1952 Conference on Graduate Psychiatric Education, the agenda stressed training for greater knowledge of psychodynamics, while the 1962 Conference emphasized sound clinical training. The latter report stated: "Efforts of the training program should also be directed toward striking a proper balance between the psychiatrist's specific skills, as in psychotherapy, and other skills which will equip him to meet his wider social responsibilities." Even though little specific attention was given to training in consultation and liaison activities, these were mentioned as residency requirements. The primary characteristic of the psychiatrist was described: "He needs, first and foremost, to be a physician with the knowledge, ethics, values, and codes expected of a member of the medical profession." The same report recommended that the psychiatrist should have a biologic, socioanthropologic, and psychologic understanding of his patients.

Other factors influence the demand for the psychiatrist trained in consultation-liaison work: a greater medical awareness of psychogenic variables in all illness; an emphasis on the early return of the mentally ill patient to the community; the inclusion of psychiatric services in the general hospital; and lastly, a public health orientation which stresses prevention of mental illness.

GOALS

With this background, our faculty saw the need to combine the traditional patient-physician centered curriculum with a collaboration-centered one. Specific training goals for psychiatric residents were established. As early as 1950, Lidz and Fleck recognized that training goals were lacking and stated further that psychiatric treatment in a liaison service cannot follow preconceived or standardized methods but must offer a challenge to the adaptability of the staff. Specifying educational and training goals for a program makes it possible to scrutinize objectively the accomplishments or lack thereof.

The broad educational goals, revealing the philosophy of our program, are to enable the resident to become a specialist in comprehensive medicine, and to promote his development as a teacher of medical psychology. To these we add the more specific training goals:

1. To practice as a psychiatric consultant with medical and surgical patients. The resident sees by daily practice that his specialized skills and knowledge enhance patient care and that his work is valued by the consultees, nurses, and other personnel.

2. To be comfortable on medical and surgical units in general hospitals. Too often, the psychiatric resident experiences acute discomfort on returning to active work with medically ill patients. Extensive consultative experience reinforces his identity as a physician; one who has devoted almost a decade of his life, through premedical college, medical school, and internship, to this profession. Thus, he is able to take his rightful place as a medical specialist.

3. To gain experience working with many patients whom he would seldom see in the more conventional psychiatric inpatient units and outpatient clinics: patients with both acute and chronic medical and surgical illnesses; management problems; critical illnesses; and, very importantly, certain types of illnesses such as conversion phenomena, now found infrequently in psychiatric outpatient clinics (Ziegler and Imboden, 1960).

4. To acquire proficiency in formulating case dynamics, making rapid diagnoses, and designing treatment programs. This necessitates a steady increase in: a) his knowledge of basic psychiatry including the origins, development, and expressive modes of psychopathology; b) his ability to communicate by perfecting interviewing techniques and understanding sociocultural differences; c) his skills for patient management which involve the intricacies of transference and countertransference; and d) his self-awareness of his own reactions to patients and staff, and his sensitivity to his impact upon them.

IMPLEMENTING THE GOALS

Five major factors facilitate the attainment of the goals. These are: 1) the timing of the consultation rotation, 2) the variety of consultation experiences, 3) the individual supervision, 4) the didactic program, and 5) the routine operations of the service.

CONSULTATION ROTATION IN THE SECOND YEAR

The psychiatric resident works six months, one-half time, on the consultation-liaison program during his second year of residency. At this time, his attitudes are still malleable, not as structured as they become during the latter phases of training.

Too frequently, consultation work is provided for the resident only in the third year when he is approaching the completion of his training. Then, his view of what he wishes to do as a psychiatrist, and his attitudes toward how he will practice, are crystallized; consultation activities are merely an exercise in using his skills on a service basis, and the experience is not a formative one. We, and others, experimented with scheduling the resident's consultation rotation in the first year. When he begins the residency with consultation work, the experience should be formative; however, at this early stage of training, the new resident is usually so beset by anxieties about his lack of knowledge, that his abilities as a consultant are limited. This obstacle can be overcome by very intensive supervision; but too intensive supervision is a handicap which may hinder development. Consequently, we think that timing the rotation for the second year combines the advantages but not the liabilities of the first- and third-year rotations.

There are other advantages of the second-year rotation; the resident has had only one year's training, usually on an inpatient or an outpatient service, and he is not so far removed in time from his internship that he is estranged from the medical atmosphere. Yet, his one year of specialized training gives him skills which need to be used; he is not a neophyte.

VARIETY IN THE CONSULTATION EXPERIENCE

The intensive experience gained by the resident while working as a consultant is crucial.

He sees many patients. During the rotation, he answers about 100 consultation requests from the various medical, surgical, and obstetric-gynecologic services; both the number and type of his clinical experiences are regulated. During the first three to four months he is not permitted to become a "favorite" consultant to one service; however, during the last two months, he is allowed to develop a more intensive liaison with a particular service.

He sees a variety of illnesses. Patients with emotional reactions to medical and surgical illness, those suffering from reactions to medications, those with delirium, and those who are management problems, are referred. The resident also works with dying patients. His understanding of personality disorders deepens as he sees all the variations of dependency, compulsivity, and suspicion. Thus, he obtains valuable experience in caring for "garden variety" problems: the admixtures of concurrent psychiatric illness and medical disease (Schwab et al., 1964–1965).

He sees the varied reactions to illness. The resident learns that psychologic reactions to illness are variable and that, indeed, every sick person has his own style of reacting, adaptive or nonadaptive. Further, he studies the influence of previous medical illness, family difficulties, and everyday problems of living, on the production, course, and treatment of disease. Of special value is the resident's growing awareness that positive findings, on either the physical or the psychiatric examination, do not indicate that the patient has to be categorized exclusively as either medically or psychiatrically ill.

SUPERVISION

Both quantitatively and qualitatively, supervision is essential if the resident is to develop his proficiency as a consultant.

CLINICAL CONFERENCES. At the beginning of the rotation, all cases are reviewed during three clinical conferences each week. Two members of the faculty meet with the three or four residents and other personnel on the service. Special emphasis is placed on the physical and psychiatric findings as well as on the delineation of the patient's life style, personality type, and characteristic mode of reacting to stress. A resident presents the patient's medical history, summarizes his physical status, and reports the results of laboratory procedures, as well as his findings from the consultation. This is mandatory. When we do not know about a new diagnostic procedure, or when the medical data are very complicated, we turn to the standard texts on medicine or ask a medical or surgical colleague to provide an explanation. A modified form of the Meyerian Life Chart is used as a model, and the dynamics, a concise formulation of the conflict, and the diagnoses are explicated. Thus, there is diagnosis by inclusion of all the facts. Diagnoses are viewed as hypotheses either to be confirmed or rejected by the data. We use the APA *Diagnostic and Statistical Manual of Mental Disorders* (1952). Once the diagnosis has been made, treatment plans are outlined.

During the early weeks of the rotation, the supervisor teaches the basic aspects of consultation work: how to approach the patient and how to interview effectively. Obviously, the resident's relationships with the medical and surgical staff are continuously evaluated. The consultant's report is analyzed for style and content. Emphasis is given to the resident's teaching capabilities; the faculty insist that every consultation is an opportunity for teaching the medical staff and nurses.

PERSONAL SUPERVISION. In addition to the case conferences, each resident is given individual supervision by one of the three faculty members in charge of this program. Supervision is informally arranged and is more intensive at the beginning of the rotation. Together, the supervisor and the resident discuss the approach to the patient and the consultee, conferences with the nursing staff, and the resident's special problems. In many instances, the supervisor and the resident interview patients together. One faculty member is always available for assistance; short, impromptu supervisory sessions are encouraged. When he is having a problem, the resident is expected to find a supervisor and present specific questions; in these sessions a "give and take" atmosphere prevails.

ENCOURAGING INDEPENDENCE.   One of the supervisor's greatest tasks is to limit his instruction so that while the resident is assisted with the problem, he will still develop his own resources for coping with it. Excessive supervision is contraindicated; it can diminish the learning experience for the resident and deprive him of the feeling that he is becoming an effective consultant. Consequently, as he gains experience, supervision is gradually reduced.

SEMINARS: THE DIDACTIC PROGRAM

There are weekly seminars throughout the resident's six-month consultation-liaison rotation. Participation is obligatory. These seminars are attended by the residents, Psychosomatic Fellows, the two externs, the social worker, the research associate, and faculty members. The curriculum stresses concepts. Readings are assigned for critical study. They are selected to increase the resident's knowledge, stimulate discussion, and encourage expression. To ensure that these seminars do not deteriorate into "canned" reviews of books and journals, the residents are expected to correlate the seminar topics with their daily work. For at least one session per month there is no assigned reading; instead, the resident is given some general references to use as he wishes. During these less structured seminars, he is expected to raise questions and to develop his own ideas about this work.

THE FIRST TWO MONTHS.   During the first two months, the seminars cover the nature of psychiatric consultation work and the role of the consultant. These topics are explored in depth in order to provide the resident with a conceptual basis for his training in this field. Without concepts, there is only training and service; education is neglected. This segment of the didactic program covers the following areas:

Development of Consultation-Liaison Psychiatry.   We review the historical background for the development of consultation-liaison psychiatry, its emergence as an outgrowth of the psychosomatic movement of the last few decades, and the sociocultural and scientific changes which necessitate the integration of psychiatry and medicine. Key writings by Kaufman and Margolin (1948), Cushing (1950), Kaufman (1953), Grinker (1953, 1965), Bibring (1956), and others (Beigler et al., 1959; Hackett and Weisman, 1960) are used to illustrate patient-oriented consultation. The limitations of this earlier approach are revealed by the change to consultee-oriented consultations first advocated by Balint (1957), Grotjahn and Treusch (1957), and others (Bartemeier, 1955), and later discussed by Schiff and Pilot (1959). After a few sessions, the seminar material considers the third and current stage of this work, the situation-oriented consultations which were described by Meyer and Mendelson (1961), Greenberg (1960), and others (Bursten, 1963).

Evaluation of Theoretical Models. Specifically, we study three conceptual models intensively: Hackett and Weisman's "Therapeutic Consultation" (1960b), Meyer and Mendelson's "Psychiatric Consultation with Patients on Medical and Surgical Wards" (1961), and Sandt and Leifer's "The Psychiatric Consultation" (1964).

Concepts of Disease. As we outlined in Chapter I, concepts of disease have changed. At present they are controversial; however, this is salutary. When concepts ossify, they lose their value. The acceptance of one concept does not necessarily signify the rejection of another. Therefore, our seminars consider the applicability, as well as the limitations, of mechanistic, biologic, psychosomatic, and field theories of illness. The works of Halliday (1948), Lewin (1951), Wittkower and Cleghorn (1954), Gregg (1956), and Hinkle and Wolff (1957) are reviewed. We emphasize a comprehensive-ecologic concept of illness and the necessity for a holistic approach to the patient.

The Consultant's Special Problems. We focus on the relationship between the consultant and the patient, transference and countertransference phenomena (Orr, 1954; Mendelson and Meyer, 1961), and the role of the psychiatric consultant.

THE SECOND TWO MONTHS. The seminars take up the relationships between psychiatry, the other medical specialties, and the problems unique to each.

Differential Approach. Much time is devoted to examining the necessity for differential approaches to the specialties. For example, techniques for consultations with surgical patients and staff must differ from those used in a medical situation. For these sessions we use Titchener and Levine's book *Surgery as a Human Experience* (1960), Hackett and

Weisman's two-part paper on "Psychiatric Management of Operative Syndromes" (1960b, 1960c) and selected writings from the voluminous literature on plastic surgery (Meyer et al., 1960; Meyer, 1964; Hill and Silver, 1950) as well as Paul Schilder's, *The Image and Appearance of the Human Body* (1950).

Because of time limitations the special problems with pediatric and obstetrical consultations are covered only briefly. Rather than review the entire field of consultation work, we prefer to study a few areas in depth, thus providing a base for the resident's work with the many differing consultation situations.

Hospitalization as a Process.   We study the special features of hospitalization and their influence on the patient. The hospital environment with its social organization and staff expectations creates adaptation problems for patients. We emphasize that consultants must be prepared to evaluate the meaning of hospitalization for each patient.

The Last Two Months.   These sessions are used to study the more traditional subject matter of psychosomatic medicine, with emphasis on therapy. During a few sessions, we review the works of Alexander (1950), Deutsch (1953), Dunbar (1954), and others (Engel, 1962, Lief et al., 1963). In the remaining time we discuss the treatment of psychosomatic disorders. The residents are encouraged to present comparative evaluations of various types of treatments: brief psychotherapy, sleep therapy, anaclitic therapy, group therapy, and others. By the time the resident approaches the end of his rotation, he has had an opportunity to use many of these treatments, and an open discussion of their indications, effectiveness, and limitations is fruitful.

ROUTINE OPERATIONS

Lastly, the routine operations of the service are designed to implement the training goals.

Appointment System.   All consultation requests are sent to a central office where they are assigned to the residents in rotation. The secretary in charge sets up definite appointments for the resident consultant. The appointment system has many advantages. Too often, when there is not an appointment, the patient will not be available; he may be undergoing a diagnostic procedure or be elsewhere in the hospital. Also, appointments enhance the importance of the consultation for both the consultant and the patient.

Consultant-Consultee Conferences. Our routine procedure calls for the resident's meeting with the consultee both before and after he sees the patient. This promotes communication and improves the relationship between the consultants and the referring staff.

In addition, the residents make early morning work-rounds, once or twice a week, with one of the services. At first, they accompany a faculty member, but as they acquire greater proficiency, they are permitted to choose a specific service on which they will make rounds without a supervisor.

DISCUSSION

Obviously, it is difficult to evaluate the extent to which educational goals are met. Results usually defy accurate measurement. Although goals should change as warranted, setting goals has a distinct purpose: it provides specific objectives for both the trainee and the faculty. Since this program has been established, there is much indirect and some direct evidence that it is successful and that setting distinct goals contributes to this success.

Some results can be measured. There has been a steady increase in the number of consultations since the liaison program was instituted. In the past, almost 25 percent of the consultations were requested during the last 48 hours of hospitalization; now less than 10 percent of the referrals are made this late. More importantly, about two thirds of the referrals are made within the first two days after admission to the hospital. Earlier consultations potentiate effective collaboration between the consultant and his medical colleagues, and serve to minimize diagnosis by exclusion. The incidence of delirium has been markedly reduced, and the severe psychiatric emergency is now a rarity.

In the past, psychiatric residents often regarded consultation activities as a chore, one of the necessary burdens of residency; now, although both their time commitments and their efforts are extensive, they state that this is the single most valuable learning experience of their three years. They say that productive consultation work contributes to patient care and morale throughout the hospital and they indicate that it enhances their self-esteem. They feel that they are no longer looked upon as members of an esoteric specialty removed from the practice of medicine (Schwab and Clemmons, 1966). Instead, we have noted that the resident's identity as a psychiatrist and a physician is crystallized; colleagues in other specialties hold him in respect as a member of the medical team.

The residents obtain additional benefits. They report that their skills in case-formulation and diagnosis and their ability to provide concrete recommendations for treatment and disposition are of tremendous help when they appear in court or meet with community agencies. Their approaches to therapy are more flexible; the residents generate treatment programs on an experimental basis. Familiarity with group therapy, sleep therapy, brief psychotherapy, environmental manipulation, and the combined team approach with social workers and nurses is the fruit of their experience.

At the same time, the residents encounter problems. There is pressure from the amount of work. In addition to answering new requests, the resident usually has three or four patients whom he follows on a daily basis. Also, consultation work is variable in terms of the amount of work that is required on a particular day. The resident has to learn to adapt to these uncertainties. However, assigning consultations in rotation and establishing appointments has ameliorated these pressures.

The residents feel anxiety arising from the necessity for making rapid formulations, specific diagnoses, and exact recommendations for treatment. Although some anxiety is always engendered by these demands, it is alleviated by experience. Also, anxiety is reduced by the supervisory program.

There is frustration because of problems with disposition. The shortage of psychiatric facilities, and the long waiting periods for appointments in clinics or with psychiatrists in practice, leave the trainee with a feeling that much of his work is wasted or never brought to fruition. This, of course, is a chronic problem which can be met only by an increase in personnel and facilities on a national basis. Part of the trainee's frustration is diminished, however, when his liaison with the referring staff and his achievements with patients during brief consultations are pointed out by the supervisor.

Interpersonal difficulties with one or more members of a referring staff crop up. These problems can be alleviated by the supervisor's support of the resident, and his insistence that the resident develop his own skill as a specialist in human relations.

Notwithstanding these difficulties, intensive training on an established consultation-liaison program which has specific objectives is necessary. It offers opportunities for learning and self-development which cannot be found in other phases of the psychiatric residency. The resident is trained for his decisive role in teaching medical psychology to the house staff, students, nurses, and paramedical personnel.

Lastly, opportunities for research abound. To develop consultation work, comparative studies are necessary. Through all the phases of this program, the resident is shown where gaps in knowledge exist and how he can fill them by participating in our ongoing research, by independently following up others' studies, or by his own endeavors.

Henry Sigerist (1960) once said, "All education presupposes an educational ideal." We have had fears that our structured program with its defined content might be an obstacle for the realization of the ideal: the consultant as the specialist in comprehensive medicine. Yet, this entire area is still in its infancy, only now receiving attention. We think that there are too few established consultation-liaison programs and that unless they are developed and unless goals are specified, we will never know whether the programs are too rigid, whether they promote, or whether they obstruct the attainment of the ideal.

REFERENCES

ALEXANDER, F. Psychosomatic Medicine. New York, W. W. Norton & Company, Inc., 1950.

American Psychiatric Association Conference on Graduate Psychiatric Education. The Psychiatrist, His Training and Development, 1952. Washington, 1953.

American Psychiatric Association. Training the Psychiatrist to Meet Changing Needs, 1962. Washington, 1964.

American Psychiatric Association Annual Meeting, 1965.

American Psychiatric Association Meeting in Washington, 1966.

BALINT, M. The Doctor, His Patient, and the Illness. New York, International Universities Press, Inc., 1957.

BARTEMEIER, L. H. Psychiatric consultations. Amer. J. Psychiat., 111:364, 1955.

BEIGLER, J. S. et al. Report on liaison psychiatry at Michael Reese Hospital. AMA Arch. Neurol. Psychiat., 81:733, 1959.

BIBRING, G. L. Psychiatry and Medical practice in a general hospital. New Eng. J. Med., 254:366, 1956.

BURSTEN, B. The psychiatric consultant and the nurse. Nurs. Forum, 2:7, 1963.

CUSHING, J. G. N. Role of the psychiatrist as a consultant. Amer. J. Psychiat., 106:861, 1950.

DEUTSCH, F. The Psychosomatic concept in Psychoanalysis. With contributions by Bernard Bandler (and others). New York, International Universities Press, Inc., 1953.

Diagnostic and Statistical Manual of Mental Disorders. Washington, American Psychiatric Association, 1952.

DUNBAR, F. Emotions and Bodily Changes, 4th ed. New York, Columbia University Press, 1954.

ENGEL, G. L. Psychological Development in Health and Disease. Philadelphia, W. B. Saunders Co., 1962.

EWALT, J. R. Programs for residents in psychiatry. In Kaufman, M. R., ed. The Psychiatric Unit in a General Hospital. New York, International Universities Press, Inc., 1965, pp. 307–314.

GREENBERG, I. M. Approaches to psychiatric consultation in a research hospital setting. Arch. Gen. Psychiat. (Chicago), 3:691, 1960.

GREGG, A. What is the meaning of disease? Challenges to Contemporary Medicine. New York, Columbia University Press, 1956, pp. 25–48.

GRINKER, R. R. Psychotherapy in medical and surgical hospitals. Dis. Nerv. Syst., 13:269, 1953.

———— Research potentials of departments of psychiatry in general hospitals. *In* Kaufman, M. R., ed. The Psychiatric Unit in a General Hospital. New York, International Universities Press, Inc., 1965, pp. 405–413.

GROTJAHN, M., and TREUSCH, J. V. A new technique of psychosomatic consultations: Some illustrations of teamwork between an internist and a psychiatrist. Psychoanal. Rev., 44:176, 1957.

HACKETT, T. P., and WEISMAN, A. D. Organization and function of a psychiatric consultation service. Internat. Rec. Med., 173:306, 1960a.

———— WEISMAN, A. D. Psychiatric management of operative syndromes: I. The therapeutic consultation and the effect of non-interpretive intervention, Psychosom. Med., 22:267–282, 1960b.

———— WEISMAN, A. D. Psychiatric management of operative syndromes: II. Psychodynamic factors in formulation and management. Psychosom. Med., 22:356, 1960c.

HALLIDAY, J. L. Psychosocial Medicine: A Study of a Sick Society. New York, W. W. Norton & Company, Inc., 1948, pp. 17, 26.

HILL, G., and SILVER, G. Psychodynamic and esthetic motivations for plastic surgery. Psychosom. Med., 12:345, 1950.

HINKLE, L. E., and WOLFF, H. G. Health and the social environment: Experimental investigations. *In* Leighton, A., Clausen, J., and Wilson, R., eds., Explorations in Social Psychiatry. New York, Basic Books, Inc., Publishers, 1957, pp. 105–137.

KAUFMAN, M. R. The role of the psychiatrist in a general hospital. Psychiat. Quart., 27:367, 1953.

———— ed. The Psychiatric Unit in a General Hospital. New York, International Universities Press, Inc., 1965.

———— MARGOLIN, S. Theory and practice of psychosomatic medicine in a general hospital. Med. Clin. N. Amer., 32:611, 1948.

LEWIN, K. Field Theory in Social Science: Selected Theoretical Papers. New York, Harper & Row, Publishers, 1951.

LIDZ, T., and FLECK, S. Integration of medical and scientific methods and objectives on a medical service. Psychosom. Med., 12:103, 1950.

LIEF, H. I., LIEF, V. F., and LIEF, N. R. The Psychological Basis of Medical Practice. New York, Harper & Row, Publishers, 1963.

LIPOWSKI, Z. J. Review of consultation psychiatry and psychosomatic medicine. I. General principles. Psychosom. Med., 28(2):153, 1966.

———— Review of consultation psychiatry and psychosomatic medicine. II. Clinical aspects. Psychosom. Med., 28(3):201, 1966.

MENDEL, W. M. and SOLOMON, P. The Psychiatric Consultation. New York, Grune and Stratton, 1968.

MENDELSON, M., and MEYER, E. Countertransference problems of the liaison psychiatrist. Psychosom. Med., 23:115, 1961.

MEYER, E. Psychiatric aspects of plastic surgery. *In* Reconstructive Plastic Surgery, Vol. 1. J. M. Converse, ed. Philadelphia, Saunders, 1964, pp. 365–384.

———— JACOBSON, E. W., EDGERTON, M. T., and CANTER, A. Motivational patterns in patients seeking elective plastic surgery: I. Women who seek rhinoplasty. Psychosom. Med., 22:193, 1960.

———— and MENDELSON, M. Psychiatric consultation with patients on medical and surgical wards: Patterns and processes. Psychiatry, 24:197, 1961.

ORR, D. W. Transference and countertransference: A historical survey. J. Amer. Psychoanal. Ass., 2:621, 1954.

SANDT, J. J., and LEIFER, R. The psychiatric consultation. Compr. Psychiat., 5:409, 1964.

SCHIFF, S. K., and PILOT, M. L. An approach to psychiatric consultation in the general hospital. Arch. Gen. Psychiat. (Chicago), 1:349, 1959.

SCHILDER, P. The Image and Appearance of the Human Body. New York, International Universities Press, Inc., 1950.

SCHWAB, J. J., CLEMMONS, R. S., FREEMON, B. S., and SCOTT, M. L. Problems in psychosomatic diagnosis: I. A controlled study of medical in-patients. Psychosomatics, 5:369, 1964. II. Severity of medical illness and psychiatric consultations. Psychosomatics, 6:69, 1965. III. Physical examinations, laboratory procedures, and psychiatric consultations. Psychosomatics, 6:147, 1965. IV. A challenge to all physicians. Psychosomatics, 6:198, 1965.

——— and CLEMMONS, R. S. Psychiatric consulttaions with medical patients: The interface between psychiatry and medicine. Arch. Gen. Psychiat. (Chicago), 14:504, 1966.

SIGERIST, H. On the Sociology of Medicine. Roemer, M. J., ed. New York, MD Publications, Inc., 1960.

Symposium on Comprehensive Medical Care and the Psychiatric Consultation. University of California Medical Center, November, 1965.

TITCHENER, J. L., and LEVINE, M. Surgery as a Human Experience. New York, Oxford University Press, Inc., 1960.

WITTKOWER, E. D., and CLEGHORN, R. A., eds. Recent Developments in Psychosomatic Medicine. Philadelphia, J. B. Lippincott Co., 1954, pp. 3–28.

ZIEGLER, F., and IMBODEN, J. B. Contemporary conversion reactions. Amer. J. Psychiat., 116:901, 1960.

ZINBERG, N. E., ed. Psychiatry and Medical Practice in a General Hospital. New York, International Universities Press, Inc., 1964.

BIBLIOGRAPHY

ABRAHAMS, D., and GOLDEN, J. Psychiatric consultations on a medical ward. Arch. Intern. Med. (Chicago), 112:766, 1963.

ABRAM, H. S. The psychiatrist, the treatment of chronic renal failure, and the prolongation of life. Amer. J. Psychiat., 124(10):1351, April, 1968.

——— The psychiatrist, the treatment of chronic renal failure, and the prolongation of life. II. Delivered at the 124th Annual Meeting of the American Psychiatric Association, May 15, 1968, Boston.

ACKNER, B., et al. Acute porphyria: A neuropsychiatric and biochemical study. J. Psychosom. Res., 6:1, 1962.

ADAMS, R. D., and HOPE, J. M. The anxiety state and psychasthenia. In Harrison, T. R., et al., eds. Principles of Internal Medicine. New York, McGraw-Hill Book Company, 1962, pp. 390-397.

——— RESNIK, W. H. Cardinal manifestations of disease: Pain. In Harrison, T. R., et al, eds. Principles of Internal Medicine. 5th ed. New York, McGraw-Hill Book Company, 1966, pp. 10-17.

ADAMSON, J. D., and SCHMALE, A. H. Object loss, giving up, and the onset of psychiatric disease. Psychosom. Med., 17(6):557, 1965.

ALDRICH, C. K. Psychiatric teaching on an inpatient medical service. J. Med. Educ., 28:36, 1953.

——— The dying patient's grief. J.A.M.A., 184:329, 1963.

——— Discussion. GAP Report, 5(9):645, 1965.

ALEXANDER, F. Psychosomatic Medicine. New York, W. W. Norton & Company, Inc., 1950.

ANDRÉSON, A. F. R. A practical approach to anxiety reactions. New York J. Med., 63:1144, 1963.

ANGYAL, A. Neurosis and Treatment. New York, John Wiley & Sons, Inc., 1965, p. 246.

ALTROCCHI, J., and EISDORFER, C. Changes in attitudes toward mental illness. Ment. Hyg., 45:563, 1961.

American Psychiatric Association Annual Meeting, 1965.

American Psychiatric Association Conference on Graduate Psychiatric Education. The Psychiatrist, His Training and Development, 1952. Washington, 1953.

American Psychiatric Association Meeting in Washington, 1966.

American Psychiatric Association. Training the Psychiatrist to Meet Changing Needs, 1962. Washington, 1964.

ANSHIN, R. N. Emotional problems of the chronically ill. J. Amer. Geriat. Soc., 10:447, 1962.

ARONSON, G. T. Treatment of the dying person. In Feifel, H., ed. The Meaning of Death. New York, McGraw-Hill Book Company, 1959, pp. 251-8.

BACKNER, B., and KISSINGER, R. D. Hospitalized patients' attitudes toward mental health professionals and mental patients. J. Nerv. Ment. Dis., 136:72, 1963.

BALINT, M. The Doctor, His Patient, and the Illness. New York, International Universities Press, Inc., 1957.

BARD, M., and DYK, R. B. Psychodynamic significance of beliefs regarding the cause of serious illness. Psychoanal. Rev., 43:146, 1956.

BARNES, R. H., et al. The training of psychiatric residents in consultative skills. J. Med. Educ., 32:124, 1957.

BARRY, M. J. Psychiatric aspects of the eye, ear, nose and throat. Int. Rec. Med., 10:170, 1957.

BARTEMEIER, L. H. Psychiatric consultations. Amer. J. Psychiat., 111:364, 1955.

――― On referring patients to other physicians. Northwest Med., 56:312, 1957.

――― Psychiatric aspects of medical practice; emotional reactions to illness. Maryland Med. J., 10:240, 1961.

BECK, A.T. Depression: Clinical, Experimental, and Theoretical Aspects. New York, Harper & Row, 1967.

――― WARD, C. H., MENDELSON, M., MOCK, J., and ERBAUGH, J. An inventory for measuring depression. Arch. Gen. Psychiat., 4:561, 1961.

BEIGLER, J. S., ROBBINS, F. P., LANE, E. W., MILLER, A. A., and SAMELSON, C. Report on liaison psychiatry at Michael Reese Hospital, 1950–58. AMA Arch. Neurol. Psychiat., 81:733, 1959.

BELLAK, L. Psychology of Physical Illness. New York, Grune & Stratton, Inc., 1952.

BERBLINGER, K. W. Psychiatric perspectives in medicine, part II. Psychosomatics, 3(2):42, 1962.

――― Brief psychotherapy and the psychiatric consultation. Psychosomatics, 8(1):6, 1967.

BERES, D., and BRENNER, C. Mental reactions in patients with neurological disease. Psychoanal. Quart., 19:170, 1950.

BERGER, F. M. The treatment of anxiety: A critical review. J. Neuropsychiat., 98:103, 1962.

BERNSTEIN, S., and KAUFMAN, M. R. The psychiatrist in a general hospital: His functional relationship to the non-psychiatric service. J. Mount Sinai Hosp. N.Y., 29:385, 1962.

BIBRING, G. L. Preventive psychiatry in a general hospital. Bull. World Fed. Ment. Health, 3:224, 1951.

――― Psychiatry and medical practice in a general hospital. New Eng. J. Med., 254:366, 1956.

――― Psychiatry and Medical Practice in a General Hospital. Zinberg, N. E., ed. New York, International Universities Press, Inc., 1964.

BILOON, S., and KARLINER, W. The clinical picture of manic-depressive equivalents. New Eng. J. Med., 259:684, 1958.

BINDER, H. J. Helping your patient accept psychiatric referral. J. Okla. Med. Ass., 45:279, 1952.

BINGER, C. The two faces of medicine. New Eng. J. Med., 275(4), 1966.

BITTNER, E. Social institutions and medical care. Psychosomatics, 8(3):126, 1967.

BLACHLY, P. H. Management of the opiate abstinence syndrome. Amer. J. Psychiat., 122:742, 1966.

――― Procedure for withdrawal of barbiturates. Amer. J. Psychiat., 120:894, 1964.

BLEULER, E. Textbook of Psychiatry, 10th ed. Springer-Verlag New York Inc., 1960.

BLEULER, M. Akute Psychische Veränderungen bei Akuten Körpererkran-
kungen. Schweiz Med. Wschr., 92:1521, 1962.

───── et al. Akute Psychische Begleiterscheinungen Körperlicher Krank-
heiten. Thieme, Stuttgart, 1966.

───── Investigations from the borderline of psychopathology and endocrinology. Arch. Psychiat. Nervenkr., 118:271, 1948.

BONHOEFFER, K. Zur Frage der Klassification der Symptomatischen Psychosen. Berlin Klinik Wschr., 14:2257, 1908.

BOYD, W. Pathology for the Physician, 7th ed. Philadelphia, Lea & Febiger,
1965, p. 4.

BRADLEY, J. J. Severe localized pain associated with the depressive syndrome. Brit. J. Psychiat., 109:741, 1963.

BRADY, J. P., et al. Attitudinal factors influencing outcome of treatment of
hospitalized psychiatric patients. J. Clin. Exp. Psychopath., 20:326, 1959.

───── REZNIKOFF, M., and ZELLER, W. W. The psychiatric attitudes
battery: A procedure for assessing attitudes toward psychiatric treatment
and hospitals. J. Clin. Psychol., 15:260, 1959.

BRAIN, W. R. Clinical Neurology, 2nd ed. London and New York, Oxford
University Press, Inc., 1964, p. 463.

BRENNEMAN, J. The menace of psychiatry. Amer. J. Dis. Child., 42:376,
1931.

BREUER, J., and FREUD, S. Studies on hysteria, standard edition. Complete
Psychological Works of Freud. London, Hogarth Press, 1955.

BROCK, S., and KRIEGER, H. The Basis of Clinical Neurology, 4th ed.
Baltimore, The Williams & Wilkins Co., 1963.

BRODMAN, K., ERDMANN, A. J., LORGE, I., GERSHENSON, C., and
WOLFF, H. G. The Cornell medical index health questionnaire, III. The evaluation of emotional disturbances. J. Clin. Psychol., 8:119, 1952.

BRODSKY, C. A social view of the psychiatric consultation. Psychosomatics,
8(2):61, 1967.

BROSIN, H. W. Discussion. GAP Report, 5(9):642, 1965.

───── Communication systems of the consultation process. In The Psychiatric
Consultation. Mendel, W. M., and Solomon, P., eds. New York, Grune and
Stratton, 1968.

BROWN, J. R. The holistic treatment of neurologic disease. Med. Clin. N.
Amer., p. 1019, July 1950.

BROWN, W., and PISETSKY, J. E. Suicidal behavior in a general hospital.
Amer. J. Med., 29:307, 1960.

BURSTEN, B. The psychiatric consultant and the nurse. Nurs. Forum, 2(4):7,
1963.

BURTON, R. The Anatomy of Melancholy. New York, Tudor Publishing
Co., 1927.

BURTON, R. Symptomatology—organic or psychogenic. New York J. Med.,
66:1304, 1966.

BUTLER, R. N., and PERLIN, S. Psychiatric consultations in a research
setting. Med. Ann. D.C., 27:503, 1958.

BINDER, H. Physicians choose psychiatrists: Medical social structure and
patterns of choice. J. Health Hum. Behav., 6:83, 1965.

CAIRNS, H. W. B. Observations on the localization of intracranial tumors.
Arch. Surg., 18:1936, 1929.

CAMPBELL, A. D. Consultations then and now. Canad. Med. Ass. J., 89:1030, 1963.

CANNON, W. B. Bodily Changes in Pain, Hunger, Fear, and Rage. New York, Appleton-Century Co., 1939.

CANTOR, A. J., and BAILEY, C. P., eds. Psychosomatic Aspects of Surgery. New York, Grune & Stratton, Inc., 1956.

CAPLAN, G. An Approach to Community Mental Health. New York, Grune & Stratton, Inc., 1961, pp. 20–23.

——— Types of mental health consultation. Amer. J. Orthopsychiat., 33:470, 1963.

——— Principles of Preventive Psychiatry. New York, Basic Books, Inc., Publishers, 1964, p. 41.

CARLSON, C. C. How to refer a psychosomatic patient to a psychiatric specialist. G.P., 18(6):105, 1958.

CATTELL, R. B., and SCHEIER, I. H. The Meaning and Measurement of Neuroticism and Anxiety. New York, The Ronald Press Company, 1961.

CHALGREN, W. Physical symptoms of depression. Minn. Med., 36:148, 1953.

CHAPMAN, L. F., and WOLFF, H. G. Disease of the neopallium. Med. Clin. N. Amer., May 1958.

CHODOFF, P. Re-examination of some aspects of conversion hysteria. Psychiatry, 17:75, 1954.

——— When should the physician refer a patient to a psychiatrist? Med. Ann. D.C., 23:313, 1954.

CLAUSEN, J. A. The sociology of mental illness. In Merton, R. K., Broom, L., and Cottrell, L. S., Jr., eds. Sociology Today: Problems and Prospects. New York, Basic Books, Inc., publishers, 1959, pp. 485–508.

CLEGHORN, R. A., and CURTIS, G. C. Psychosomatic accompaniments of latent and manifest depressive affect. Canad. Psychiat. Ass. J., 4(Suppl.):13, 1959.

——— Depression: mood, symptom, syndrome. Acta Psychosomatica Documenta Geigy, No. 2, North American Series, 1959.

CLYNE, M. B. Undergraduate teaching in psychological medicine as applicable to general practice. J. Med. Educ., 38:961, 1963.

CONRAD, K. Die symptomatischen Psychosen. In Gruhle, H. W., ed. Psychiatrie der Gegenwart, Bd. 2. Springer, Berlin, 1960.

COOPER, I. S., and BRACELAND, F. J. Psychosomatic aspects of pain. Med. Clin. N. Amer., p. 981, 1950.

CORSELLIS, J. A. N. Mental Illness and the Aging Brain. London, Oxford University Press, Inc., 1962.

COSER, R. L. The adjustment of patients. In Life in the Ward. East Lansing, Mich., Michigan State University Press, 1962.

COURT, J. H. Anxiety among acute schizophrenics and temporal lobe patients. Brit. J. Soc. Clin. Psychol., 4:254, 1965.

CULPAN, R., and DAVIS, B. Psychiatric illness at medical and surgical outpatient clinic. Compr. Psychiat., 1:228, 1960.

CUSHING, J. G. N. The role of the psychiatrist as a consultant. Amer. J. Psychiat., 106:861, 1950.

CUTSHALL, B. J. The Saunders-Sutton syndrome: An analysis of delirium tremens. Quart. J. Stud. Alcohol, 26:423, 1965.

DAVIES, E. B., Depression. Cambridge, Cambridge University Press, 1964.

DEAN, E. S. Writing psychiatric reports. Amer. J. Psychiat., 119:759, 1963.

DENNEY, D. A record keeping system for a psychiatric consultation service. J. Nerv. Ment. Dis., 141:474, 1965.

────── et al. Psychiatric patients on medical wards. Arch. Gen. Psychiat. (Chicago), 14:530, 1966.

DEUTSCH, F. Psychoanalysis at the bedside. Int. J. Psychoanal., 5:394, 1924.

────── The choice of the organ in organ neurosis. (Read before the Amer. Psychiat. Assoc., Chicago, May 8, 1939), Int. J. Psychoanal., 20:3, 1939.

────── The Psychosomatic Concept in Psychoanalysis. New York, International Press, Inc., 1953.

────── et al., eds. Training in Psychosomatic Medicine. New York, Hafner Publishing Co., Inc., 1964.

DEVINE, R., and MERSKEY, H. The description of pain in psychiatric and general medical patients. J. Psychosom. Res., 9:311, 1965.

DEWAN, J. G. Mild depressions. Med. Clin. N. Amer., March:527, 1952.

────── and SPAULDING, W. B. The Organic Psychoses. Toronto, University of Toronto Press, 1958.

Diagnostic and Statistical Manual of Mental Disorders. Washington, American Psychiatric Association, 1952.

DICKEL, H. A. The physician and the clinical psychologist. J.A.M.A., 195(5):365, 1966.

DOUST, B. C. Anxiety as a manifestation of pheochromocytoma. Arch. Intern. Med. (Chicago), 102:811, 1958.

DOVENMUEHLE, R. H. Affective response to life-threatening cardiovascular disease. In Death and Dying. GAP Report, 5(9):607, 1965.

────── and VERWOERDT, A. Physical illness and depressive symptomatology. 1. Incidence of depressive symptoms in hospitalized cardiac patients. J. Amer. Geriat. Soc., 10:932, 1962.

DUNBAR, F. Emotions and Bodily Changes, 4th ed. New York, Columbia University Press, 1954.

EATON, J. W., et al. Resistance to psychiatry in a general hospital. Ment. Hosp., 16:156, 1965.

EBAUGH, F. The depressed patient. In Liebman, S., ed. Management of Emotional Problems in Medical Practice. Philadelphia, J. B. Lippincott Co., 1956.

EDITORIAL. Psychological tests and medical prognosis. Ann. Intern. Med., 56(3):524, 1962.

EDITORIAL. Psychosom. Med., 5(1):3, 1939.

EDITORIAL. Science and psychiatry. Canad. Med. Ass. J., 89:902, 1963.

EDITORIAL. Southern Med. J., 59:979, 1966.

EDMONDS, E. P. Psychosomatic pain—articular rheumatism. Ann. Rheum. Dis., 6:36, 1947.

EHRENTHEIL, O. F. Some remarks about somato-psychic compared to psychosomatic relationships. Psychosom. Med., 21:1, 1959.

EILENBERG, M. D. Psychiatric illness and pernicious anemia. A clinical re-evaluation. J. Ment. Sci., 106:1539, 1960.

────── Survey of inpatient referrals to an American psychiatric department. Brit. J. Psychiat., 111:1211, 1965.

EINHORN, E. H. Recognition of symptomatology based on emotional and mental disturbances. New York Med. J., 57(15):2509, 1957.

EISSLER, K. R. The Psychiatrist and the Dying Patient. New York, International Universities Press, Inc., 1955, pp. 1–86.

ELMS, R., and DIERS, D. The patient comes to the hospital. Nurs. Forum, 2:89, 1963.

ENGEL, F. General concepts of adrenocortical function in relation to response to stress. Psychosom. Med., 15:565, 1953.

ENGEL, G. L. Homeostasis, behavioral adjustment and the concept of health and disease. In Grinker, R., ed. Mid-Century Psychiatry. Springfield, Ill., Charles C Thomas, Publisher, 1953.

——— "Psychogenic" pain. Med. Clin. N. Amer., 1491, November, 1958.

——— "Psychogenic" pain and the pain-prone patient. Amer. J. Med., 26:899, 1959.

——— Anxiety and depression-withdrawal: The primary affects of unpleasure. Int. J. Psychoanal., 43:89, 1962.

——— Psychological Development in Health and Disease. Philadelphia, W. B. Saunders Co., 1962.

——— Psychological processes and gastrointestinal disorder. In Paulson, M., ed. Gastroenterologic Medicine. Philadelphia, Lea & Febiger, 1967.

——— et al. A graduate and under graduate teaching program on the psychological aspects of medicine. J. Med. Educ., 32:859, 1957.

——— REICHSMAN, F. Spontaneous and experimentally induced depressions in an infant with gastric fistula: A contribution to the problem of depression. J. Amer. Psychoanal Ass., 4:428, 1956.

——— ROMANO, J. Delirium, a syndrome of cerebral insufficiency. J. Chronic Dis., 9:260, 1959.

——— SCHMALE, A. H. Psychoanalytic theory of somatic disorder: Conversion, specificity, and the disease onset situation. J. Amer. Psychoanal. Ass., 15(2):344, 1967.

ENGLISH, J. Mental Health consultation with a government agency. In The Psychiatric Consultation, Mendel, W. H., and Solomon, P., eds. New York, Grune and Stratton, 1968.

ESSIG, C. F. Newer sedative drugs that can cause intoxication and dependence of barbiturate type. J.A.M.A., 196:714, 1966.

EWALT, J. R. Somatic equivalents of depression. J. Mich. Med. Soc., 59(9), 1960.

——— Programs for residents in psychiatry. In Kaufman, M. R., ed. The Psychiatric Unit in a General Hospital. New York, International Universities Press, Inc., 1965, pp. 307–314.

EYSENCK, H. J. The Scientific Study of Personality. London, Routledge and Kegan Paul, 1952.

FAUCETT, R. L. Psychiatric interview as tool of medical diagnosis. J.A.M.A., 162:537, 1956.

FEDER, S. L. Attitudes of patients with advanced malignancy. GAP Report, 5(9):614, 1965.

FEIFEL, H., ed. The Meaning of Death. New York, McGraw-Hill Book Company, 1959.

——— Death-relevant variable in psychology. In May, R., ed. Existential Psychology. New York, Random House, 1961, pp. 61–74.

——— The function of attitudes toward death. GAP Report, 5(9):632, 1965.

FENICHEL, O. The Psychoanalytic Theory of the Neuroses. New York, W. W. Norton & Company, Inc., 1945.

FERENCZI, S. Disease or patho-neuroses. *In* Further Contributions to the Theory and Technique of Psycho-Analysis. London, Hogarth Press, 1926.

—— Further contributions to the theory and technique of psychoanalysis. *In* Selected Papers. New York, Basic Books, Inc., Publishers, 1952.

FEVRIER, F. Metamorphosis: on becoming a doctor. (poem) University of Florida Medical School, Class of 1968.

FINN, R., and HUSTEN, P. E. Emotional and mental symptoms in private medical practice. J. Iowa Med. Soc., 56(2):138, 1966.

FISCHER, K. H. The hospital bedside interview. Psychosomatics, 2:445, 1961.

FLACH, F. F., and REGAN, P. Chemo-Therapy in Emotional Disorders. New York, McGraw-Hill Book Company, 1960, p. 225.

FLECK, U. Symptomatische Psychosen (1941–1957). Fortschr. Neurol. Psychiat., 1:28, 1960.

FLEMINGER, J. J., and MALLETT, B. L. Psychiatric referrals from medical and surgical wards. J. Ment. Sci., 108:183, 1962.

FOX, H. M. Psychiatric consultation in general medical clinics; an experiment in postgraduate education. J.A.M.A., 185:999, 1963.

—— Psychiatric residency on a medical service. Arch. Gen. Psychiat., 11:19, 1964.

FRANK, L. K. Society as the Patient: Essays on Culture and Personality. New Brunswick, Rutgers University Press, 1948.

FRANKEL, F. H., CHAFETZ, M. E., and HOWARD, T. B. The treatment of psychosocial crises in the emergency service of a general hospital. J.A.M.A., 195(8):626, 1966.

FREEMAN, W. Psychosurgery. *In* Arieti, S., ed. American Handbook of Psychiatry. New York, Basic Books, Inc., Publishers, 1959, pp. 1521–1540.

FREUD, S. Three essays on the theory of sexuality. *In* The Complete Psychological Works of Sigmund Freud. London, The Hogarth Press, 1905, Vol. VII, pp. 123–245.

—— The Complete Psychological Works of Sigmund Freud. Strachey, J., ed. London, The Hogarth Press, 1921, Vol. XX, p. 132.

—— The Problem of Anxiety. New York, W. W. Norton & Company, Inc., 1936.

—— The justification for detaching from neurasthenia a particular syndrome: The anxiety-neurosis. *In* Collected Papers. New York, Basic Books, Inc., Publishers, 1959, Vol. 1, p. 76.

—— The Ego and the Id, Vol. XIX. Complete Psychological Works. Strachey, J., and Freud, A. (translators and editors). London, The Hogarth Press, 1961.

FRIEDMAN, J. H., and CANCELLIERI, R. Suicidal risk in a municipal general hospital. Dis. Nerv. Syst., 19:556, 1958.

GAP Report No. 2, p. 1, Jan. 1948.

GATFIELD, P. D., and GUZE, S. B. Prognosis and differential diagnosis of conversion reactions. Dis. Nerv. Syst., 23:623, 1962.

GEOCARIS, K. Psychotic episodes heralding the diagnosis of multiple sclerosis. Bull. Menninger Clin., 21:107, 1957.

GOLDMAN, J., and SCHWAB, J. J. Medical illness and patients' attitudes: Somatopsychic relationships. J. Nerv. Ment. Dis., 141(6):678, 1965.

GOLDSTEIN, K. Functional disturbances in brain damage. *In* Appel, et al., eds. American Handbook of Psychiatry. New York, Basic Books, Inc., Publishers, 1959, Vol. I, pp. 770–796.

GOULD, J. Virus disease and psychiatric ill-health. Brit. J. Clin. Pract., 11:1, 1957.

———— The assessment of pain in clinical practice. Brit. J. Clin. Pract., 16:31, 1962.

GREENBERG, I. M. Approaches to psychiatric consultation in a research hospital setting. Arch. Gen. Psychiat. (Chicago), 3:691, 1960.

GREENHILL, M. H., and KILGORE, S. R. Principles of methodology in teaching the psychiatric approach to medical house officers. Psychosom. Med., 12:38, 1950.

GREGG, A. What is the meaning of disease? *In* Challenges to Contemporary Medicine. New York, Columbia University Press, 1956, pp. 25–48.

GRINKER, R. R. Psychosomatic Research. New York, W. W. Norton & Company, Inc., 1953, pp. 159–160, 165.

———— Psychotherapy in medical and surgical hospitals. Dis. Nerv. Syst., 13:269, 1953.

———— Psychosomatic approach to anxiety. Amer. J. Psychiat., 113:443, 1956.

———— Anxiety as a significant variable for a unified theory of human behavior. Arch. Gen. Psychiat., 1:537, 1959.

———— Research potentials of departments of psychiatry in general hospitals. *In* Kaufman, M. R., ed. The Psychiatric Unit in a General Hospital. New York, International Universities Press, Inc., 1965, pp. 405–413.

———— MILLER, J., SABSHIN, M., NUNN, R., and NUNNALLY, J. C. The Phenomena of Depressions. New York, Paul B. Hoeber, Inc., 1961.

GRODDECK, G. Psychische Bedingtheit und Psychoanalytische Behandlung Organischer Leiden. (Psychic conditioning and the psychoanalytic treatment of organic disorders.) Leipzig, Hirzel, 1917.

———— Psychical treatment of organic disease. Brit. J. Med. Psychol., 9:179, 1929.

———— Book of the It. New York, Vintage, 1961.

GROTJAHN, M., and TREUSCH, J. V. A new technique of psychosomatic consultations: Some illustrations of teamwork between an internist and a psychiatrist. Psychoanal. Rev., 44:176, 1957.

Group for Advancement of Psychiatry: Committee on Child Psychiatry. Contribution of child psychiatry to pediatric training and practice. Report #21, 1952.

GUZE, S. B. A formulation of principles of comprehensive medicine with special reference to learning theory. J. Clin. Psychol., 9:127, 1953.

———— CANTWELL, D. P. The prognosis in organic brain syndromes. Amer. J. Psychiat., 120:878, 1964.

GYNTHER, M. D., REZNIKOFF, M., and FISHMAN, M. Attitudes of psychiatric patients toward treatment, psychiatrists, and mental hospitals. J. Nerv. Ment. Dis., 136:68, 1963.

HABERLAND, C. Psychiatric manifestations in brain tumors. Akt Fragen Psychiat. Neurol., 2:65, 1965.

HACKETT, T. P., and WEISMAN, A. D. Organization and function of a psychiatric consultation service. Internat. Rec. Med., 173:306, 1960.

———— Psychiatric management of operative syndromes: I. The therapeutic consultation and the effect of non-interpretive intervention. Psychosom. Med., 22:267, 1960.

———— Psychiatric management of operative syndromes: II. Psychodynamic factors in formulation and management. Psychosom. Med., 22:356, 1960.

HALL, C. S., and LINDZEY, G. Theories of Personality. New York, John Wiley & Sons, Inc., 1957, p. 240.

HALLIDAY, J. L. Psychosocial Medicine: A Study of the Sick Society. New York, W. W. Norton & Company, Inc., 1948, pp. 17, 26.

HALLORAN, H. M. The role of the caseworker. In Kaufman, M. R., ed. The Psychiatric Unit in a General Hospital. New York, International Universities Press, Inc., 1965.

HAMILTON, M. A rating scale for depression. J. Neurol. Neurosurg. Psychiat., 23:56, 1960.

HARDY, J. D. Pharmacodynamics of human disease: 3. The pain threshold and the nature of pain sensation. Postgrad. Med., 34:579, 1963.

HART, H. Displacement of guilt and pain. Psychoanal. Rev., 34:259, 1947.

HAYLETT, C. H., and RAPOPORT, L. Mental health consultation. In Bellak, L., ed. Handbook of Community Psychiatry. New York, Grune & Stratton, Inc., 1964, pp. 319–340.

HAYMAKER, W. Bing's Local Diagnosis in Neurological Diseases. St. Louis, The C. V. Mosby Co., 1956, p. 293.

HELSBORG, H. C. Psychiatric investigations of patients in a medical department. Acta Psychiat. Neurol. Scand., 33:303, 1958.

HENDERSON, D., GILLESPIE, R., and BATCHELER, I. A Textbook of Psychiatry, 8th ed. London, Oxford University Press, Inc., 1956.

HENRY, D. W., and MANN, A. M. Diagnosis and treatment of delirium. Canad. Med. Ass. J., 93:1156, 1965.

HERON, M. J. Functions and problems of psychiatric units in general hospitals. Brit. Med. J., 2:1529, 1962.

HERRICK, C. J. Brains of Rats and Men. New York, Hafner Publishing Co., Inc., 1963.

HILKEVITCH, A. Psychiatric disturbances in outpatients of a general medical outpatient clinic. Int. J. Neuropsychiat., 1:371, 1965.

HILL, G., and SILVER, G. Psychodynamic and esthetic motivations for plastic surgery. Psychosom. Med., 12:345, 1950.

HINKLE, L. E. Ecological observations of the relation of physical illness, mental illness, and the social environment. Psychosom. Med., 23:289, 1961.

———— WOLFF, H. G. Health and the social environment: Experimental investigations. In Leighton, A., Clausen, U., and Wilson, R., eds. Explorations in Social Psychiatry. New York, Basic Books, Inc., Publishers, 1957, pp. 105–137.

HOCH, A. Psychogenesis in dementia praecox. Med. Rec., 73:452, 1908.

———— Review of Bleuler's schizophrenia. Rev. Neurol. Psychiat., 10:259, 1912.

HOCKADAY, W. J. Experiences of a psychiatrist as a member of a surgical faculty. Amer. J. Psychiat., 117:706, 1961.

HOLLENDER, M. H. The Psychology of Medical Practice. Philadelphia, W. B. Saunders Co., 1958.

––––––– Ambulatory schizophrenia. J. Chronic Dis., 9:249, 1959.

HOLLINGSHEAD, A. B., and REDLICH, F. C. Social Class and Mental Illness: A Community Study. New York, John Wiley & Sons, Inc., 1958.

HOLLISTER, L. E. Psychopharmacologic drugs. J.A.M.A., 196(5):125, 1966.

HOLLISTER, W. G. The psychiatrist as a consultant to the school. In The Psychiatric Consultation, Mendel, W. M., and Solomon, P., eds. New York, Grune and Stratton, 1968.

HOLSTEIN, S., and SCHWAB, J. J. A coordinated consultation program for nurses and psychiatrists. J.A.M.A., 194:491, 1965.

HOPE, J. M. The anxiety state. Med. World News, 96:99, 1962.

HUNTER, R. C. A., et al. Nosophobia and hypochondriasis in medical students. J. Nerv. Ment. Dis., 139:147, 1964.

INGLE, D. The role of adrenal cortex in homeostasis. J. Endocrinol., 8:22, 1952.

JACKSON, H. Selected Writings of John Hughlings Jackson. New York, Basic Books, Inc., Publishers, 1958.

JACO, E. G., ed. Patients, Physicians, and Illness. New York, The Free Press of Glencoe, 1958.

JAFFEE, M. Psychiatric referral. Rocky Mountain Med. J., 60:26, 1963.

JANIS, I. L. Psychological Stress. New York, John Wiley & Sons, Inc., 1958.

JASPERS, K. General Psychopathology, 7th ed. Hoenig, J., and Hamilton, M. W., trans. Manchester, Manchester University Press, 1963.

JOHNSON, B. S. Psychiatric nurse consult in a general hospital. Nurs. Outlook Forum, 11:728, 1963.

JONAS, A. D. Ictal and Subictal Neurosis. Springfield, Ill., Charles C Thomas, Publisher, 1965.

JONES, D., and HALL, S. B. Significance of somatic complaints in patients suffering from psychotic depression. Acta Psychother. (Basel), 11:193, 1963.

JONES, N., KAHN, M., and MacDONALD, J. Psychiatric patients' views of mental illness, hospitalization, and treatment. J. Nerv. Ment. Dis., 136:82, 1963.

JOURARD, S. M. The Transparent Self. Princeton, D. Van Nostrand Co., Inc., 1964.

KAHANA, R. J. Teaching medical psychology through psychiatric consultation. J. Med. Educ., 34:1003, 1959.

––––––– BIBRING, G. L. Personality types in medical management. In Zinberg, N. E., ed. Psychiatry and Medical Practice in a General Hospital. New York, International Universities Press, Inc., 1964.

KANE, F. J., Jr., and EWING, J. A. Iatrogenic brain syndrome. Southern Med. J., 58:875, 1965.

KAPLAN, A. H. Social work therapy and psychiatric psychotherapy. Arch. Gen. Psychiat. (Chicago), 9:497, 1963.

KAPLAN, D. M. Why I am not a psychiatrist. Harpers Magazine, Feb. 1967, p. 45.

KAPLAN, S. M. Laboratory procedures as an emotional stress. J.A.M.A., 161:677, 1956.

KASPER, A. M. The doctor and death. In The Meaning of Death. New York, McGraw-Hill Book Company, 1959.

KAUFMAN, M. R. The role of the psychiatrist in a general hospital. Psychiat. Quart., 27:367, 1953.

———— A psychiatric unit in a general hospital. J. Mount Sinai Hosp. N.Y., 24:572, 1957.

———— ed. The Psychiatric Unit in a General Hospital. New York, International Universities Press, Inc., 1965.

———— et al. The emotional impact of ward rounds. J. Mount Sinai Hosp. N.Y., 23:782, 1956.

———— et al. Psychiatric findings in admissions to a medical service in a general hospital. J. Mount Sinai Hosp. N.Y., 26:160, 1959.

———— BERNSTEIN, S. A psychiatric evaluation of the problem patient. J.A.M.A., 163:108, 1957.

———— MARGOLIN, S. G. Theory and practice of psychosomatic medicine in a general hospital. Med. Clin. N. Amer., 32:611, 1948.

KENYON, F. E. Hypochondriasis: A clinical study. Brit. J. Psychiat., 110:467, 1964.

———— Hypochondriasis: A survey of some historical, clinical, and social aspects. Brit. J. Med. Psychol., 38:117, 1965.

———— RUTTER, M. L. The psychiatrist and the general hospital. Compr. Psychiat., 4:80, 1963.

KEPECS, J. G. Some patterns of somatic displacement. Psychosom. Med., 15:425, 1953.

KEYES, J. W. Iatrogenic heart disease. J.A.M.A., 192:951, 1965.

KIELHOLZ, P. Diagnosis and therapy of the depressive state. Acta Psychosomatica Documenta Geigy No. 1, North American Series, 1959.

KISSEN, D. M. The significance of syndrome shift and late syndrome association in psychosomatic medicine. J. Nerv. Ment. Dis., 136:34, 1963.

KLEE, G. D., et al. Pain and other somatic complaints in a psychiatric clinic. Maryland Med. J., 8:188, 1959.

KLEIN, D. C., and LINDEMANN, E. Preventive intervention in individual and family crisis situations. In Caplan, G., ed. Prevention of Mental Disorders in Children. New York, Basic Books, Inc., Publishers, 1961, pp. 283–306.

KLOPFER, W., WYLIE, A., and HILLSON, J. Attitudes toward mental hospitals. J. Clin. Psychol., 12:361, 1956.

KNIGHT, J. A. Epidemic hysteria: A field study. Amer. J. Public Health, 55:858, 1965.

KOLB, L. C. Anxiety and the anxiety states. J. Chronic Dis., 9:199, 1959.

KOUMANS, A. J. R. Psychiatric consultation in an intensive care unit. J.A.M.A., 194:163, 1965.

KORNFELD, D. S., and FELDMAN, M. The psychiatric service in the general hospital. New York J. Med., 65:1332, 1965.

———— et al. Psychiatric complications of open-heart surgery. New Eng. J. Med., 273:287, 1965.

KRAEPELIN, E. Psychiatry, 8th ed. Leipzig, 1909–13.

KRAINES, S. H. Mental Depressions and Their Treatment. New York, The Macmillan Company, 1957.

KREITMAN, N. Hypochondriasis and depression in out-patients at a general hospital. Brit. J. Psychiat., 111:476, 1965.

KROGER, W. S., ed. Psychosomatic Obstetrics, Gynecology, and Endocrinology. Springfield, Ill., Charles C Thomas, Publishers, 1962.

KRUG, O. M., ed. Career Training in Child Psychiatry. Washington, D.C., American Psychiatric Association, 1964.

KUBIE, L. S. The future of preventive psychiatry. Ment. Hyg. News (NH Conn.), 24:1, 1948.

—— Practical and Theoretical Aspects of Psychoanalysis. New York, International Universities Press, Inc., 1950.

—— A school of psychological medicine within the framework of medical school and university. J. Med. Educ., 39:476, 1964.

LANGNER, T. S., and MICHAEL, S. T. The Midtown Manhattan Study. Life Stress and Mental Health. New York, McGraw-Hill Book Company, 1963, Vol. II, pp. 61, 407, 462.

LEDLEY, R. S., and LUSTIG, L. B. Reasoning foundations of medical diagnosis. Science, 130:9, 1959.

LeSHAN, L. L. Psychosomatic Aspects of Neoplastic Disease. Kissen, D. M., and LeShan, L. L., eds. Philadelphia, J. B. Lippincott Co., 1964.

LEVIN, M. Delirium: A gap in psychiatric teaching. Amer. J. Psychiat., 107:689, 1951.

LEVINE, M. A. Psychotherapy in Medical Practice. New York, The Macmillan Company, 1942.

—— Psychosomatic medicine. J. Kentucky Med. Ass., 43:39, 1945.

LEVINSON, H. Psychiatric consultation in industry. In The Psychiatric Consultation, Mendel, W. M., and Solomon, P., eds. New York, Grune and Stratton, 1968.

LEWIN, K. Field Theory in Social Science: Selected Theoretical Papers. New York, Harper & Row, Publishers, 1951.

LEWIS, B. I. A psycho-medical survey of a private out-patient clinic in a university hospital. Amer. J. Med., 14:586, 1953.

—— The hyperventilation syndrome. Ann. Intern. Med., 38:918, 1953.

LEWIS, W. C., and BERMAN, M. Studies of conversion hysteria. Arch. Gen. Psychiat. (Chicago), 13:275, 1965.

LIDZ, T., and FLECK, S. Integration of medical and scientific methods and objectives on a medical service. Psychosom. Med., 12:103, 1950.

LIEF, H. I., et al. The Psychological Basis of Medical Practice. New York, Paul B. Hoeber, Inc. 1963.

LINDEMANN, E. Hysteria as a problem in a general hospital. Med. Clin. N. Amer., May 1938.

—— The meaning of crisis in individual and family living. Teachers College Rec., 57:310, 1956.

—— Symptomatology and management of acute grief. Amer. J. Psychiat., 101:141, 1944.

LINN, L., ed. Frontiers in General Hospital Psychiatry. New York, International Universities Press, Inc., 1961.

LIPIN, T. Psychic functioning in patients with undiagnosed somatic symptoms. A.M.A. Arch. Neur. and Psychiat., 73:239, 1955.

LIPOWSKI, Z. J. Review of consultation psychiatry and psychosomatic medicine. I. General principles. Psychosom. Med., 28(2):153, 1966.

—— Review of consultation psychiatry and psychosomatic medicine. II. Clinical aspects. Psychosom. Med., 28(3):201, 1966.

—— Review of consultation psychiatry and psychosomatic medicine. III. To be published in Psychosom. Med.

—— Psychopathology as a science: Its scope and tasks. Compr. Psychiat. In press.

LIPSITT, D. R. Integration clinic: An approach to the teaching and practice of medical psychology in an outpatient setting. *In* Zinberg, N. E., ed. Psychiatry and Medical Practice in a General Hospital. New York, International Universities Press, Inc., 1964.

LITIN, E. M. Preoperative psychiatric consultation. J.A.M.A., 170:1369, 1959.

LOURIE, R. S. The teaching of child psychiatry in pediatrics. J. Amer. Acad. Child Psychiat., 1:477, 1962.

LOVETT DOUST, J. W. Psychiatric aspects of somatic immunity: Differential evidence of physical disease in histories of psychiatric patients. Brit. J. Prev. Soc. Med., 6(49), 1952.

LOWY, F. The neuropsychiatric complications of viral hepatitis. Canad. Med. Ass. J., 92:237, 1965.

LUSTMAN, S. L., and RICHMOND, J. B. On the acceptance of realistic goals in medicine. *In* Solnit, A. J., and Provence, S. A., eds. Modern Perspectives in Child Development. New York, International Universities Press, Inc., 1963, pp. 558–574.

MABRY, J. H. Lay concepts of etiology. J. Chron. Dis., 17:371, 1964.

MacDONALD, J. M. The Murderer and His Victim. Springfield, Ill., Charles C Thomas, Publisher, 1961.

MACKEITH, R., and SANDLER, J., eds. Psychosomatic Aspects of Pediatrics. New York, Pergamon Press, Inc., 1961.

MACRAE, D. Isolated fear. A temporal lobe aura. Neurology (Minneap.), 4:497, 1954.

MAGRAW, R. M. The patient's presenting complaint—signpost or goal. Univ. Minn. Med. Bull., 29:329, 1958.

—— Psychosomatic medicine and the diagnostic process. Postgrad. Med., 25:639, 1959.

MALITZ, S. and WHARTON, R. "Lithium in manic-depressive psychosis." *In* American Handbook of Psychiatry, III (Arieti, S., Ed.), Basic Books, Inc., New York, 1966, pp. 509–512.

MALMO, R. B., et al. Specificity of bodily reactions under stress. *In* Wolff, H. G., ed. Life Stress and Bodily Disease. Assoc. Research Nervous Mental Disease. Baltimore, The Williams & Wilkins Co., 1950.

MASSERMAN, J. The Practice of Dynamic Psychiatry. Philadelphia, W. B. Saunders Co., 1955.

MATARAZZO, R. G., MATARAZZO, J. D., and SASLOW, G. The relationship between medical and psychiatric symptoms. J. Abnorm. Soc. Psychol., 62(1):55, 1961.

MAY, R. The Meaning of Anxiety. New York, The Ronald Press Company, 1950.

—— The existential approach. *In* Ariete, S., ed. American Handbook of Psychiatry. New York, Basic Books, Inc., Publishers, 1967, pp. 1348–1361.

MAYER-GROSS, W., SLATER, E., and ROTH, M. Clinical Psychiatry, 2nd ed. Baltimore, The Williams & Wilkins Co., 1960.

McWHIRTER, D. P. Consultation with the clergy. *In* The Psychiatric Consultation, Mendel, W. H., and Solomon, P., eds. New York, Grune and Stratton, 1968.

MECHANIC, D. The concept of illness behavior. J. Chron. Dis., 15:189, 1962.

MEERLOO, J. A. M. Illness and Cure. New York, Grune & Stratton, Inc., 1964, p. 44.

MENDEL, W. M., and SOLOMON, P., eds. The Psychiatric Consultation. New York, Grune and Stratton, 1968.

MENDELSON, J., et al. Hallucinations of poliomyelitis patients during treatment in a respirator. J. Nerv. Ment. Dis., 126:421, 1958.

MENDELSON, M., and MEYER, E. Countertransference problems of the liaison psychiatrist. Psychosom. Med., 23:115, 1961.

MENNINGER, K. A. Psychological aspects of the organism under stress: Part I: The homeostatic regulatory function of the ego. J. Amer. Psychoanal. Ass., 2:67, 1954.

MERING and EARLEY, Human Organization, 25(1):20, 1966.

MERSKEY, H. The characteristics of persistent pain in psychological illness. J. Psychosom. Res., 9:291, 1965.

MEYER, W. E. Disturbed behavior on medical and surgical wards: A training and research opportunity. In Masserman, J. H., ed. Science and Psychoanalysis: Psychoanalytic Education. New York, Grune & Stratton, Inc., 1962, Vol. 5.

——— Psychiatric aspects of plastic surgery. In Converse, J. M., ed. Reconstructive Plastic Surgery. Philadelphia, W. B. Saunders Co., 1964, Vol. 1, pp. 365–384.

——— JACOBSON, E. W., EDGERTON, M. T., and CANTER, A. Motivational patterns in patients seeking elective plastic surgery: I. Women who seek rhinoplasty. Psychosom. Med., 22:193, 1960.

——— MENDELSON, M. The psychiatric consultation in postgraduate medical teaching. J. Nerv. Ment. Dis., 130:78, 1960.

——— MENDELSON, M. Psychiatric consultation with patients on medical and surgical wards: Patterns and processes. Psychiatry, 24:197, 1961.

MILLER, M. H. The borderline psychotic patient: The importance of diagnosis in medical and surgical practice. Ann. Intern. Med., 46:736, 1957.

MITFORD, J. The American Way of Death. New York, Simon and Schuster, Inc., 1963.

MITTLEMAN, B., WEIDER, A., BRODMAN, K., WECHSLER, D., and WOLFF, H. G. Personality and psychosomatic disturbances in patients in medical and surgical wards. Psychosom. Med., 7:220, 1945.

MOWRER, O. H. Learning Theory and Personality Dynamics. New York, The Ronald Press Company, 1950.

NOYES, A., and KOLB, L. Modern Clinical Psychiatry, 6th ed. Philadelphia, W. B. Saunders Co., 1963, p. 135.

NUNNALLY, J. The communication of mental health information: A comparison of the opinions of experts and the public with mass media. Behav. Sci., 2:222, 1957.

——— KITTROSS, J. M. Public attitudes toward mental health professions. Amer. J. Psychol., 13:589, 1958.

NUSSBAUM, K. Somatic complaints and homeostasis in psychiatric patients. Psychiat. Quart., 34:311, 1960.

O'CONNOR, J. F., and MUSHER, D. M. Central nervous system involvement in systemic lupus erythematosus. Arch. Neurol. (Chicago), 14:157, 1966.

OFFENKRANTZ, W. Multiple somatic complaints as a precursor of schizophrenia. Amer. J. Psychiat., 119:258, 1962.

OBERMAYER, M. E. Psychocutaneous Medicine. Springfield, Ill., Charles C Thomas, Publisher, 1955.

O'LEARY, J. P., COLUMBARO, R. L., SCHWAB, J. J., and McGINNIS,

N. H. Cardiac anxiety: A comparative study of medical inpatients. In Press, J. Dis. Nerv. Sys., 1967.

ORLAND, F. The general practitioner and the psychiatric referral. Med. Times, 88:1426, 1960.

ORR, D. W. Transference and countertransference: A historical survey. J. Amer. Psychoanal. Ass., 2:621, 1954.

OVERLEY, T. M. Discovering the functional illness in interview. J.A.M.A., 186(8):776, 1963.

PALAREA, E. P. Medical evaluation of the psychiatric patient. J. Amer. Geriat. Soc., 13:14, 1965.

PARSONS, T. Definitions of health and illness in the light of American values and social structure. In Social Structure and Personality. New York, The Free Press of Glencoe, 1964, pp. 258–291.

PAYSON, H. E., et al. Recognition and referral of psychiatric illness on a university medical inpatient service. Scientific Proceedings of the 117th Annual Meeting of the American Psychiatric Association, Washington, 1961.

PERLAS, A. P., and FAILLACE, L. A. Psychiatric manifestations of carcinoma of the pancreas. Amer. J. Psychiat., 121:182, 1964.

PETROVITCH, D. V. A survey of painfulness concepts. J. Clin. Psychol., 14:288, 1958.

PILLERSDORF, L. The psychiatric referral: When and how? Ohio Med. J., 47:527, 1951.

PITTS, F. N., and WINOKUR, G. Affective disorder, III: Diagnostic correlates and incidence of suicide. J. Nerv. Ment. Dis., 139:176, 1964.

POE, R. O., et al. Depression, J.A.M.A., 195:345, 1966.

POLLACK, I. W., OCHBERG, F. M., and MEYER, E. Effect of deprivation of sight of subjective time sense. Psychosom. Med., 27:71, 1965.

POLLACK, S. Consultation with the courts. In The Psychiatric Consultation, Mendel, W. M., and Solomon, P., eds. New York, Grune and Stratton, 1968.

PROCTOR, R. C. Consultative psychiatry. Med. Times, 86:1043, 1958.

QUARTON, G. C., et al. Mental disturbances associated with ACTH and cortisone: A review of explanatory hypotheses. Medicine (Balt.), 34:13, 1955.

QUERIDO, A. Forecast and follow-up: An investigation into the clinical, social and mental factors determining the results of hospital treatment. Brit. J. Prev. Soc. Med., 13:33, 1959.

RACHLIN, H. A follow-up study of Hoch's benign stupor cases. Amer. J. Psychiat., 92:531, 1935.

RANGELL, L. Psychiatric aspects of pain. Psychosom. Med., 15:22, 1953.

REDING, G. R., and DANIELS, R. S. Organic brain syndromes in a general hospital. Amer. J. Psychiat., 120:800, 1964.

REID, D. D. Epidemiological Methods in the Study of Mental Disorders. Geneva, World Health Organ., 1960.

REISER, M. F. Cardiovascular disorders. In Freedman, A. M., Kaplan, H. I., and Kaplan, H., eds. Comprehensive Textbook of Psychiatry. Baltimore, The Williams & Wilkins Co., 1967.

RENNIE, T. A. C. Anxiety states: Their recognition and management. Med. Clin. N. Amer., p. 597, May 1948.

REZNIKOFF, M., BRADY, J. P., ZELLER, W. W., and TOOMEY, L. C. Attitudinal change in hospitalized psychiatric patients. J. Clin. Exp. Psychopath., 21:309, 1960.

RICE, D. Somatic syndromes causing depressive state. Practitioner, 183:49, 1959.

RICHARDSON, C. Psychic aspects of cerebral attacks. Med. Clin. N. Amer., March:557, 1952.

RICHMAN, A., et al. Symptom questionnaire validity in assessing the need for psychiatrists' care. Brit. J. Psychiat., 112:549, 1966.

RICHMOND, J. B. Relationship of the psychiatric unit to other departments of the hospital. In Kaufman, M. R., ed. The Psychiatric Unit in a General Hospital. New York, International Universities Press, Inc., 1965.

RIPLEY, H. Depressive reactions in a general hospital: A study of one hundred and fifty cases. J. Nerv. Ment. Dis., 105:607, 1947.

ROBERTS, B. H., and NORTON, N. M. The prevalence of psychiatric illness in a medical out-patient clinic. New Eng. J. Med., 246:82, 1952.

ROBINSON, W. G., Jr. The toxic delirious reactions of old age. In Kaplan, O. J., ed. Mental Disorders in Later Life. Stanford, Stanford University Press, 1956.

ROESSLER, R., and GREENFIELD, N. S. Incidence of somatic disease in psychiatric patients. Psychosom. Med., 23:413, 1961.

ROMANO, J., and ENGEL, G. L. Physiologic and psychological considerations of delirium. Med. Clin. N. Amer., p. 629, May, 1944.

ROME, H. P., et al. Symposium on automation technique in personality assessment. Mayo Clin. Proc., 37:61, 1962.

ROSENBAUM, M., and COHEN, Y. A. Psychological preparation of the individual for medical and surgical care. In Liebman, S., ed. Understanding Your Patient. Philadelphia, J. B. Lippincott Co., 1957.

ROSS, J. A. Social class and medical care. J. Health Hum. Behav., III:35, 1962.

ROSSMAN, P. L. Organic diseases simulating functional disorders. GP, 28:78, 1963.

ROTHENBERG, A. Psychological problems in terminal cancer management. Cancer, 14:1063, 1961.

RUD, F. Psychiatric activities and instruction at a general hospital. J. Clin. Exper. Psychopath., 14:139, 1953.

RUESCH, JURGEN. Comprehensive medical care and the psychiatric consultation. Psychosomatics, 8(3):119, 1967.

—— et al. Psychiatric Care. New York, Grune & Stratton, Inc., 1964.

SAND, P., et al. Psychological assessment of candidates for a hemodialysis program. Ann. Intern. Med., 64:602, 1966.

SANDT, J. J., and LEIFER, R. The psychiatric consultation. Compr. Psychiat., 5:409, 1964.

SARBIN, T. R. Anxiety: Reification of a metaphor. Arch. Gen. Psychiat. (Chicago), 10:630, 1964.

SAUNDERS, L. Cultural Differences and Medical Care. New York, Russel Sage Foundation, 1954.

SCHEIER, I. H. Experimental results to date from the standpoint of the clinician. Ann. N.Y. Acad. Sci., 93:840, 1962.

SCHIFF, S. K., and PILOT, M. L. An approach to psychiatric consultation in the general hospital. Arch. Gen. Psychiat. (Chicago), 1:349, 1959.

SCHILDER, P. The Image and Appearance of the Human Body. New York, International Universities Press, Inc., 1950.

SCHIMMELL, E. M. The hazards of hospitalization. Ann. Intern. Med., 60:100, 1964.

SCHLAEGEL, T. F. Psychosomatic Ophthalmology. Baltimore, The Williams & Wilkins Co., 1957.

SCHMALE, A. H. Relationship of separation and depression to disease. I. A report on a hospitalized medical population. Psychosom. Med., 20(4):259, 1958.

——— Object loss, "giving up" and disease onset: An overview of research in progress. Walter Reed Army Institute of Research, p. 433, 22–24 April, 1964.

——— A genetic view of affects with special reference to the genesis of helplessness and hopelessness. Psychoanal. Stud. Child, 19:287, 1964.

——— IKER, H. P. The psychological setting of uterine cervical cancer. Ann. N.Y. Acad. Sci., 125:807, 1966.

——— IKER, H. P. The affect of hopelessness and the development of cancer. I. Identification of uterine cervical cancer in women and atypical cytology. Psychosom. Med., 28(5):714, 1966.

SCHOTTSTAEDT, W. W. Psychophysiologic Approach in Medical Practice. Chicago, Year Book Medical Publishers, Inc., 1960.

——— et al. Sociologic, psychologic, and metabolic observations on patients in the community of a metabolic ward. Amer. J. Med., 25:248, 1958.

SCHWAB, J. J. The treatment of delirium. In Conn, H. F., ed. Current Therapy. Philadelphia, W. B. Saunders Co., 1966.

——— BARROW, M. V. A reaction to organic fluorides simulating classical catatonia. Amer. J. Psychiat. 120(12):1196, 1964.

——— CLEMMONS, R. S., BIALOW, M., DUGGAN, V., and DAVIS, B. A study of the somatic symptomatology of depression in medical inpatients. Psychosomatics, 6:273, 1965.

——— CLEMMONS, R. S., FREEMON, B. S., and SCOTT, M. L. Problems in psychosomatic diagnosis: I. A controlled study of medical inpatients. Psychosomatics, 5:369, 1964. II. Severity of medical illness and psychiatric consultations. Psychosomatics, 6:69, 1965. III. Physical examinations, laboratory procedures, and psychiatric consultations. Psychosomatics, 6:147, 1965. IV. A challenge to all physicians. Psychosomatics 6:198, 1965.

——— CLEMMONS, R. S., SCOTT, M. L., and FREEMON, F. R. Differential characteristics of medical inpatients referred for psychiatric consultation: A controlled study. Psychosom. Med., 27:112, 1965.

——— CLEMMONS, R. S., VALDER, M. J., and RAULERSON, J. D. Medical inpatients reactions to psychiatric consultations. J. Nerv. Ment. Dis., 14(3), 1966.

——— CLEMMONS, R. S., VALDER, M. J., and RAULERSON, N. D. Patients' reactions to referring physicians. J.A.M.A., 195:1120, 1966.

——— BIALOW, M. R., BROWN, J. M., and HOLZER, C. E. Diagnosing depression in medical inpatients. Ann. Intern. Med., 67:695, 1967.

——— BIALOW, M. R., HOLZER, C. E., BROWN, J. M., and STEVENSON, B. E. Sociocultural aspects of depression in medical inpatients. I. Frequency and social variables. II. Symptomatology and class. Arch. Gen. Psychiat. (Chicago), 17:533, 539, 1967.

——— BROWN, J. M., and HOLZER, C. E. Depression in medical inpatients with gastrointestinal diseases. Amer. J. Gastroent., 49(2):146, 1967.

——— BROWN, J. M., HOLZER, C. E., and SOKOLOF, M. T. Current concepts of depression: The sociocultural. Int. J. Soc. Psychiat. In Press.

——— BROWN, J. M. The treatment of anxiety and depression. Postgrad. Med. In Press.

——— BROWN, J. M., and HOLZER, C. E. Depression in medical inpatients: Sex and age differences. Ment. Hyg., in press, 1968.

——— CLEMMONS, R. S. Psychiatric consultations with medical patients: The interface between psychiatry and medicine. Arch. Gen. Psychiat. (Chicago), 14:504, 1966.

——— HARMELING, J. D., and McGINNIS, N. H. Anxiety, self concept, and body image: Psychosomatic correlations, I. A preliminary report. Presented at the IV World Congress of Psychiatry in Madrid, Spain, Sept. 5–11, 1966, in press.

——— MARDER, L., CLEMMONS, R. S., and McGINNIS, N. H. Anxiety, severity of illness, and other medical variables. J. Psychosom. Res., 10:291, 1966.

——— McGINNIS, N. H., and HARMELING, J. D. Anxiety in medical patients. Excerpta Medica International Congress Series No. 134. Psychosom. Med., Proceedings of the First International Congress of the Academy of Psychosomatic Medicine: 229, Palma de Mallorca, Spain, Sept. 1966.

——— McGINNIS, N. H., MARDER, L., and CLEMMONS, R. S. Evaluating anxiety in medical patients. J. Chronic Dis., 19:1049, 1966.

——— and McGINNIS, N. H. The treatment of anxiety. Medical College of Virginia Quarterly, 3(2):101, Summer, 1967.

——— Evaluating psychiatric consultation work. Psychosomatics, 8:309, 1967.

SCHWARTZ, L. A. Application of psychosomatic concepts by a liaison psychiatrist on a medical service. J. Mich. Med. Soc., 57:1547, 1958.

SCOTT, W. A. Social, psychological correlates of mental illness and mental health. Psychol. Bull., 55(2):65, 1958.

SEITZ, P. F. D. Symbolism and organ choice in conversion reactions. Psychosom. Med., 13:254, 1951.

SELYE, H. The concept of stress in experimental physiology. In Tanner, J. M., ed. Stress and Psychiatric Disorder. Oxford, Blackwell Scientific Publications, 1960.

SENESCU, R. A. The development of emotional complications in the patient with cancer. J. Chron. Dis., 16:813, 1963.

SHEPHERD, M., et al. Psychiatric illness in the general hospital. Acta. Psychiat. Neurol. Scand., 35:518, 1960.

SIGERIST, H. E. A History of Medicine. London, Oxford University Press, 1951.

——— On the Sociology of Medicine. Roemer, M. J. ed. New York, MD Publications, Inc., 1960.

SIMON, A., and CAHAN, R. B. The acute brain syndrome in geriatric patients. Psychiat. Res. Rep. Amer. Psychiat. Ass., May 16, 1963.

SLATER, E. Diagnosis of "hysteria." Brit. Med. J., 1:1395, 1965.

SMALL, I. F., et al. Organic cognates of acute psychiatric illness. Amer. J. Psychiat., 122:790, 1966.

SPENCER, R. F. Medical patients: Consultation and psychotherapy. Arch. Gen. Psychiat. (Chicago), 10:270, 1964.

STARR, A. M. Personality changes in Cushing's syndrome. J. Clin. Endocr., 12:502, 1952.

STARRETT, D. Psychiatric mechanisms in severe disability. Rocky Mountain Med. J., 58:42, 1961.

STEIGER, W. A. Medical science and things. Health Hum. Behav., 5(1), Spring 1964.
STENBÄCK, A., and RIMON, R. Hypochondria and paranoia. Acta Psychiat. Scand., 49:379, 1964.
STENGEL, E. Pain and the psychiatrist. Brit. J. Psychiat., 111:795, 1965.
STEWART, M. A., TUASON, V. B., GUZE, S. B., and SATTERFIELD, J. H. A study of psychiatric consultations in a general hospital. J. Chron. Dis., 15:331, 1962.
———— et al. Depression among medically ill patients. Dis. Nerv. Syst., 26:479, 1965.
STOECKLE, J. D., and DAVIDSON, G. E. Bodily complaints and the other symptoms of a depressive reaction, its diagnosis and significance in a medical clinic. J.A.M.A., 180:134, 1962.
———— and DAVIDSON, G. E. The use of "crisis" as an orientation for the study of patients in a medical clinic. J. Med. Educ., 37:604, 1962.
———— et al. The quantity and significance of psychological distress in medical patients. J. Chronic Dis., 17:959, 1964.
STOLLER, R. J., and ESTESS, F. M. Suicides in medical and surgical wards of general hospitals. J. Chronic Dis., 12:592, 1960.
STRECKER, E. A. Contributions of psychiatry to medical theory and practice. Med. Clin. N. Amer., July 1957, p. 1123.
SULLIVAN, P. Is this symptom functional. J.A.M.A., 185(10):747, 1963.
Symposium on Comprehensive Medical Care and the Psychiatric Consultation. University of California Medical Center, November 1965.
SWIFT, N. I. Psychological reactions to illness. Physiotherapy, 48:172, 1962.
SZASZ, T. S. Pain and Pleasure. New York, Basic Books, Inc., Publishers, 1957.
———— Language and pain. In Arieti, S., ed. American Handbook of Psychiatry. New York, Basic Books, Inc., Publishers, 1959, pp. 982–999.
———— The Myth of Mental Illness. New York, Paul B. Hoeber, Inc., 1961, p. 297.
TAVEL, M. E. Hyperventilation syndrome with unilateral somatic symptoms. J.A.M.A., 187:301, 1964.
TEITELBAUM, H. A. Psychosomatic Neurology. New York, Grune & Stratton, Inc., 1964.
TITCHENER, J. L. Problems of delay in seeking surgical care. J.A.M.A., 160:1187, 1956.
———— LEVINE, M. Surgery as a Human Experience. New York, Oxford University Press, Inc., 1960.
Training the Psychiatrist to Meet Changing Needs. Amer. Psychiat. Assoc., Washington D.C., 1963.
TREUSCH, J. V., and GROTJAHN, M. Psychiatric family consultations. Ann. Intern. Med., 66(2):295, February, 1967.
TROTTER, T. A View of the Nervous Temperament. London, Longsman, Hurst, Rees, and Orme, 1807.
UNGERLEIDER, J. T. The psychiatric emergency, analysis of six month's experience of a university hospital's consultation service. Arch. Gen. Psychiat. (Chicago), 3:593, 1961.
VEITH, I. Hysteria. The History of a Disease. Chicago, University of Chicago Press, 1965.

WAHL, C. W. The medical management of acute anxiety states. New Physician, 2(12):430, 1962.

―――― ed. New Dimensions in Psychosomatic Medicine. Boston, Little, Brown and Company, 1964.

―――― GOLDEN, J. S. The psychodynamics of the polysurgical patient: Report of 16 patients. Psychosom. Med., 7(2), 1966.

WALTERS, A. Psychogenic regional pain alias hysterical pain. Brain, 84:1, 1961.

WATTERS, T. A. Certain pitfalls and perils in psychiatric referral. Amer. Practit. Digest of Treatment, 3:198, 1952.

WEDGE, B. M. Discussion. GAP Report, 5(9):648, 1965.

WEINBERG, J. Discussion. GAP Report, 5(9):643, 1965.

WEINSTOCK, H. I. Discussion of schizophrenia in: Early recognition and management of psychiatric disorders in general practice. J. Mount Sinai Hosp. N.Y., 25:137, 1958.

WEISMAN, A. D. Psychodynamic formulation of conflict. Arch. Gen. Psychiat. (Chicago), 1:288, 1959.

―――― HACKETT, T. P. Psychosis after eye surgery. New Eng. J. Med., 258:1284, 1958.

―――― HACKETT, T. The organization and function of a psychiatric consultation service. Int. Record Med., 173:306, 1960.

―――― HACKETT, T. Predeliction to death: Death and dying as a psychiatric problem. Psychosom. Med., 23:232, 1961.

WEISS, E., and ENGLISH, S. O. Psychosomatic Medicine. Philadelphia, W. B. Saunders Co., 1957.

WEST, L. J. Psychophysiology. In Lief, H. I., Lief, V. F., and Lief, N. R., eds. The Psychological Basis of Medical Practice. New York, Harper & Row, Publishers, 1963.

What are the Facts About Mental Illness. Washington, The National Committee Against Mental Illness, Inc., p. 1, 1964.

WHITTINGTON, H. G. Consultation practice in colleges and universities. In The Psychiatric Consultation, Mendel, W. M., and Solomon, P., eds. New York, Grune and Stratton, 1968.

WILSON, M. S., and MEYER, E. Diagnostic consistency in a psychiatric liaison service. Amer. J. Psychiat., 119:207, 1962.

WILSON, M., and MEYER, E. The doctors' vs. the nurses' view of emotional disturbances. Canad. Psychiat. Ass. J., 10:212, 1965.

WITTKOWER, E., and CLEGHORN, R. A. Basic concepts of psychosomatic medicine. In MacLeod, A. W., Wittkower, E. D., and Margolin, S. G., eds. Recent Developments in Psychosomatic Medicine. Philadelphia, J. B. Lippincott Co., 1954, pp. 3–28.

WITTKOWER, E. D., and LIPOWSKI, Z. J. Recent developments in psychosomatic medicine. Psychosom. Med., in press.

WOHLRABE, J. C., et al. Delirium and complex electrolyte disturbance. Dis. Nerv. Syst., 26:44, 1965.

WOLFE, H. E. Consultation: Role, function, and process. Ment. Hyg., 50:132, 1966.

WOLFF, H. Concepts of disease. Psychosom. Med., 24(1), 1962.

―――― CURRAN, D. Nature of delirium and allied states, dysergastic reaction. Arch. Neurol. Psychiat., 33:1175, 1935.

WORTIS, S. B., and HALPERN, F. Psychological tests and indications for their use. Med. Clin. N. Amer., May:741, 1958.

WRIGHT, R. G., and HOLMES, T. H. Psychological aspects of hospitalization. *In* Lief, H., Lief, V., and Lief, N., eds. The Psychological Basis of Medical Practice. New York, Harper & Row, Publishers, 1963, pp. 219–231.

ZBOROWSKI, M. Cultural components in responses to pain. J. Social Issues, XIII:16, 1952.

ZIEGLER, J. J., IMBODEN, J. B., and MEYER, E. Contemporary conversion reactions. A clinical study. Amer. J. Psychiat., 116:901–909, 1960.

ZIEGLER, F. J., and IMBODEN, J. B. Contemporary conversion reactions. II. A conceptual model. Arch. Gen. Psychiat. (Chicago), 6:279, 1962.

ZIEGLER, F. J., et al. Contemporary conversion reactions. III. Diagnostic considerations. J.A.M.A., 186:307, 1963.

ZINBERG, N. E., ed. Psychiatry and Medical Practice in a General Hospital. New York, International Universities Press, Inc., 1964.

ZWERLING, I., TITCHENER, et al. Personality disorder and the relationships of emotion to surgical illness in 200 surgical patients. Amer. J. Psychiat., 112:270, 1955.

SECTION EIGHT   Appendices

A. DIFFERENTIAL DIAGNOSIS OF THE ACUTE
   PSYCHIATRIC DISORDERS

B. POSSIBLE MEDICAL SOURCES OF EMOTIONAL
   SYMPTOMS

C. PSYCHIATRIC SYMPTOMS ACCOMPANYING
   MEDICAL ILLNESS

D. MEDICATIONS

APPENDIX A

Differential Diagnosis of the Acute Psychiatric Disorders*

	CATATONIC EXCITEMENT	ACUTE, SCHIZO-PHRENIC REACTION	THE MANIC STATE
APPEARANCE	Grossly disturbed	Apprehensive, fearful, excited, on edge, suspicious. May be bizarre	Extremely excited, disheveled
SPEECH	Rapid, explosive, incoherent	Loose, rambling	Very rapid, forceful, flighty
MOTOR ACTIVITY	Overactive, extremely violent, dangerous	Slightly overactive, or impulsive but may be apathetic	Extremely overactive
MENTAL ACTIVITY	Completely disorganized	Ranges from fear to suspicion, loose associations. May be hallucinating or delusional.	Extremely distractible, scattered, may be hostile. No delusions or hallucinations, grandiose
AFFECT AND MOOD	Completely inappropriate, extremely excited	Inappropriate, usually fearful and guarded, but often "depressed"	Buoyant, cheerful, changing, irritable, hostile
INSIGHT	None	Poor	Poor, uncooperative

ACUTE BRAIN SYNDROME	DISSOCIATIVE REACTION	ANXIETY STATE	CONVERSION REACTION
Apprehensive, fearful, distressed	Usually bewildered, may be dazed, dreamy, or panicky	Tense, restless	Usually calm— inappropriately so—but may be overreactive, flighty
Rambling or tense, vague in later stages, delirious	Slow, vague	Slightly increased, or tremulous	Calm, usually undertalkative
Aimless, clumsy	Usually normal but may be overactive	Normal to restless	Normal, or paralyzed, or twitching, or "convulsive"
Disoriented in time, later in place, confused, delusions and hallucinations in later stages	Confused, slightly disoriented, loose associations	Preoccupied with physical condition and mental state	Focused on complaints, but may be detached
Fearful, looks severely ill	Inappropriate, dreamy, frightened or depressed	Frightened but otherwise normal	Inappropriately flat and may be "depressed"
Poor, gives impression cannot cooperate	Poor, but accepts help	Good, very cooperative	Accepts help

* A medical history and physical examination is essential. Besides the more common diseases, the following should be kept in mind:

> Hypoglycemia
> Drug Intoxication
> Head Trauma
> Brain Tumor
> Porphyria (after taking barbiturates)
> Epilepsy

APPENDIX B

Possible Medical Sources of Emotional Symptoms

ANXIETY

Hyperthyroidism (Thyrotoxicosis)
Hyperinsulinism (Insulinoma, Exogenous Insulin)
Pheochromocytoma
Carcinoid syndrome
Porphyria
Menopause

CONVERSION

Epilepsy
Brain tumor presenting with convulsions or focal seizures
Hyperinsulinism (Insulinoma, Exogenous Insulin)
Hypoparathyroidism (Tetany may occur years after thyroidectomy or be precipitated by pregnancy or lactation)
Neurologic syndromes
Chorea
Ménière's syndrome
Parkinsonism (Tremors in hands of the young, Stiffness of legs in the more elderly)
Peripheral neurological disorders (Root compression, Cord compression)

DEPRESSION

Severe anemia
Hypothyroidism
Diabetes mellitus
Brucellosis
Carcinoma of pancreas
Adrenal cortical insufficiency (Addison's disease)
Intestinal parasites
Preceding onset of many serious illnesses

DISSOCIATIVE REACTIONS

Drug intoxications
Hyperinsulinism (Insulinoma, Exogenous Insulin)
Metabolic encephalopathies
Severe hyperthyroidism
Chemical poisoning (especially industrial, agricultural and pest control chemicals)

LOSS OF LIBIDO

Adrenal cortical insufficiency
Hypothyroidism
Diabetes mellitus
Acromegaly
Hypopituitarism
Cirrhosis
Leriche syndrome
Any medical illness in which "depressive syndrome" is present
Exogenous sex hormones of the opposite sex

SCHIZOPHRENIA

Acute brain syndromes
Drug intoxications
Epilepsy
Hypoglycemia (Insulinoma, Exogenous Insulin)
Congestive heart failure or emphysema in the elderly with arteriosclerotic vascular disease
Chemical poisoning (agricultural, industrial, and pest control chemicals)

WEAKNESS-FATIGUE

Adrenal cortical insufficiency
Aldosteronism
Amyotrophic lateral sclerosis
Cirrhosis
Diabetes mellitus
Hyperparathyroidism
Hyperthyroidism
Hypokalemia (Chlorothiazide and other diuretics)
Hypothyroidism
Lupus erythematosus
Myasthenia gravis
Progressive muscular dystrophy
Renal insufficiency
Severe anemia (of any etiology)
Hypoxia (of any cause)
Congestive heart failure
Chronic pulmonary failure (Emphysema)

APPENDIX C

Psychiatric Symptoms
Accompanying Medical Illnesses

DISEASE	PSYCHIATRIC MANIFESTATIONS
Acromegaly	headache +++ fatigue ++ muscular weakness ++ visual difficulty ++ withdrawal + shyness +
Acute Porphyria	confusion +++ "hysterical" crying ++ hallucinations + convulsions +
Adrenal Cortical Insufficiency (Addison's disease)	weakness +++ fatigue ++ nervousness ++ anorexia ++ depression + nausea and vomiting +

+++ Frequent, may be severe
++ Occurs sometimes, moderate severity
+ Occurs occasionally, severity variable

277

DISEASE	PSYCHIATRIC MANIFESTATIONS
Aldosteronism	headaches +++ fatigue ++ weakness ++ nocturia ++ lethargy + tetany +
Anoxia	headache ++ anxiety ++ transient confusion ++ impairment of judgment + decreased attention span + weakness + anorexia +
Brucellosis	fatigue ++ apathy ++ irritability ++ depression ++ weakness ++
Carcinoid syndrome	acute anxiety attacks with suffocation ++ flushing of trunk, neck, and face with hot feeling in above areas +
Carcinoma of Pancreas	indigestion +++ weight loss ++ depression +
Chronic Renal Insufficiency	fatigue +++ weakness +++ brain syndrome (developing gradually) ++ anorexia ++
Costochondritis (Tietze's syndrome)	chest pain near sternum +++ negative laboratory work-up +++ anxiety about heart disease +++ acute form misdiagnosed

DISEASE	PSYCHIATRIC MANIFESTATIONS
Cushing's syndrome	fatigue +++ weakness +++ personality change (usually from neat and orderly to careless and sloppy) ++ irritability ++ tension +
Diabetes Mellitus	weakness +++ depressive syndrome ++ fatigue ++ loss of libido ++
Epilepsy	fugue state or stupor + psychomotor automatisms + rage state + local motor (Jacksonian) seizures + sensory seizures (auditory, visual, and uncinate hallucinations) +
Functioning Ovarian Tumors	feminizing or masculinizing increased libidinal drive in early stages +
Hyperinsulinism (Insulinoma)	weakness +++ anxiety attacks +++ fainting ++ extreme hunger ++ confusion ++ apprehension + convulsions (late)
Hyperparathyroidism	patients appear to be "functional" +++ weakness +++ anorexia +++ nausea ++ constipation ++ delirium (late)

DISEASE	PSYCHIATRIC MANIFESTATIONS
Hyperthyroidism	insomnia +++ anxiety +++ nervousness +++ personality change with increased emotional lability +++ palpitations ++ fatigue ++ depression (late)
Hyperventilation	paresthesias, especially hands and feet +++ fear +++ simulates neurological or cardiovascular illness + neuromuscular irritability with hand and foot cramping + myalgia + precordial pain + palpitations + aerophagy (shortness of breath)
Hypoparathyroidism	neuromuscular irritability +++ irritability ++ anxiety + depression + delirium (late)
Hypopituitarism	weakness +++ fatigue +++ anorexia ++ weight loss ++ multiple complaints in review of symptoms ++
Hypothyroidism	depression +++ weakness ++ nonspecific symptoms ++ nervousness ++

DISEASE	PSYCHIATRIC MANIFESTATIONS
Multiple Sclerosis	bizarre complaints +++ depression seen early ++ personality change ++ emotional lability + euphoria (late) +
Narcolepsy	passive aggressive characteristics +++ hypnagogic hallucinations + anxiety + tachycardia +

Neurological

ANTERIOR CEREBRAL ARTERY	frontal lobe syndrome (impairment of judgment and intellectual acuity, personality change)
ENCEPHALOPATHIES	metabolic-acute brain syndrome (higher functions—memory, orientation, mood —affected first) emotional lability in postanoxic states—chronic brain syndrome with impairment of mental functions, particularly reasoning ability
FRONTAL LOBE SYNDROME	personality change, often with euphoria, dullness, childishness, and lack of concern, attention, and judgment no neurological signs until late
INTRACRANIAL NEOPLASMS	mental symptoms almost always prominent, depression personality change and headache are usually the presenting symptoms convulsion may be the presenting symptom late—hallucinations (gustatory) acute brain syndrome

DISEASE	PSYCHIATRIC MANIFESTATIONS
PITUITARY OR III VENTRICLE TUMOR	apathy, alternating with periods of ir-ritability or hyperactivity ++ dullness ++ difficulty with concentration ++ decreased or increased libido +
POSTENCEPHALITIC	myriad complaints +++ drowsiness ++ detachment + carelessness + emotional lability +
TEMPOROPARIETAL SYNDROME	difficult to diagnose early, anxiety ++ low frustration tolerance + irritability + depression + visual or auditory hallucinations
VASOSPASM OF BASILAR-VERTEBRAL ARTERIAL SYSTEM	unusual complaints of loss of vision in one or both eyes ++ clouded vision—may vary from side to side + "dizziness" +
Parkinsonism	personality change ++ depression ++ emotional lability with heightened emo-tional stress ++ apathy +
Pernicious Anemia	increased fatigue +++ weakness ++ anorexia ++ depression ++ irritability + sensory disturbances (tingling and numb-ness in extremities) +

DISEASE   PSYCHIATRIC MANIFESTATIONS

                                ataxia
                                failing memory

Pheochromocytoma   acute "anxiety" attacks +++
                                palpitation ++
                                tachycardia ++
                                headache ++
                                fear ++

Pulmonary Insufficiency and   dyspnea +++
   Respiratory Disease   lethargy ++
   (Chronic)   hyperventilation +
                                anxiety +
                                confusion
                                decreased attention span

Pulmonary Tuberculosis   depression +++
                                insomnia +++
                                weakness +++
                                nervousness ++
                                vague complaints ++
                                lassitude ++
                                fatigue +

Tetany   spasms
                                tremors
                                mentally clear

Uremia   in florid stage, onset of acute brain syn-
                                    drome, may appear to be sudden,
                                    headaches
                                liver disease: coma or convulsions (late)

Wilson's Disease (Hepatolen-   may first appear in adolescence as schiz-
   ticular Degeneration)   ophrenia

APPENDIX D

Medications

GUIDELINES

Since the introduction of the psychopharmacologic agents in 1952, psychiatrists have been working with an overwhelming number of these medications. Although a great deal is still unknown about their pharmacologic activity, particularly specific mechanisms, the following generalizations can be made about their use.

First, they are more effective in severe mental illness; their effectiveness is definitely limited in the treatment of the neuroses and psychophysiologic reactions; they are only slightly, if at all, useful for the treatment of patients with personality disorders.

Second, these medications are not panaceas or "cure-alls"; when used discriminately, however, they act with varying degrees of effectiveness by stimulating or suppressing various target symptoms such as anxiety, aggressiveness, sexual unrest, depression, and so on.

Third, target symptoms are handy guides for their use, but they cannot be used as the sole index to indications and contraindications. The physician must also acquire a working knowledge of the patient's personality pattern and the meaning of the symptom(s) to obtain optimal benefits from the use of these agents.

Fourth, the great numbers of these medications have produced confusion; many physicians, who rely upon them excessively and whose expectations of them are too great, switch quickly and hopefully from one new medication to another. Although the consultant must be familiar with the indications, dosage, and side effects of many drugs, he should have extensive clinical experience with a limited number of medications and understand them thoroughly.

Fifth, in general, although there has been a great hubbub about the side effects of these medications, as the years go on the incidence of verified adverse reactions is decreasing.

Sixth, these medications cannot be used specifically to do the therapeutic task. They do not "purge" the patient of symptoms. Rather, they can be used to alleviate distressing symptoms, thereby enabling the patient to order his world about him more appropriately, to engage in a therapeutic dialogue with his physician, and to promote communication with his family and other members of society. Redlich and Freedman (1966) emphasize: "No drug acts directly on behavior, and no behavioral pattern can be entirely determined by drug action. Behavior, whether that of an isolated organ or of an organism, is influenced by the surrounding conditions; in the case of psychotropic compounds, these are psychosocial conditions."

TARGET SYMPTOMS STIMULATED OR SUPPRESSED

1. Anxiety	
2. Hostility	
3. Aggressiveness	Diminished by the major
4. Sexual Unrest	tranquilizers but some-
5. Agitation	times stimulated by the
6. Confusion	antidepressants
7. Disturbed Thinking	
8. Insomnia	

9. Depression	Diminished by the anti-
10. Fatigue	depressants but may be
11. Helplessness—Hopelessness	increased by the major
	tranquilizers

CLASSIFICATION

These drugs are conventionally classified as the major tranquilizers, minor tranquilizers, and the antidepressants. To these are added sedatives and hypnotics which are frequently used by consultants.

A. Major Tranquilizers
    1. Phenothiazine compounds
    2. Rauwolfia

B. Minor Tranquilizers
 1. Meprobamate (Miltown, Equanil)
 2. Chlordiazepoxide-HCl (Librium)
 3. Diazepam (Valium)
 4. Oxazepam (Serax)
 5. Barbiturates
C. Antidepressants
 1. Direct Stimulating—Amphetamines
 2. Indirect Stimulating—Marplan, Nardil.
 3. Bimodal Stimulating—Parnate.
 4. Suppressant—Related to Phenothiazines
  (a) Tofranil, Pertofrane, Norpramin
  (b) Elavil, Aventyl
D. Sedatives and Hypnotics

The Major Tranquilizers

Action on subcortical structures, probably hypothalamus, reticular activating system, basal ganglia.

A. Phenothiazines—use for schizophrenia and target symptoms 1–8.
 1. Dimethyl group
    chlorpromazine (Thorazine) 25–200 mg q.i.d.
    promazine (Sparine) 50–100 mg q.i.d.
    triflupromazine (Vesprin) 10–30 mg q.i.d.
 2. Piperidyl group
    Thioridazine (Mellaril) 25–200 mg q.i.d.
 3. Piperazine group
    Fluphenazine (Prolixin, Permitil) 1–4 mg q.i.d.
    Trifluoperazine (Stelazine) 2–5 mg q.i.d.
    Perphenazine (Trilafon) 2–10 mg q.i.d.
    Prochlorperazine (Compazine) 5–10 mg q.i.d.
B. Rauwolfia
   Use only if phenothiazines are contraindicated; sedation may still be preferred.

(left margin: SEDATION | EXTRAPYRAMIDAL)

SIDE EFFECTS OF MAJOR TRANQUILIZERS

A. Phenothiazines
 1. Transient Hypotension [Do not treat with epinephrine, use levarterenol (Levophed) if necessary]
 2. Extrapyramidal
  (a) tremors
  (b) muscular weakness

      (c) dyskinesias

      (d) akithisia (the jitters—reduce phenothiazine)

      (e) dystonias [do not mistake for conversion—use diphenhy-dramine (Benadryl) 50 mg parenterally and discontinue phenothiazine]

      (f) Parkinsonism—Most of the extrapyramidal symptoms respond to concurrent use of one of the following anti-Parkinson agents:

          Benztropine (Cogentin) 3 mg/day
          Trihexyphenidyl (Artane) 10 mg/day
          Biperidin (Akineton) 6 mg/day

  3. Blood Dyscrasias—check blood count at regular intervals

  4. Jaundice—now very rarely reported; discontinue phenothiazines

  5. Photosensitivity and dermatitis

  6. Eye: Granular opacities of cornea and lens; also do not use with glaucoma

  7. Epileptogenic—particularly chlorpromazine; discontinue chlorpromazine, substitute thioridazine and give Dilantin

  8. Miscellaneous: dry mouth, drowsiness, weakness

 B. Rauwolfia—used very rarely

  1. Depression—Suicide

  2. Cardiovascular—Hypotension

  3. Gastrointestinal—Upper GI Distress; Peptic Ulcer

Minor Tranquilizers and Related Compounds

The minor tranquilizers, barbiturates, and a few related compounds are widely used for the symptomatic treatment of anxiety, tension, and depression. These medications have limited effectiveness; their placebo effect is great; they seem to act as sedatives; they have little specific action. Habituation, sensitivity, paradoxical reactions, and withdrawal reactions may occur with most of these medications.

MEDICATION	DOSE	SIDE EFFECTS AND CONTRA-INDICATIONS	COMMENTS
Meprobamate Miltown Equanil	400 mg t.i.d. or q.i.d.	Habituation Sensitivity Drowsiness Withdrawal	A mild sedative with a wide margin of safety.
Chlordia-zepoxide-HCl Librium	10–20 mg t.i.d. or q.i.d.	Habituation Paradoxical reactions with ataxia or excitement	Probably more potent than meprobamate.

MEDICATION	DOSE	SIDE EFFECTS AND CONTRA-INDICATIONS	COMMENTS
Diazepam Valium	5–10 mg t.i.d. or q.i.d.	Fatigue Drowsiness Ataxia	Comparable to Librium.
Oxazepam Serax	10–15 mg t.i.d. or q.i.d.	Drowsiness Dizziness Excitement	Comparable to Librium.
Hydroxyzine Vistaril Atarax	25 mg t.i.d. or q.i.d.	Drowsiness	Safe, nonspecific. Probably less likely to be habituating.
Amobarbital Amytal	30 mg t.i.d. or q.i.d.	Drowsiness Habituation Withdrawal reactions	Do not use for longer than 2–3 weeks. Discontinue gradually.
Butabarbital Sodium Butisol	30 mg t.i.d. or q.i.d.	Drowsiness. Same as amobarbital.	Same as amobarbital.

Antidepressant Medications

If depression is moderate or severe, or if the patient with mild depression does not respond to sedation at bedtime and a small dose of amphetamine during the day, use Elavil or Aventyl as a first choice and Parnate as a last resort. Heed precautions to interrupt medications for 7 to 14 days before and after switching among and from the MAO inhibitors and the Dibenzazepine derivatives.

MEDICATION	DOSE	SIDE EFFECTS AND CONTRA-INDICATIONS	COMMENTS
Amphetamines Dexedrine	5 mg in morning and at noon	Sympathomimetic action. Cardiovascular disease with hypertension is a contraindication.	Occasionally beneficial for mildly depressed or for the elderly. Also, use for narcolepsy and for agitated behavioral disorders in children.
Dexamyl	5 mg in morning and at noon		

MEDICATION	DOSE	SIDE EFFECTS AND CONTRA-INDICATIONS	COMMENTS
Deprol	1 tab. q.i.d.	Habituation Withdrawal reactions	Specific effect doubtful; occasional patient reports a good response; a relatively wide margin of safety.

Dibenzazepine Derivatives

These medications appear to have both a phenothiazine (tranquilizing) and antidepressant actions.

Amitriptyline Elavil	25 mg t.i.d. or q.i.d. (range 40–150 mg/day)	Drowsiness Dizziness Occasional agitation. Atropine-like effects	Generally effective and safe; preferred if anxiety and agitation are present. Do *not* use with MAO inhibitors. See Parnate.
Imipramine Tofranil	25 mg t.i.d. or q.i.d. Maintenance may be as low as 25–50 mg/day	Atropine-like effects; Hypotension; Agitation; Glaucoma Urinary retention	Generally effective. Do not use with MAO inhibitors (See Parnate). Allow 1 week free of other antidepressants before and after beginning treatment. Slow onset of action; raise dose at 14 days if necessary. Discontinue if no response in 21 days.
Desipramine HCl Norpramin or Pertofrane	50 mg t.i.d. Maintenance 100 mg/day	Atropine-like side effects. Occasional agitation	Reported to have a more rapid onset than other compounds; not proved to be superior.

MEDICATION	DOSE	SIDE EFFECTS AND CONTRA-INDICATIONS	COMMENTS
Nortriptyline HCl Aventyl	10 mg t.i.d.; increase to 25 mg t.i.d., then reduce to desired maintenance level.	Atropine-like side effects. Occasional stimulation and confusion reported	Reported to be as rapid and as safe as similar compounds. May be preferred if there is anxiety with the depression. Do not use until patient has been off MAO inhibitors 10 days.

Mono-Amine Oxidase Inhibitors (MAO)

Marplan	10 mg t.i.d. Maintenance dose may be 20 mg/day.	Generally the same as listed for Parnate, but not so marked.	Occasionally, specifically effective, but dangerous. Use same precautions with all MAO inhibitors.
Nardil	15 mg t.i.d. Maintenance may be 15–30 mg/day.	Hypotension, liver disease, and agitation have been reported. Do not use with other drugs, or cheese.	Patient should be free of drugs 7 days before and after using MAO drugs. See Parnate. Use only if other medications fail.
Parnate Tranylcypromine	10 mg b.i.d. or t.i.d.	Hypotension or hypertensive crises. Cardiovascular disease, cerebrovascular disease, or over age of 60 are contraindications. Do not use with other antidepressants or sympathomimetics. Cheese and alcohol prohibited.	Dangerous, specific but limited effectiveness. Use only if other antidepressants fail and if patient is in hospital. Allow 7 drug-free days before changing to or from Parnate and other antidepressants. Discontinue if no response in 14 days. Use only after other R_x fail. See warnings in *Physician's Desk Reference*.

Sedatives and Hypnotics

Adequate night-time sedation is usually essential. In itself, effective sedation is curative for many patients with mild depression and those with minor anxiety states; it is mandatory for most acutely and chronically disturbed patients.

MEDICATION	DOSE	CONTRA-INDICATIONS	COMMENTS
Pentobarbital	100 mg HS	Habituation	Usually preferred for most patients but not for the elderly or others who have to get up at night. To increase effectiveness add 50 mg diphenhydramine (Benadryl) or 50 mg Chlorpromazine (Thorazine)
		Sensitivity	
Secobarbital	100 mg HS	Overdosage	
		Suicide	
Diphenhydramine (Benadryl)	50 mg	Minor atropine-like action	Preferred medication for *mild* sedation, for the elderly, and for those who react poorly to sedatives with a hangover.
Chloral Hydrate	0.5–1.0 g	Long-term use inadvisable— some patients develop "intoxication"	Quite safe; should be used more often, particularly for 5–10 days or while the patient is in the hospital.
Sodium amytal barbital combination	200 mg sodium amytal and 200 mg barbital can be given orally (in liquid form) at bedtime to a disturbed patient who		

MEDICATION	DOSE	CONTRA- INDICATIONS	COMMENTS
	needs 8–10 hours of sleep.		
Paraldehyde	10–15 ml	Respiratory insufficiency	Useful for treatment of acute alcoholism.

GENERAL REFERENCES FOR PSYCHOPHARMACOLOGIC AGENTS

AINSLIE, J. D., JONES, M. B., and STIEFEL, J. R. A practical drug evaluation method: Imipramine in depressed outpatients. Arch. Gen. Psychiat. (Chicago), 12:368, 1965.

———— The use of newer psychiatric drugs in medical practice. Their specificity of action in relation to target symptoms and dynamic situations. J. Florida Med. Ass. 47:901, 1961.

COLE, J. O. Evaluation of drug treatments in psychiatry. Psychopharmacology Service Center Bulletin, 2:28, 1962.

———— Therapeutic efficacy of anti-depressant drugs. J.A.M.A., 190:448, 1964.

———— et al. Phenothiazine treatment in acute schizophrenia: Effectiveness. Arch. Gen. Psychiat. (Chicago), The National Institute of Mental Health Psychopharmacology Service Center Collaborative Study Group, 10:246, 1964.

ENELOW, A. J., and WEXLER, M. Psychiatry in the Practice of Medicine, New York, Oxford University Press, Inc., 1966, pp. 210–247.

GREENBLATT, M., GROSSER, G. H., and WECHSLER, H. A comparative study of selected antidepressant medications and EST. Amer. J. Psychiat., 119:144, 1962.

HOLLISTER, L. E. Complications from psychotherapeutic drugs—1964. Clin. Pharmacol. Ther., 5:322, 1964.

———— Drugs and emotional disorders: Past and present. Ann. Intern. Med., 51:1032, 1959.

———— Toxicity of psychotherapeutic drugs. Practitioner, 194:72, 1965.

JONES, M. B., and AINSLIE, J. D. Value of placebo wash-out. Dis. Nerv. Syst., 27:393, 1966.

KURLAND, A. K. Placebo effect. In Uhr, L., and Miller, J. G., eds. Drugs and Behavior. New York, John Wiley & Sons, Inc., 1960.

LANGSLEY, D. G., et al. A comparison of chlorpromazine and EST in treatment of acute schizophrenic and manic reactions. A.M.A. Arch. Neurol. Psychiat., 81:384, 1959.

LESSE, S. Electroshock therapy and tranquilizing drugs. J.A.M.A., 170:1791, 1959.

Psychopharmacology Service Center Bulletin, NIMH, Bethesda, Maryland, 2(1), 1962.

MALITZ, S. and WHARTON, R. "Lithium in manic-depressive psychosis." In American Handbook of Psychiatry, III, Arieti, S., Ed., New York, Basic Books, Inc., 1966, pp. 509–512.

REDLICH, F. K., and FREEDMAN, D. X. Theory and Practice of Psychiatry. New York, Basic Books, Inc., Publishers, 1966, pp. 306–332.

RICKELS, K. Psychopharmacologic agents: A clinical psychiatrist's individualistic point of view: Patient and doctor variables. J. Nerv. Ment. Dis., 136:540, 1963.

SCHIELE, B. C. Newer drugs for mental illness. J.A.M.A., 181:126, 1962.

SCHWAB, J. J., and BROWN, J. M. The limitations of drug therapy. Psychosomatics, 8(2), 1967.

SHAPIRO, A. K. The placebo effect in the history of medical treatment. Amer. J. Psychiat., 116:298, 1959.

STEINBOOK, R. M., JONES, M. B., and AINSLIE, J. D. Suggestibility and the placebo response. J. Nerv. Ment. Dis., 140:87, 1965.

AUTHOR INDEX

SUBJECT INDEX